KNOWLEDGE DEVELOPMENT IN NURSING
THEORY AND PROCESS

KNOWLEDGE DEVELOPMENT IN NURSING

THEORY AND PROCESS

Tenth Edition

PEGGY L. CHINN, RN, PhD, FAAN

Professor Emerita,
School of Nursing,
University of Connecticut,
Storrs, Connecticut

MAEONA K. KRAMER, APRN, PhD

Professor Emerita,
College of Nursing,
University of Utah,
Salt Lake City, Utah

ELSEVIER

ELSEVIER

3251 Riverport Lane
St. Louis, Missouri 63043

Notices

Knowledge and best practice in this field are constantly changing. As new research and experience broaden our understanding, changes in research methods, professional practices, or medical treatment may become necessary.

Practitioners and researchers must always rely on their own experience and knowledge in evaluating and using any information, methods, compounds, or experiments described herein. In using such information or methods, they should be mindful of their own safety and the safety of others, including parties for whom they have a professional responsibility.

With respect to any drug or pharmaceutical products identified, readers are advised to check the most current information provided (i) on procedures featured or (ii) by the manufacturer of each product to be administered and to verify the recommended dose or formula, the method and duration of administration, and contraindications. It is the responsibility of practitioners, relying on their own experience and knowledge of their patients, to make diagnoses, to determine dosages and the best treatment for each individual patient, and to take all appropriate safety precautions.

To the fullest extent of the law, neither the Publisher nor the authors, contributors, or editors assume any liability for any injury and/or damage to persons or property as a matter of products liability, negligence or otherwise, or from any use or operation of any methods, products, instructions, or ideas contained in the material herein.

Library of Congress Cataloging-in-Publication Data
Names: Chinn, Peggy L., author. | Kramer, Maeona K., author.
Title: Knowledge development in nursing : theory and process / Peggy L.
   Chinn, RN, PhD, FAAN, Professor Emerita, School of Nursing, University of
   Connecticut, Storrs, Connecticut, Maeona K. Kramer, APRN, PhD, Professor
   Emerita, College of Nursing, University of Utah, Salt Lake City, Utah.
Description: Tenth edition. | St. Louis, Missouri : Elsevier, Inc., [2018] |
   Includes bibliographical references and index.
Identifiers: LCCN 2017042494 | ISBN 9780323530613 (paperback)
Subjects: LCSH: Nursing--Philosophy.
Classification: LCC RT84.5 .C49 2018 | DDC 610.7301--dc23 LC record available at
   https://lccn.loc.gov/2017042494

Content Strategist: Kristin Geen
Content Development Manager: Lisa Newton
Publishing Services Manager: Deepthi Unni
Project Manager: Apoorva V
Design Direction: Ashley Miner

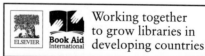

Working together
to grow libraries in
developing countries

www.elsevier.com • www.bookaid.org

Printed in United States of America

Last digit is the print number: 9   8   7   6   5   4   3   2

Preface

When we composed the first edition of this book in the early 1980s we could not have envisioned a 10th edition, even if we had been inclined to do so! We wrote this book initially with the simple expectation to complete a book on nursing theory and how it is developed. We had each completed our doctoral degrees with emphases on theory and knowledge development during an era of significant growth in nursing scholarship that yielded advancements in nursing research, establishment of new nursing journals focused on nursing scholarship, and the emergence of theories developed by nurses. The early theories focused broadly on the nature of nursing and the role of nurses in care management. We had every reason to expect that our book could contribute to the discourse in nursing about the nature and development of theory in nursing, but we did not envision the book evolving to a 10th edition, with vastly different content.

From the beginning we were committed to a broad view of theory and theory development processes. Our first two editions anchored nursing theory development, in a broad range of scholarly activities, beyond empiric research, that we felt were required to develop adequate and useful nursing knowledge. In the 1st edition (1983), titled "Theory and Nursing: A Systematic Approach," we used a four-quadrant model depicting four equally important processes in the development of theory: concept analysis, construction of theoretical relationships, testing of theoretical relationships, and practical validation of theory. These four processes remain as significant features of our text.

The 2nd edition (1987) introduced the four fundamental patterns of knowing identified by Barbara Carper (1978). In the 3rd edition (1991), we made significant revisions in language to reflect our growing feminist and critical awareness of ways in which language itself perpetrated limited views of science and theory development that have significant relevance for how nursing knowledge is developed. We continued to develop our ideas related to nursing's patterns of knowing, and the ways in which nursing's disciplinary knowing and knowledge is shaped (and limited) by the dominance of empiric thought.

The 5th edition (1999), titled "Theory and Nursing: Integrated Knowledge Development," was the first to present our conceptual extension of Carper's fundamental patterns of knowing. We retained Carper's early conceptualizations of each of the four patterns, but added description of the ways in which each pattern can be developed, how each pattern is uniquely expressed in a way that can be taught and communicated, and finally ways for authenticating each pattern's expression. Our aim in doing so was to acknowledge that while empiric approaches are important and useful, nursing requires more. This shift continued to evolve in the 6th edition (2004), titled "Integrated Knowledge Development in Nursing."

In the 7th edition (2008), we formulated our conceptualization of emancipatory knowing based on a growing body of nursing literature that reflected a greater emphasis on the social and political core from which nursing practice emerged. Emancipatory knowing reflected the historical commitment of nurses, to address "upstream" factors that shape health and well-being. The title of the 9th edition (2015), "Knowledge Development in Nursing: Theory and Process," reflected our growing intention to view knowing and knowledge as a whole—a whole with distinct parts that reflect the whole, and that cannot be separated from the whole. In this, the 10th edition, we have made significant revisions that reflect our attempt to represent knowing and knowledge as a whole.

Over the years the core purpose of this text has remained—to examine the roots of nursing knowledge and how nursing's values define its very nature. We have consistently paid attention to how and why carefully considering nursing knowledge and its nature is critically important for practice, and we have always recognized and appreciated the vital role that all nurses play in the evolution of the discipline. The content of the text fundamentally reflects our own unique perspectives on these processes, but our ideas and perspectives have been shaped and influenced by the remarkable works of many other nurse scholars who have articulated nursing theories and philosophies, and who have interrogated the trends, assumptions, and practices of the discipline. See in particular the works of Sally Thorne and her colleagues (Thorne, 2014; Thorne & Sawatzky, 2014; Thorne, Stephens, & Truant, 2016).

The remarkable body of scholarly literature that has influenced our own work has emerged despite the fact that in recent years, nursing education has moved away from a focus on theory and philosophic thought. This transition has many roots, including the limited time educators have to provide nursing education in the face of a limited time frame, as well as the shifting role of advanced practice nurses to provide more and more medical care. We believe that sacrificing theoretic and philosophic foundations in graduate education is a detriment to the discipline, and that practice itself can and will be enhanced if this trend can take a new direction.

Recent trends that emphasize the importance of reliable evidence for practice have also created significant changes in education. Doctoral education has traditionally been founded on standards of quality that highlight scientific rigor and quality. The Doctorate of Nursing Practice was introduced to underscore greater emphasis on advanced practice roles, leadership in practice that promotes high standards of quality in nursing care, and scholarship that provides evidence for practice. We believe that a broad understanding of knowledge and knowing is essential for preparation of advanced practice nurses and research scholars. This broad understanding that encompasses the aesthetic, personal, ethical, and emancipatory patterns of knowing is crucial for defining nursing in practice and in knowledge development. Whether consciously recognized or not, those who practice nursing use these patterns, and acknowledging and attending to them can only enhance care. If patients and clients are to be better served by their health care providers, it is essential that educators understand and help learners deliberatively develop and assess knowledge within all patterns of knowing.

The very fact that we now have a 10th edition of this book affirms a growing recognition of the importance of nursing's history and the early theoretical roots in defining our disciplinary core. We are more convinced than ever that realizing nursing's potential depends on a strong grounding in the foundational values and concepts of the discipline. In this edition we have retained our focus on the early works that established nursing's core concepts and values. We have returned to the book the Appendix titled "Interpretive Summary: Examples of Broad Theoretic Frameworks Defining the Scope, Philosophy, and General Characteristics of Nursing." We have also retained nursing's patterns of knowing as the conceptual framework of the book, a framework now widely recognized as facilitating a broad commitment to the wholeness of the human health experience in nursing practice and in the development of nursing knowledge.

However, in this edition, we have reorganized the content to reach toward the wholeness of knowing and knowledge. We recognize that wholeness just "is"—but the human mind perceives parts, not the whole. Early chapters address each pattern as it relates to the dimensions of critical questions, creative processes, and formalized expressions. Later chapters detail authentication processes across all patterns and finally we focus on the integrated expressions in practice as well as the broader context within which care is rendered. With these changes we believe the patterns are treated more equally than in prior editions reflecting their equal importance in care provision. In this edition we have added even more examples as well as enhanced prompts to engage the reader with the ideas in the book by inserting features labeled "Think about it . . .," "Why is this important?," "Consider this . . .," "Imagine this . . .," and "Discuss this . . .." Rather than interrupting the flow of the text, these are stand-out features that flow with the text to draw the reader into interacting with the ideas. We have added and updated references from literature published since the last edition—an impressive body of literature that is consistent with the ideas and intentions of our text. Here are specific changes that you will find in each chapter:

Chapter 1 continues to overview nursing's patterns of knowing, inclusive of the four fundamental patterns identified by Barbara Carper, and emancipatory knowing introduced in the 8th edition. We present our model of the essential interrelationships between knowing and knowledge in nursing for each pattern and as a whole. Chapter 1 strengthens content related to the "authentication" and "integration in practice" dimensions.

Chapter 2 retains our overview of the historical development of nursing with a particular focus on the story of knowledge development. We integrate new information on current knowledge development trends, including translational research, evidence-informed practice, practice-based evidence, and intersectionality. This chapter reinforces our conviction that appreciation of our history is vital to the continuing evolution of the discipline.

Chapters 3, 4, 5, 6 and 7 are devoted to each of the patterns of knowing—emancipatory, ethical, personal, aesthetic, and empiric. However, each of these chapters is limited to explanation of the pattern's development of formal expressions of knowledge, leaving the authentication and practice integration processes to the last three chapters.

Chapter 8 addresses the description and critical reflection of empiric theory, a chapter that remains important in the process of acquiring an understanding of the nature of empiric theory.

Chapters 9, 10, and 11 deal with the authentication of nursing knowledge and integration in practice processes that were previously discussed in the chapters focused on the individual patterns. In this edition, we emphasize that in fact, knowing and the development of knowledge must reflect the whole of knowing, not any one pattern of knowing alone.

Chapter 9 focuses on authentication of knowledge and it's importance for strengthening Nursing's knowledge base. Chapter 10 develops how the integration of knowledge forms a whole of knowing that directs care as well as ongoing knowledge development. We have reconceptualized these processes to emphasize the importance of practice in forming and shaping the whole of nursing knowledge.

The new Chapter 11 details the broader conceptualization of nursing "practice" to include nursing management, administration and leadership, nursing education, public advocacy and policy, and community organizing. Each of these areas of practice contribute in significant ways to the overall development of nursing knowledge and to the evolution of nursing as a discipline. We continue to emphasize the importance of nursing foundational values in all places where nurses practice.

This text can be used by all "levels" of learners. As was our intention with the very first edition of this text, we believe that this knowledge is basic nursing knowledge and as such is essential for entry-level learners. However, the fact remains that most learners are introduced to this material in graduate education, and we fully endorse the use of this text for graduate learners. We think it is particularly important for those enrolled in programs culminating in the practice doctorate. If these practitioners are the refiners and users of knowledge that is "developed" by nursing scholars, their level of sophistication and success in validating, confirming, and refining knowledge will be directly related to how well they understand how personal, aesthetic, and ethical knowing affect those processes. Additionally, without understanding the nature and need for emancipatory knowing, practitioners and researchers alike will be less effective in their efforts to engender real praxis in our health care system.

It is our passion for the best nursing care and best nursing education possible that has energized us to produce this work; it is why we have labored to make it understandable and accessible for the beginner as well as the seasoned practitioner. Many users of this text have told us that as they have grown in their nursing experience and education, their reading and understanding of the text has markedly changed. Although what they found in the text was useful as a beginning learner, as they understood more about nursing, they understood the text in deeper and more meaningful ways.

Finally, practitioners who are focused on (and rightfully so) using best evidence to inform their practice must understand how the utilization of that "best evidence" is both facilitated and impeded by the state of knowledge and the disciplinary foundation of knowing within all patterns. For these reasons, we believe a work such as this is important for all of nursing.

IN THANKS

When we first conceived the essential elements of this book, we had both recently completed our doctoral programs and were beginning our academic careers. During a 2-year period of our early academic lives, we were both employed at the University of Utah, where we collaborated professionally and discovered our mutual interests in theory and knowledge development. Despite living in different geographic locations, we have since maintained an ongoing professional association. We now have completed our active teaching careers and continue our personal growth as we begin to experience our "resignation" from formally appointed academic life. We owe so much of our ability to change and mature in our thinking to those who enrolled in our classes and labored with us to push the edges of knowledge and venture into that which is possible but not yet fully real. It is to each of you who have worked with us in classrooms that we owe our greatest debt of gratitude. Without your continual prodding for clearer explanations, your challenges to our ideas, and your insistence that we make matters of theory, knowledge, and philosophy pertinent to practice by pushing us beyond our preconceived notions, much of what has emerged in this book would not have been possible. Indeed, in the classroom you became our teachers, and we give to you our deepest appreciation. Our many academic colleagues—within the institutions where we taught and studied as well as those around the world—have contributed to our thinking by being an informed, critical, and thoughtful audience. We also owe much to those who early on negated and challenged our radical ideas. These challenges to our way of thinking about nursing knowledge in a time where such ideas were considered liberal and unfounded strengthened our resolve to clarify and make our thinking meaningful in relation to nursing practice.

Our close friends and chosen families, especially Karen and Sue, have continued to provide the love and support so essential to this type of work—our deepest thanks and gratitude to you.

To the formal reviewers who thoughtfully read and commented on the 9th edition, we are grateful. Each of you provided insights that were helpful in this revision. We made many of the changes you suggested. We feel confident that your careful critique, both positive and negative, has produced a stronger volume. We truly appreciate your effort.

As much as we feel deeply the ways in which this work depends on our interactions with each of our colleagues, we acknowledge that the content of this book remains our own doing and our own responsibility. We have taken the responsibility to represent and acknowledge the work of others as openly and honestly as possible. We hope there are no errors in the text, yet we expect there will be; we are learners and make no claim to having final answers. We ask that you understand and honor our wish not to be seen as an authoritative voice, but rather a voice among many to be challenged and moved beyond. We began our professional collaboration in 1972 and continue to provide for one another the challenges and the grounding that are inherent in conceptualizing and co-writing a work of this type. It is our mutual respect and appreciation for one another, as well as our inherent differences, that sustain this type of relationship over time. We are grateful to each other for these mutual gifts. We offer this work, always in progress, to you with hope that it will continue to provide a perspective that is worthy of critique and that deepens your understanding and inspires your own thoughts and actions.

References

Carper, B. A. (1978). Fundamental patterns of knowing in nursing. *ANS. Advances in Nursing Science,* *1,* 13–23.

Thorne, S. (2014). Nursing as social justice: a case for emancipatory disciplinary theorizing. In P. Kagan, M. Smith, & P. Chinn (Eds.), *Philosophies and practices of emancipatory nursing: Social justice as praxis* (pp. 79–90). New York, NY: Routledge Taylor & Francis Group.

Thorne, S., & Sawatzky, R. (2014). Particularizing the general: Sustaining theoretical integrity in the context of an evidence-based practice agenda. *ANS. Advances in Nursing Science, 37,* 1–10.

Thorne, S., Stephens, J., & Truant, T. (2016). Building qualitative study design using nursing's disciplinary epistemology. *Journal of Advanced Nursing, 72*(2), 451–460. https://doi.org/10.1111/jan.12822.

Reviewers

Sally Dampier, RN, BScN, MMedSc, DNP
Nursing
Confederation College
Thunder Bay, Ontario, Canada

Gwen Keeler, BA, BScN, RN
Senior Lab Instructor
School of Nursing
University of Northern British Columbia
Prince George, British Columbia

Jeanette McNeill, DrPH, RN, MSN, CNE, ANEF
Associate Professor
School of Nursing, College of Natural and Health Sciences
University of Northern Colorado
Greeley, Colorado

Table of Contents

Nursing's Fundamental Patterns of Knowing

What is nursing science? The definition, I propose, must be broad enough to encompass all disciplinary knowledge and cannot focus on only one paradigm. Nor can the primary focus be on the activities of our science, such as theory development and research; rather, the essential focus is on knowledge.

Elizabeth Ann Manhart Barrett (2002, p. 56)

It is the general conception of any field of inquiry that ultimately determines the kind of knowledge that field aims to develop as well as the manner in which that knowledge is to be organized, tested and applied.... Such an understanding... involves critical attention to the question of what it means to know and what kinds of knowledge are held to be of most value in the discipline of nursing.

Barbara A. Carper (1978, p. 13)

These quotes from Elizabeth Barrett and Barbara Carper underscore the importance of a broad disciplinary focus of nursing. Barrett and Carper suggest that what we value as nurses is centrally important, determining the methods we use for developing knowledge, and ultimately the scope and the essence of what we claim as the underlying knowledge foundation for nursing practice.

This text challenges you to think broadly, to consider deliberately what you need to know to be an effective nurse, and to think about the values that ground what you know. This chapter examines five patterns of knowing as a basis for considering the value of multiple forms of knowledge and knowing in nursing. It provides an overview of four fundamental patterns of knowing originally developed by Carper (1978). This text expands on Carper's conceptualization and includes a discussion of knowing and knowledge within the pattern of emancipatory knowing, a pattern of knowing that is now widely recognized as equally foundational for nursing practice. These patterns of knowing, while distinct and equally essential, are vital parts of the whole of nursing knowledge—a concept that we return to throughout the text but emphasize in Chapters 9 through 11, where we examine ways to authenticate and integrate nursing knowledge through scholarly approaches, including research and in practice. In fact, in this edition, we provide substantial revisions that reflect a growing shift toward integration of theory and practice, art and science, knowing and doing—a shift that Margaret Newman (2003) described in her article, "A World of No Boundaries." This shift is one of thinking and action that better coincides with the experience of nursing—experience that is complex, shaped by the environmental context, and calls forth a unified understanding of the general and specific demands inherent in being a nurse (Bliss, Baltzly, Bull, Dalton, & Jones, 2017; Hartrick Doane, Reimer-Kirkham, Antifeau, & Stajduhar, 2015; Jacobs, 2013; Kangasniemi, Kallio, & Pietilä, 2014; Linderman, Pesut, & Disch, 2015; Terry, Carr, & Curzio, 2016; Thorne, Stephens, & Truant, 2016).

 Think About It...

- What do you believe nurses need to know?
- Do you find your answer to be related to what you value or what the profession values? Or both sets of values?
- If you believe that nurses need to know more than what they learn in books and articles, where does that knowledge come from?

KNOWLEDGE FOR A PRACTICE DISCIPLINE

The patterns of knowing identified by Carper (1978) include traditional ideas of empiric knowledge as well as knowledge that is personal, ethical, and aesthetic in nature. The pattern of emancipatory knowing, initially developed by Chinn and Kramer (2007), focuses on developing an awareness of social problems and taking action to create social change (see Chapter 3). Although we believe that knowledge and knowing within all patterns are required for effective nursing care, empirics has been and continues to be a major focus for all health care disciplines, including nursing (Archibald, 2012; Bliss et al., 2017; Mantzorou & Mastrogiannis, 2011; Paley, Cheyne, Dalgleish, Duncan, & Niven, 2007; Porter, 2010; Satterfield et al., 2009; Thorne, 2014; Thorne & Sawatzky, 2014). Understanding knowledge for nursing practice as something more inclusive and broader than empirics is, in our view, critical for a practice discipline.

Nursing involves processes, dynamics, and interactions that are most effective when the five knowing patterns of empirics, ethics, aesthetics, personal knowing, and emancipatory knowing come together. Praxis is possible when all patterns of knowing are integrated in a way that supports social justice. The term *praxis* is not just a fancy word for "practice." A nurse who follows orders and thoughtfully completes an ordered treatment such as wound irrigation is practicing and indeed may be practicing well. To be engaged in praxis, however, the nurse moves beyond the isolated performance of tasks, to engage in processes that address social inequities in which the task is embedded, asking, for example, how and why gunfights occur in this community.

 Consider This...

Consider a young woman—we'll call her Nayan—who sustained a gunshot wound that requires extensive management, including painful cleansing irrigation. In the context of this treatment, the nurse will surely be thinking about more than just aseptically irrigating this young woman's wound (a procedure grounded in empirics). He might be wondering whether he should advise Nayan to get rid of her pistol (a move with moral/ ethical implications). He questions the ethics of this because Nayan lives in a tough neighborhood where her life is endangered. Although his day is rushed because another nurse called in sick, the nurse certainly cannot in good conscience (ethics) omit this treatment any more than he can shortcut aseptic procedures. He may be keeping his feelings about guns in check, because he realizes that his biases (personal knowing) may affect his approach and the subsequent trust that Nayan has in him. This nurse is probably also considering how to finesse or carry out the treatment in the way that makes it as pain free but effective as possible, which falls within the realm of aesthetics. Aesthetic knowing would guide how vigorously he tends to the wound and how he will modify his technique in response to how Nayan responds.

Emancipatory knowing requires the nurse to reflect thoughtfully and to act in relation to a treatment and its implications in a way that makes things better for the future, not just for Nayan at this particular moment but for society in general. It is this reflection and action that we call *praxis*. In this example, the very existence of a needless gunshot wound that requires extensive care and that involves lost wages and additional expenses for this young woman is considered. Praxis means that the nurse considers the situation and does something about it. Praxis may come in the form of political action, such as joining in a letter-writing campaign or lobbying about limiting or not limiting access to guns; working to increase the safety of neighborhoods so that guns are not needed; or championing programs to promote the safe handling of guns. Thus, emancipatory knowing would lead this nurse to do something broader about gunshot wounds in an effort to stop them from occurring in the first place. We do not mean to imply that praxis should come out of each and every nursing encounter. What we do imply is that, in the context of practice and within the professional community, it is important to be aware of situations of injustice, to raise everyone's awareness of injustices, and to reflect on these situations and act to improve them whenever possible.

In the remainder of this chapter, we provide more detail about the nature of knowledge forms and about the knowing processes that are unique to each pattern. Each pattern involves distinct processes for developing knowledge. These processes are located within five dimensions: (1) critical questions, (2) creative processes that initiate and generate knowing and knowledge, (3) formal expressions, (4) integrated practice expressions of knowledge and knowing, and (5) authentication processes that are used to examine and improve knowledge for the discipline.

Although a complete understanding requires that each pattern be considered separately, we return again and again to the complementarity of the processes within each pattern and their contribution to the whole of knowing. We also shun the unquestioned use of rules, methods, and principles often associated with knowledge development and embrace perspectives that value knowledge development that is grounded in creating an envisioned future—a future that is shaped by nursing values of health and wellness.

KNOWING AND KNOWLEDGE

In the context of this text, the term *knowing* refers to ways of perceiving and understanding the Self and the world. The term *knowledge* refers to knowing that is expressed in a form that can be shared or communicated with others. The "knowledge of a discipline" is knowledge that has been collectively judged by standards shared by members of the disciplinary community and that is taken to be a valid and accurate understanding of elements and features that comprise the discipline. The *epistemology* of a discipline refers to the ways in which knowledge is developed. Epistemology is the "how to" of knowledge development. The types of knowledge that are taken to be most important for the discipline of nursing are epistemologic concerns (Thorne et al., 2016).

Knowing is a more elusive concept. Knowing is fluid, and it is internal to the knower. People know things as a result of interactions with multiple sources: from what they are taught by others, from books, from their own thinking and experiential processes, from the subconscious absorption of background societal directives (e.g., the nature of personal space), and from many other sources. People "know" more than they can ever express formally as knowledge. For example, try to explain what an onion tastes like to someone who has never eaten onions, or try to explain fully how you, as an expert nurse, managed a difficult clinical situation. Not only is your experience of onions or nursing expertise personal to you, but you also cannot fully impart the nature of these experiences to others. However, you do know what an onion tastes like, and you know that you managed a difficult nursing situation well. In this way, knowing is a concept linked to ontology, or a way of being; knowing is particular and unique to our existence and to each individual's personal reality.

As they practice, nurses make use of insights and understandings gained from a variety of sources that they often take for granted and that they do not consciously think about. Much of what they know is expressed through actions, movements, or sounds in a fluid nursing situation. What is conveyed in a nurse's actions is a simultaneous wholeness or "whole of knowing" that textbooks and theories can never portray. This whole of knowing that happens in practice can only exist in the moment, and it is typically not available to a broader audience.

To summarize, knowing is a particular and unique awareness that grounds and expresses the being and doing of a person, whereas knowledge is knowing that can be expressed and communicated to others in many forms, including principles of practice, works of art, stories, and theories. *Disciplinary* knowledge is knowledge that has been judged to be pertinent to the focus of a discipline by its members.

! Why Is This Important?

We believe that much of what nurses know has the potential to be more fully expressed and communicated than it has been in the past, and that this can happen when all patterns of knowing are valued. Formal descriptions and theories that are used to convey empiric knowledge will only partially reflect the whole. However, when you move beyond the traditional limits of empirics and consider representing knowing within the aesthetic, ethical, personal, and emancipatory patterns, it is possible to convey a more complete picture of what is known within the discipline as a whole. When the knowledge picture is more complete, its value can be more openly assessed and embraced.

Sharing knowledge is important because it creates a disciplinary community beyond the isolation of individual experience. When this happens, social purposes form, and knowledge development and shared social purposes can form a cyclic interrelationship that moves us toward the prospective, value-grounded change that emerges from praxis.

OVERVIEW OF NURSING'S PATTERNS OF KNOWING

Since Florence Nightingale first established formal secular education for nurses, nursing has depended on formal knowledge as a basis for practice (see Chapter 2). The nature of knowledge changes with time, but the fundamental values that guide nursing practice have remained remarkably stable (Adams & Natarajan, 2016; Clements & Averill, 2006; Fawcett, 2006; Fawcett, Watson, Neuman, Walker, & Fitzpatrick, 2001; Gallagher, 2013; Thorne & Sawatzky, 2014).

Carper's (1978) examination of the early nursing literature resulted in the naming of four fundamental and enduring patterns of knowing. Carper called the familiar and respected pattern of *empirics* the science of nursing. She described *ethics* as the component of moral knowledge in nursing; *personal knowing* as knowledge of the Self and others in relationship; and *aesthetics* as the art of nursing. As noted, we have developed the pattern of *emancipatory knowing* as a fifth pattern. The fundamental patterns of knowing as identified by Carper were valuable in that they conceptualized a broad scope of knowing that acknowledged knowing patterns beyond the limited boundaries of empirics.

The empiric knowing pattern has been a central focus for knowledge development within the nursing discipline. The emancipatory, ethical, personal, and aesthetic patterns have not been as well developed, which reflects a neglect of these patterns of knowing and an overvaluing of empirics as the knowledge of the discipline (Fawcett, 2006; Fawcett et al., 2001; Thorne & Sawatzky, 2014). However, methods for developing knowledge related to emancipatory, ethical, personal, and aesthetic knowledge are beginning to be systematically described. The appearance of a literature devoted to additional knowing patterns underscores the value of a broader scope of knowing and knowledge in practice (Archibald, 2012; Clements & Averill, 2006; Cloutier, Duncan, & Bailey, 2007; Galuska, 2012; Gramling, 2006; Lane, 2006; Mantzorou & Mastrogiannis, 2011; Porter & O'Halloran, 2009; Thorne et al., 2016; Weis, Schank, & Matheus, 2006; Wittmann-Price & Bhattacharya, 2008). Because of this shift, in this and subsequent chapters, we first discuss emancipatory knowing, followed by ethics, personal knowing, and aesthetic knowing.

We provide an overview of our conceptualization of each of the patterns of knowing in nursing in the following sections. We have expanded Carper's descriptions of the nature of each pattern. Expansions include development of creative processes, formal expressions, authentication processes, and integrated expressions in practice for each pattern. These expansions are based on our ideas, research, and the insights of other nursing scholars. In addition, the overview of each pattern introduces the methods that we propose for the ongoing development of knowledge within each of the patterns.

Emancipatory Knowing: The Praxis of Nursing

Emancipatory knowing is the human capacity to be aware of and critically reflect on the social, cultural, and political status quo and to determine how and why it came to be that way. Emancipatory knowing calls forth action in ways that reduce or eliminate inequality and injustice. Awareness and critical reflection are essential to identify the inequities that are embedded in social and political institutions, as well as to identify the cultural values and beliefs that need to change to create fair and just conditions for all. Emancipatory knowing requires an understanding of the power dynamics that create knowledge and of the social and political contexts that shape and influence prevailing epistemologies of knowledge and knowing. Emancipatory knowing seeks freedom from institutional and institutionalized social and political contexts that sustain advantage for some and disadvantage for others.

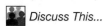 *Discuss This...*

> Cherise, a nurse practitioner in a wellness clinic, becomes aware of the extent to which overweight children are seen in her practice. Emancipatory knowing would focus on understanding the social and political processes that have contributed to the problem of childhood obesity, such as understanding how lack of regulation of the food industry with regard to labeling or use of harmful food ingredients is linked to capitalistic profit motives for large corporations that market to children. Discuss what nursing actions Cherise might consider based on her awareness of these social and political processes.

Emancipatory knowledge, as an expression of emancipatory knowing, begins with being aware of social problems such as injustices and questioning why these exist. This questioning leads to critiques of the status quo. These critiques lead to imagining the changes that are needed to create equitable and just conditions that support all humans in reaching their full potential. Formal written expressions of emancipatory knowledge (e.g., action plans, manifestoes, critical analyses, vision statements) describe the conditions that limit human potential, the circumstances that create and sustain those conditions, what is required to change the status quo, and what needs to be created in place of the status quo. Emancipatory knowledge is also expressed in activist projects directed toward changing existing social structures and establishing practices and structures that are more equitable and favorable to human health and well-being.

The integrated expression of emancipatory knowing is praxis, which produces changes that are intended for the benefit of all. We emphasize "integrated," because the action and reflection of true praxis must be grounded in all knowing patterns to be effective.

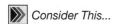 *Consider This...*

> To illustrate further, we return to the nurse caring for the young woman with a gunshot wound. To have had some awareness that this situation was not only unnecessary but also unjust, the nurse had to be aware that Nayan's need for aseptic wound irrigation (which requires empiric knowing) was in part the result of the city shifting police resources from poorer to wealthier neighborhoods (an ethical issue). The nurse would have also had to know that—if he were going to have any influence on this young woman with regard to the safe handling and use of guns, removing guns from the home, or encouraging Nayan to speak out politically—his counsel and teaching would have to be performed with a consideration of Nayan's and her family's feelings about weapons (aesthetic knowing), and his own bias regarding gun control (personal knowing).
>
> Although this is a simple example, it illustrates that emancipatory knowing is integrated with the four knowing patterns when the nurse encourages the young woman

to speak out politically about the situation in her neighborhood. In addition, praxis at the community level would occur when the nurse teams up with friends and peers to work with community leaders to improve police patrol in underserved neighborhoods.

Praxis at the individual level occurs when people recognize conditions that unjustly limit their own or others' abilities and experiences, reflect on these situations with a growing realization that things could be different, and take action to change the circumstances of their own and others' lives. As actions are taken, individuals remain continually attuned to the ideals that they seek, and they continue to reflect critically and act to transform experience into the imagined ideal.

Praxis as a collective endeavor requires reflection and action in concert with others who are engaged in creating social and political change. When groups of people collectively share their individual insights and experiences, critiques and imaginings become symbiotic, and possibilities for change multiply. When members of a discipline such as nursing engage in praxis at a collective level, their cooperative reflections and actions can create substantial change. Praxis within a disciplinary collective also creates emancipatory knowledge that can be authenticated and understood by members of the discipline.

 Why Is This Important?

As a community of critical reflectors and actors, nurses can begin to act on their insights and move toward the goal of transforming nursing and health care. In this way, the critical reflections and actions that constitute praxis at the individual and collective levels continue to energize change in the direction of creating emancipatory knowledge that show how equitable and just social structures can be created. The cycle of praxis (i.e., action and reflection to undo unjust social practices) and the emancipatory changes that it produces are ongoing processes. As praxis produces change, this change undergoes further action and reflection in relation to the envisioned future.

Ethics: The Moral Component of Nursing

Ethics in nursing is focused on matters of obligation: What ought to be done. The moral component of knowing in nursing goes beyond knowledge of the norms or ethical codes of conduct: It involves making moment-to-moment judgments about what ought to be done, what is good and right, and what is responsible. Ethical knowing guides and directs how nurses morally behave in their practices, what they select as being important, where their loyalties are placed, and what priorities demand advocacy.

 Think About It...

Ethical knowing comes into play when Juan, a nurse working in rehabilitation, learns that a young man in his care travels across state lines to legally purchase marijuana for medicinal use and then uses it for pain control in his state, where marijuana is illegal. Juan must decide whether to "play dumb" or to share this knowledge with others and run the risk that his patient's pain will not be properly controlled.

Ethical knowing also involves clarifying conflicting values and exploring alternative interests, principles, and actions. There may be no satisfactory answer to an ethical dilemma or moral distress; rather, there may only be alternatives, some of which are more satisfactory than others. Ethical knowing in nursing requires an experiential knowledge of social values and mores from which ethical reasoning arises, as well as knowledge of the formal principles and codes within the discipline (Carper, 1978).

Ethical principles and codes are formal expressions of ethical knowledge that reflect the philosophic ideals on which ethical decisions rest. Ethical knowledge does not describe or prescribe what a decision or action should be. Rather, it provides insight about which choices are possible and direction with regard to choices that are sound, good, responsible, and just.

Ethical knowledge forms are similar to empiric theory and formal descriptions in that they are expressed in language, reflect some dimensions of experience, and express relationships among phenomena. However, empiric theory relies on observations that can be tested or confirmed by others in a more or less objective manner. Ethical codes and principles cannot be tested in this sense, because the relationships expressed in codes and principles rest on underlying philosophic reasoning that leads to conclusions that concern what is right, good, responsible, or just. This means that reasoning processes—rather than an appeal to facts or observational data—authenticate ethical knowledge. The reasoning can include descriptions that substantiate an argument, but the conclusions are value statements that cannot be perceived or confirmed empirically. The integrated expression of ethical knowing is moral and ethical comportment, which requires the nurse to practice in a way that integrates disciplinary knowledge and situational factors to achieve a morally acceptable result.

Personal Knowing: The Self and the Other in Nursing

Personal knowing in nursing concerns the inner experience of becoming a whole, aware, genuine Self. Personal knowing encompasses knowing one's own Self as well as the Self in relation to others. As Carper (1978, p. 18) stated, "One does not know about the Self, one strives simply to know the self." It is through knowing one's Self in a nonobjectified way that people are able to know the other. Full awareness of the Self in the moment and in the context of interaction makes possible meaningful, shared human experience. Without this component of knowing, the idea of the therapeutic use of the Self in nursing would not be possible (Carper, 1978).

 Consider This...

> Personal knowing is operating when Luella, an older nurse-midwife, recognizes that she has strong negative feelings that she must contain about young, single itinerant mothers. Raised in a staunchly religious family with conservative political views, Luella is in touch with the source of her negativity and tries to channel it into accepting and understanding the perspective and situation of her young female clients.

Personal knowing is most fully communicated as an authentic, aware, genuine Self. Other people perceive the existence of a unique person by physical characteristics, but they also come to know each person as having a unique personality. As personal knowing emerges more fully throughout life, the unique or genuine Self can be more fully expressed and thus becomes accessible as a means by which deliberate action and interaction take form. A deliberate effort to understand the Self through the cultivation of personal knowing increases personal authenticity and genuineness.

Authenticity as a person is important for the provision of sound nursing care. Authenticity requires questioning, acknowledging, and understanding such factors as personal biases, strengths and weaknesses of character, feelings, values, and attitudes. After these have been acknowledged and understood, the nurse can work toward reconciling and resolving inner conflicts of the Self that compromise best nursing practices. In this way, the inner knowing of the Self grows, and authenticity increases.

 Discuss This...

Suppose you hold a negative bias against older adults. Unless you address personal knowing by acknowledging and understanding your bias, you are forced into inauthenticity (e.g., "I'm trying to like this old person even though I don't") when in contact with frail elders. Willfully changing a bias that you have grown up with and learning to recognize actions that reflect this bias are major lifelong processes that cannot be accomplished easily. However, when you face your bias and acknowledge that it is preventing you from being genuinely present as a nurse when you care for older people, you can deliberately choose to bring forth your desire to be genuinely present with such individuals in a nursing situation. Your actions will reflect that intention, and your bias will fade into the background. When you are genuine with older people, you also come to a place where you can begin to see older people in a more positive light. You become more comfortable working with elderly persons, and as a result of your encounters with them, you continue your own self-healing journey. Self-healing might eventually lead you to a place of complete acceptance and understanding of persons you once disliked. Your actions are motivated from an intention to provide good care. In short, the key to cultivating personal knowing is to recognize your inner Self as fully as possible and to choose those aspects of the self that best serve your intentions as a nurse.

It is possible to describe certain aspects of the Self with the use of personal stories, which are written expressions of personal knowing. These descriptions provide sources for deep reflection and a shared understanding of how personal knowledge can be developed, shared, and used in deliberative ways. Descriptions of the Self portrayed in personal stories are limited in that they never fully reflect personal knowing, and they are retrospective in that they can describe only the Self that was. However, publicly expressed descriptions can be a tool for developing self-awareness and self-intimacy and for communicating to others valuable possibilities for developing personal knowing (Caughlin, 2009; Dimitroff, Sliwoski, O'Brien, & Nichols, 2016; Hagan, 1990; Nelson, 2010; Pai, 2015). In addition to public descriptions of personal knowing, the genuine Self is expressed through our daily living in the world. This in-person, ongoing type of expression defies complete description, but it is nonetheless a formal expression of personal knowing.

 Consider This...

In a sense, all knowing is personal; individuals can know only through their personal experience (Bonis, 2009). For example, empiric theories can be learned, but their meaning for the individual comes from personal meaning and experience with the concepts and ideas within the theory. Ethical codes and moral beliefs are likewise personal in nature. We recognize the broad meaning of personal knowing, but our focus is on the aspect of personal knowing that evolves from processes for knowing the Self and for developing and growing in self-knowing through healing encounters with others. It is knowing the Self that makes the therapeutic use of the self in nursing practice possible.

Aesthetics: The Art of Nursing

Aesthetic knowing in nursing involves an appreciation of the meaning of a situation and calls forth inner resources that transform experience into what is not yet real, thus manifesting something that would not otherwise be possible. Aesthetic knowing allows one to move beyond the surface to sense the meaning of the moment and to connect with human experiences that are unique for each person: sickness, suffering, recovery, birth, and death. Aesthetic knowing in practice is expressed through the actions, bearing, conduct, attitudes, narrative, and interactions of the nurse in relation to others. It also is formally expressed in art forms such as poetry, drawings, stories, and music that reflect and communicate the symbolic meanings embedded in nursing practice.

 Consider This...

> Presley works in the orthopedic clinic of a large urban hospital and uses aesthetic knowing with each young child who comes for cast removal. It is aesthetic knowing that helps him remove the cast in the least distressing way for the child. Presley understands that Ava, a 5-year-old, likely sees a large person approaching her leg with an electric cutter and other tools that resemble those in her father's woodworking shop. Presley might use a combination of distraction and humor as well as careful timing to move through the required procedure in an artful way.

Aesthetic knowing is expressed in the moment of experience-action (Benner, 1984, 1994; Benner & Wrubel, 1989) in the transformative art/act. Aesthetic knowing is what makes possible knowing what to do and how to be in the moment, instantly, without conscious deliberation. Carper (1978) characterized aesthetic knowing as "abstracted particulars." In other words, aesthetic knowing is having an understanding of those particular features of a situation that come from a direct understanding of what is significant and meaningful in the moment. The nurse's sense of meaning in the situation is reflected in the action taken. Meaning among those in the situation is often understood and shared without a conscious exchange of words, and it may not be consciously or cognitively realized or brought into awareness; rather, it may be occurring in the background of the situation and not be consciously considered.

Sometimes what a situation means to the nurse comes from the nurse's own perspectives, which makes it possible for the nurse to share new meanings and possibilities for managing a given situation with others. These new meanings and possibilities can be rehearsed, which provides experience with possible movements and verbal expressions that can be used in future situations. Within the pattern of aesthetics, the nurse's actions take on an element of artistry and create unique, meaningful, and often deeply moving interactions with others that touch the common chords of human experience. We refer to this aspect of nursing practice as the *transformative art/act*. We use the notion of art/act to convey that nursing is art in action. A nurse who practices artfully is acting in a way that transforms what is into what could be. In short, the term *art/act* is used to convey the notion that clinical nursing is simultaneously an art and acting or doing.

Aesthetic knowing is expressed in the moment of experience-action (Benner, 1984, 1994; Benner & Wrubel, 1989) in the transformative art/act. Aesthetic knowledge is formally expressed in aesthetic criticism and in works of art that symbolize experience. Aesthetic criticism is a written expression of aesthetic knowledge that conveys the artistic aspects of the art/act, the technical skill required to perform the art/act, the knowledge that informs the development of the art/act, the historical and cultural significance of specific aspects of nursing as an art, and the potential for the future development of the art form.

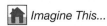 *Imagine This...*

> As an example, imagine a nurse who enters a clinic examination room and sees a young woman sitting on the examination table. Immediately, from an integration of contextual factors such as body language and facial expression, the nurse understands that the young woman is fearful; the nurse's facial expressions and movements confirm to the young woman that the nurse understands that she is afraid. The woman relaxes and looks at the nurse; the nurse places her hand on the young woman's shoulder and smiles. In this example, nothing was said, but the nurse entered the room and immediately grasped the meaning of the situation (i.e., the young woman's fear and the need to relieve it). The ongoing mutual reading of meanings that quickly occurred between the nurse and client resulted in the client's situation transforming from one of fear to one of safety. Transformative art/acts such as these constitute a form of performance art.

Empirics: The Science of Nursing

Empirics is based on the assumption that what is known is accessible through the physical senses, particularly seeing, touching, and hearing. Empirics can be traced to Florence Nightingale's precepts regarding the importance of accurate observation and record keeping. Empirics as a pattern of knowing is grounded in science and other empirically based methodologies. This means that science as a process makes use of empirically based methods to generate knowledge. Empirics assumes that an objective reality exists, and that truths about it can be understood through inferences based on observations and understandings that are verifiable or confirmable by other observers. In other words, empirics assumes that what many people observe and agree on is an objective truth.

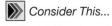 *Consider This...*

> You use empirics when you review a procedure manual and follow required aseptic procedures for inserting a urinary catheter. Empiric knowing is also used when you review a grounded theory of hopefulness as you prepare to care for a crash victim who is now

a quadriplegic patient. When you recall and use in practice what you have studied—whether about how to perform a urinary catheterization or how body language can help restore hopefulness—you are in the realm of empiric knowing.

Empiric knowing is expressed in practice as scientific competence by means of competent action grounded in empiric knowledge, including theory. Scientific competence involves conscious problem solving and logical reasoning, but much of the underlying empiric knowing that informs scientific competence remains in the background of awareness. What remains in the background usually can be brought to awareness when attention turns to the reasoning process itself. In other words, when completing the wound irrigation from our earlier example, the seasoned nurse does not consciously think about the empiric knowledge that justifies the requirement of asepsis as he performs the procedure. However, he could explain the scientific basis for asepsis if asked to do so.

Empiric knowledge is formally expressed in the form of empiric theories, statements of fact, or formalized descriptions and interpretations of empiric events or objects. The development of empiric knowledge traditionally has been accomplished by the methods of traditional science. This has often involved testing hypotheses derived from a theory that offers a tentative explanation of empiric phenomena. Many types of formal descriptions and theories that express empiric knowledge in nursing are linked to the traditional ideas about what is legitimate for developing the science of nursing. In addition, newer methods have been developed to include activities that are not strictly within the realm of traditional empiric methodologies, such as phenomenologic or ethnographic descriptions or inductive means of generating theories and formal descriptions.

> ❗ *Why Is This Important?*
>
> It is important to remember that although each of the patterns is reviewed separately in the previous sections, in clinical situations the nurse cannot be a purist with regard to using only one form of knowing or knowledge. All patterns operate, to one degree or another, in all situations of patient care. Recall a nursing care situation in which you were recently involved. How did you draw on each of the patterns of knowing as you managed the patient's care?

PROCESSES FOR DEVELOPING NURSING KNOWLEDGE

Figs. 1.1 and 1.2 illustrate the interrelationships among each of the patterns of knowing. Fig. 1.1 focuses on emancipatory knowing, whereas Fig. 1.2 details the four fundamental patterns that were originally described by Carper. As shown in Fig. 1.1, emancipatory knowing surrounds and connects with each of the four fundamental patterns of knowing. The four fundamental patterns are represented in the figure by the central, light-colored, irregular oval with praxis at its core. Because the pattern of emancipatory knowing focuses on matters of social justice and equality, it is configured as surrounding and encompassing ethical, personal, aesthetic, and empiric knowing. Embedding the four fundamental knowing patterns within emancipatory knowing also symbolizes the

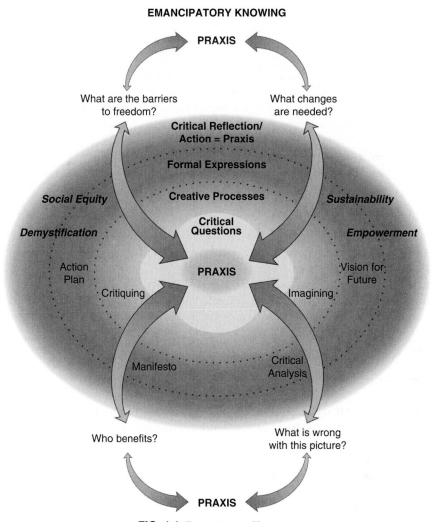

EMANCIPATORY KNOWING

PRAXIS

What are the barriers to freedom?

What changes are needed?

Critical Reflection/ Action = Praxis

Formal Expressions

Social Equity

Creative Processes

Sustainability

Demystification

Critical Questions

Empowerment

Action Plan

PRAXIS

Vision for Future

Critiquing

Imagining

Manifesto

Critical Analysis

Who benefits?

What is wrong with this picture?

PRAXIS

FIG. 1.1 Emancipatory Knowing.

need to examine and understand both practice and disciplinary approaches to knowledge development in relation to how they enable praxis and emancipatory change.

The central location of the fundamental patterns and the four large arrows that extend from the center through the outer hazy, indistinct border represent the need for an outward praxis with which the profession critically examines itself and acts in relation to the societal context in which it exists. The arrows that point inward toward the four fundamental patterns at the model's center represent the need for an inward praxis that critically reflects and acts in relation to the development of nursing knowledge and the practice of nursing. This inward view critically examines the methods used when developing and using nursing knowledge and the nature of knowledge that is considered to

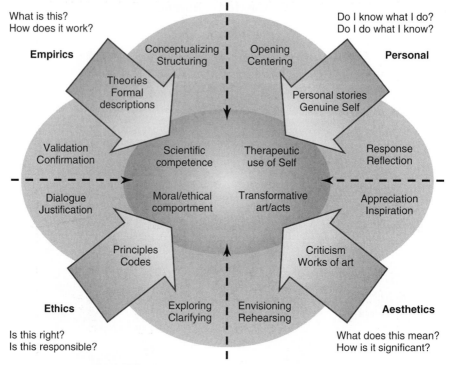

FIG. 1.2 Fundamental Patterns of Knowing.

be authenticated. The outward view considers the social and political contexts in which nursing knowledge is developed and in which nursing is practiced, the interests that nursing serves, and the ways in which nursing shapes and is shaped by its context and history.

For each pattern, we have proposed five dimensions that are shown in both figures and that are also summarized in Table 1.1:

- Critical questions
- Creative processes
- Formal expressions
- Authentication processes
- Integrated expressions in practice

It is through critical questions that creative processes for developing knowledge are initiated. Out of creative processes, knowledge is developed and can be formally expressed and shared with others for authentication. Each pattern of knowing is also associated with an integrated expression in practice. Although formal expressions of knowledge can be shared and presented for authentication, integrated practice expressions of knowing are a way of being that express in the moment of care what is known. The processes for each pattern are unique and particular to the pattern with which they are associated. To say that each process is unique to its individual pattern of knowing means that you

TABLE 1.1 Dimensions Associated With Each of the Patterns of Knowing

Dimension	Emancipatory	Ethics	Personal	Aesthetics	Empirics
Critical questions	Who benefits? What is wrong with this picture? What are the barriers to freedom? What changes are needed?	Is this right? Is this responsible?	Do I know what I do? Do I do what I know?	What does this mean? How is this significant?	What is this? How does it work?
Creative processes	Critiquing Imagining	Clarifying Exploring	Opening Centering	Envisioning Rehearsing	Conceptualizing Structuring
Formal expressions	Action plans Manifestoes Critical analyses Visions for the future	Principles and codes	Personal stories Genuine Self	Aesthetic criticism Works of art	Facts Models Formal descriptions Theories Thematic descriptions
Authentication processes	Social equity Sustainability Empowerment Demystification	Dialogue Justification	Response Reflection	Appreciation Inspiration	Confirmation Validation
Integrated expression in practice	Praxis	Moral and ethical comportment	Therapeutic use of Self	Transformative art/acts	Scientific competence

cannot create empiric theory, for example, by initiating the creative processes of ethics or personal, aesthetic, or emancipatory knowing. Processes for creating, authenticating, and expressing knowledge and knowing within each pattern are detailed next.

The critical questions of emancipatory knowing shown in Fig. 1.1 are located external to the outer boundary of the model. These queries are as follows: What are the barriers to freedom? What changes are needed? Who benefits? What is wrong with this picture? These questions focus on the social context of nursing and health care as well as on formal expressions of disciplinary knowledge and knowing in the immediate clinical situation as portrayed by the four double arrows. The critical questions awaken and sustain emancipatory awareness and suggest what needs to change. These critical questions arise from a nurse's personal experience either in practice or in some other aspect of his or her personal and professional life that affects practice. The questions are placed outside the boundaries of the model to symbolize that critical questions also come from an awareness of larger social and political contexts. The double curved configuration of the arrows also represents the ongoing, constant, and synchronous nature of praxis that arises when you or other nurses ask, reflect, and act in relation to the critical questions.

The three outer spheres that encircle the representation of the four fundamental patterns of knowing represent (1) the creative processes that are used to develop emancipatory knowledge, (2) the formal expressions of emancipatory knowledge that assist and enable praxis, and (3) the authentication processes that document emancipatory change. The creative processes within the inner sphere that surrounds the central area containing the four fundamental knowing patterns are engaged to develop emancipatory knowledge. These are critiquing the status quo and imagining what might create a world that is more equitable for all. Critique can be approached with the use of one or more of several possible lenses, including the lens of race, ethnicity, socioeconomic status, gender identity, sexual orientation, age, culture, religious beliefs, and political views. Critiques uncover the subtle ways in which injustice is sustained and deepen the awareness of what needs to change. From the critique emerges an image or imagining of what could be and ideas about the actions that are needed for change. Formal expressions of the critique are shown within the middle sphere that surrounds the fundamental patterns and include critical analyses that are published in scholarly journals, action plans that are communicated electronically or in writing, manifestoes, and vision statements. Formal expressions that are communicated as emancipatory knowledge also provide insights about the processes of praxis for emancipatory change; this knowledge is useful in other situations that call for similar forms of change.

Praxis, which is the critical action/reflection dimension of emancipatory knowing, is located both outside the porous outer sphere and centrally within our model of emancipatory knowing. The central location of praxis symbolizes the local individual expression of critical reflective nursing practice; this is a place where a new awareness of problems often begins to take shape and where consciousness shifts to a realization that your experience and your situation are problematic, and you do something to begin to change it. The outer circle of the model that is open to what is beyond symbolizes that praxis is also situated in and directed to the larger social, political, and economic contexts of nursing practice.

The discipline authenticates emancipatory knowing by demonstrating that social change—and the formal disciplinary expressions that motivate and mobilize that type of change—accomplishes imagined and intended shifts that end injustices and inequities. Authentication processes examine the sustainability of the change, the presence of social equity, to what extent the demystification of processes that sustain inequities has occurred, and the degree of empowerment for those who have been unjustly treated. These authentication processes are shown in bold black type and are primarily within the two outer spheres of Fig. 1.1, because these processes are directed toward formal expressions of emancipatory knowing that mobilize praxis. They also overlap slightly with the inner sphere of critiquing and imagining, because praxis can begin to emerge from these creative processes of emancipatory knowing.

Fig. 1.2 expands on the irregular oval at the center of Fig. 1.1 that represents the four fundamental patterns of knowing. We refer to the four patterns originally proposed by Carper as the "fundamental knowing patterns." In Fig. 1.2, each of the fundamental patterns is represented as a quadrant. At the periphery of each quadrant are the pattern's critical questions that are asked in relation to knowledge expressions as well as in the practice moment.

The large arrows that point toward the model's central core contain examples of the formal expressions of knowledge for each pattern. The central core at the tip of each large arrow contains the in-practice or integrated practice expressions of knowing associated with each pattern. The inner sphere of Fig. 1.2 is configured as a whole, without quadrant boundaries; this represents our view that, in nursing practice, knowing is experienced as an integrated whole that can never be experienced as discrete patterns. On either side of the vertical broken arrows are the creative processes for developing formal written and communicable knowledge expressions for each pattern. Above and below the broken horizontal arrows are the authentication processes used within the discipline for validating or authenticating disciplinary knowledge forms.

Knowledge and knowing come about when critical questions are asked within each of these four patterns. Personal knowing asks, "Do I know what I do?" and "Do I do what I know?" Ethics asks the critical questions "Is this right?" and "Is this responsible?" Aesthetics asks, "What does this mean?" and "How is this significant?" Finally, the critical questions for empirics are "What is this?" and "How does it work?"

These critical questions and similar queries are implicit in practice, which means that they are "asked" in the moment of care, but often not consciously or deliberately. They also are asked apart from the moment of practice to develop consciously or deliberately a better understanding of what happened in a particular situation or to initiate some form of inquiry to find an answer that seems elusive. Critical questions are also asked of the disciplinary knowledge forms located within the large arrows as a way to improve their usefulness for practice. The process of posing these questions and seeking answers or solutions improves practice and advances the knowledge on which practice is founded.

The creative processes, which are adjacent to the vertical dotted arrows in Fig. 1.2, lead to formal expressions of knowledge. Opening and centering the self creates personal knowledge. The development of ethical knowledge uses processes that clarify values, rights, and responsibilities in practice and explores alternative ethical positions and actions. Aesthetic knowledge is developed by envisioning possibilities and rehearsing art/acts that can be used to transform clinical experiences. Empiric knowledge development makes use of the reasoning processes of conceptualizing and structuring empiric phenomena.

With regard to creative inquiry processes, forms of expression evolve that can be shared with members of the discipline for authentication. The creative inquiry processes for ethics generate principles and codes as well as other expressions (e.g., precepts) that guide ethical conduct in practice. The critical questions for personal knowing generate personal stories and the lived expression of the nurse's being (i.e., who the nurse is) in nursing care situations that conveys the genuine self. Aesthetic inquiry leads to works of art that symbolize nursing experience and to aesthetic criticism that reveals deep meaning embedded in nursing art/acts. Empiric inquiry processes produce theories, formal descriptions, models, and various other constructions (e.g., facts, thematic descriptions of experience, conceptual frameworks).

The formal expressions of each pattern, after they have been made available to the members of the discipline, make possible certain formal authentication processes that depend on the collective efforts of the discipline or the community. These authentication processes, which are adjacent to the horizontal dotted lines in Fig. 1.2, begin with the critical questions for each pattern and are requisite to establishing the professional value of knowledge generated from creative inquiry processes. Ethical principles and codes are authenticated through collective dialogue and through the justification of the soundness of the principles when addressing nursing's ethical and moral dilemmas. For personal knowing, others in the discipline respond to stories and the expression of the genuine self to discern the value and adequacy of personal insights. Questioning the meaning and significance of aesthetic criticism and works of art leads to the formation of a collective appreciation of aesthetic meanings for practice and becomes a source of inspiration for the development of transformative art/acts. In the empiric pattern, formal expressions such as theories and models that are grounded in observations and perceptions of empiric events are subjected to inquiry that can be confirmed and validated in similar but different situations.

All the processes involved in developing nursing knowledge are interactive and nonlinear, and there is no single starting point. Nurses in practice and nurses who primarily engage in the formal inquiry processes all contribute to the activities that are involved in creating nursing knowledge. Each nurse engages in activities that make possible critical reflection and action, scientific competence, moral and ethical comportment, the therapeutic use of self, and transformative art/acts.

 Consider This...

The following five case problems illustrate how all of the patterns of knowing are integrated. Each case has a "starting point" arising from one of the patterns, but calls for nursing action that is grounded in the whole of knowing.

Case 1: Initial Problem, Empiric

Imagine that you have an empiric problem that involves which nursing approaches to relieving pain are effective in practice and why. You might begin to address this problem by locating evidence related to nursing approaches to pain relief and subsequently planning a research program to systematically study two different approaches to pain relief for which there are not yet sufficient evidence. You would identify the theoretic explanations associated with each approach, and develop a research plan that tests selected hypothetic relationships. Although the empiric questions are the starting point and remain the focus of your method, your approaches and methods are influenced by an awareness of social, political, and cultural attitudes and practices involved with the experience of pain and its alleviation. You realize that these practices might be reflected in ample or limited funding for your project. The aesthetic meanings of the relief of pain and suffering for the various cultural groups in your study will affect how you choose and use measurement tools. Personal meanings regarding the experience of pain will shape how you report your findings, whereas ethical values surrounding what is best or right to do when the potential for addiction arises will influence how and when pain relief is given and received.

Case 2: Initial Problem, Personal

Personal knowing is commonly the avenue through which an awareness of possibilities that are not yet fully understood emerges. For example, suppose that you come to realize and appreciate the unique perspective of an immigrant family who is receiving presurgical care in the clinic. This family has been labeled "difficult" and "uncooperative" by other nurses. As you encounter the family, you sense that something has not seemed to fit for the family and that they just have not felt right. As you open yourself to trying to understand their behavior, a growing appreciation of the family's perspective gradually brings the new insight that the entire family would like to stay with the ill family member during her hospitalization for an upcoming surgery. You share your awareness of this with the family, and the relationship shifts to bring the family's perspective to the center. Although having several family members occupy a single room during recovery is not feasible, a plan is put in place whereby one or two family members can be with the ill family member in her room, and others can occupy a nearby waiting room. Personal knowing is the starting point for bringing a situation into awareness, but, as you explore your awareness, your knowledge of the social and cultural context of an immigrant family in a hospital clinic sharpens your sensitivity to social inequities and injustices that create barriers to understanding the family's perspective. You also use empiric theories that address fear and anxiety as tools for understanding the significance of the situation within a frame of ethical principles that require both caring and justice for other hospitalized patients in the vicinity of this family's ill family member. How and when to confirm your hunches regarding the concerns of the family requires aesthetic sensibilities for discerning the meaning of the experience.

Case 3: Initial Problem, Ethical

Suppose that you want to address an ethical question that concerns what is right in a situation in which a physician asks you to withhold information related to the stage of disease from a woman who has been hospitalized for the treatment of a malignant tumor. You might begin with the focused, creative activities of making explicit the personal and group values (valuing) that should guide your actions, clarifying the positions that you find in ethical codes and principles that inform the issue, and setting forth how the application of these principles would function among the people with whom you work. These processes would lead you to a dialogue and a justification of your ideas that are primarily based in ethical reasoning. When you begin to share your ideas with colleagues, the questioning and discussion that result will bring to awareness the personal insights of others engaged in the dialogue. Your dialogue brings to light empiric evidence about what various stages of malignancy mean in relation to treatment effectiveness. You will explore the range of aesthetic significance that is possible in this and similar situations (e.g., meanings that surround treatment options related to recovery). Your dialogue will also illuminate the nature of the social processes and institutionalized values (e.g., the value of screening mammograms that may carry a risk for radiation injury) in which the ethical problem is situated.

Case 4: Initial Problem, Aesthetics

When aesthetics is the starting point, it often begins with the nurse's own awareness in much the same way that personal knowing does; however, the expression often takes an art form that shows what the nurse envisions about the situation. The art can be in the form of the nurse's actions in a situation. Suppose that you feel a connection to the experience of chronic pain in an elderly woman with dementia. During a moment of caring for the person, you act from a deeply developed knowing of the meaning of chronic pain in a way that connects with the woman's own experience. Understanding and acting aesthetically in relation to the meaning of pain require the integration of empiric knowledge of the subjective nature of the pain experience in older persons with the ethical principles related to the relief of pain as a caring act. Personal knowing that has resulted from having suffered unnecessary pain yourself also contributes to the expression of aesthetics by shaping how expressions of pain are interpreted and how you act in relation to those interpretations. Emancipatory knowing contributes to this situation when you understand that the person in pain—because she is elderly and demented—has little social value and probably is not receiving her pain medication as routinely as necessary. This understanding is important for aesthetic practice because your reflection and action in relation to this understanding (i.e., having a nursing conference that illuminates the situation of undertreated pain in demented elderly patients) enable changes that create possibilities that were not previously present (i.e., appropriately managed pain for this and other socially devalued individuals).

Case 5: Initial Problem, Emancipatory

Emancipatory knowing is a common starting point for nurses because of the value that nurses typically place on understanding the cultural and social contexts that influence people's experience of health and illness. Suppose that you become increasingly uncomfortable with the legal restrictions that influence the dispensing of medications for pain. You are aware that these restrictions are so focused on preventing drug abuse that unnecessary restrictions are being placed on legitimate uses of drugs to alleviate pain. Together with other concerned health care providers and patients, you embark on a project to change the political and legal structures so that access to pain relief is not unnecessarily limited. You draw on empiric evidence that addresses both drug misuse and pain relief, people's personal experiences and expressions of pain, aesthetic portrayals of experiences of pain and drug misuse, and ethical principles that guide decisions and actions related to drug use and misuse. You gradually form a plan of action and begin the project of changing the political and legal structures, and you continually integrate new awareness and insights and remain open to shifting the action plan as you reach toward your vision of the future.

WHY DEVELOP NURSING'S PATTERNS OF KNOWING?

Access the Model of Knowing and Knowledge Development animation by scanning the QR code on the inside front cover or by visiting http://booksite.elsevier.com/9780323530613.

As is shown in the animation, in Figs. 1.1 and 1.2, and from our discussion of the knowing patterns, the fundamental reason for developing knowledge in nursing is for the purpose of creating expert and effective nursing practice. Nursing's unique perspective and the particular contributions that nurses bring to care come from the whole of knowing; this wholeness has survived despite a cultural and contextual dominance of empiric knowing (Archibald, 2012; Betts, 2009; Billay, Myrick, Luhanga, & Yonge, 2007; Clements & Averill, 2006; Fawcett et al., 2001; Mantzorou & Mastrogiannis, 2011).

In a sense, the discipline of nursing can be viewed as the empiric pattern of "patterns gone wild" (see Chapter 10) in that most efforts in formal knowledge development have focused on empiric methods. Moreover, knowledge has been equated with empiric forms to the exclusion of any other forms of expression, and the basis for best practices in nursing has come to be associated almost exclusively with empiric evidence (Thorne & Sawatzky, 2014).

The idea that knowledge development occurs in academic settings that are separate from practice can be seen as deriving from the dominance of empirics. Empiric knowledge is inadequate to represent the complexity of the practice world. In fact, the methods of science traditionally require controlling or eliminating the uncontrolled and unpredictable contingencies in the practice realm, which makes the findings of empirics questionable when used in a practice context. The practice implications of empiric knowledge are often not direct or immediately obvious, and empiric knowledge often makes use of a different language than that used in practice.

 Think About It...

A shift to a balance in knowledge development to reflect each of the patterns of knowing in nursing holds potential to bring the realm of knowledge development and the realm of practice together. Methods for developing emancipatory, ethical, personal, and aesthetic knowing compel immersion within the realm of practice, and those nurses who hold the practice doctorate are well positioned to develop more comprehensive approaches to knowledge development. Giving attention to diverse aspects of knowledge development by focusing on all patterns of knowing shifts how empirics itself is viewed. Empirics becomes part of a larger whole, and its value takes on different meanings in this context. In addition, as greater attention is given to methods other than empirics, many of the traditions and assumptions that underlie empiric methods are challenged, thereby opening the way for creating empiric methods that better accommodate the contingencies of practice.

Formally expressed nursing knowledge provides professional and disciplinary identity, which in turn conveys to others what nursing contributes to the health care process (Adams & Natarajan, 2016; Copnell, 2008; Jackson, Clements, Averill, & Zimbro, 2009). Professional identity that evolves from distinct disciplinary knowledge provides a basis from which nurses can create certain aspects of their practice. The knowledge that forms nursing practice provides a language for talking about the nature of nursing practice and for demonstrating its effectiveness. When nursing practice is described, it is made visible. Moving to a conceptualization of knowledge that more fully reflects knowing that is required in practice will serve to impart value to what has been intangible.

In addition, when nursing's effectiveness can be shown, it can be deliberately shaped or controlled by those who practice it (Banks-Wallace, Despins, Adams-Leander, McBroom, & Tandy, 2008; Hartrick Doane et al., 2015; Linderman et al., 2015).

On an individual level, nursing knowledge can provide self-identity and confidence because you will have a firmer base when your ideas are questioned. As you become familiar with the language and processes of knowledge development, you can begin to think about how each of the patterns of knowing can be challenged. The study and understanding of knowledge development will provide a basis on which to take risks, act deliberately, and improve practice.

 Imagine This...

> Imagine yourself as a nurse who is using massage to ease chronic pain for a hospitalized person. A physician notices that you are using this method of care. Because this approach is not something the physician would customarily use, she asks you about it. You explain your reasoning, which is based on nursing knowledge. You can cite research evidence of the effectiveness of massage and how you have integrated that evidence into a clinical decision to use it. You convey to the physician information about the positive results that the person is experiencing. You explain the ethical importance of providing relief from suffering, when possible without using analgesic drugs; the aesthetic components of the meaning in the situation; and what you have learned about the therapeutic use of the self when giving a massage. You explain the societal shift toward accepting and expecting complementary therapies to be included in any approach to care and the social practices that labeled alternative practices as "quackery" that kept this valuable therapy suppressed. You also cite facts regarding the nurse practice act in your region that includes massage as a legitimate nursing care practice. Your explanation leads to an informed discussion about various approaches to caring for people with pain and why your approach seems to be effective for this person. As other practitioners learn about your knowledge in this area, they seek your consultation when caring for people with pain. Your knowledge of empiric pain theory and of what is effective when caring for people with pain—as well as your emancipatory, ethical, aesthetic, and personal knowledge—provides a valuable resource for developing and improving practice.

Nursing's formally expressed knowledge forms also provide the discipline with a coherence of purpose, and a coherence of professional purpose is closely linked to professional identity. A coherence of purpose contributes to a collective identity when nurses agree about the general practice domain. The processes for developing nursing knowledge serve as a means for resolving significant disagreements among practitioners about what is to be accomplished.

 Discuss This...

> Varying points of view that involve the general purpose of nursing are reflected in the following questions:
> - Should nurses address the prevention of illness?
> - Should nurses treat human responses to illness?
> - Should educational programs be structured around the nursing process? Nursing

diagnoses? Patterns of knowing? Critical thinking? Evidence-based nursing practices?
- Should nurses view health and illness as opposites?
- Can people with an illness or disease also be healthy?
- Is political activism part of nursing's responsibility to society?

As nurses develop individual and collective responses to questions addressing the purposes of nursing, this will help clarify our directions for developing knowledge, and in turn, our knowledge-development efforts will contribute to clarifying responses to such questions. Nursing knowledge facilitates coherence by examining such questions as a basis for deliberate choices. When nurses examine and agree about professional purposes and develop knowledge related to those purposes, the public and other practitioners will recognize nursing's expertise in relation to those arenas. The fact that nurses are responsible for certain situations will be directly and indirectly communicated to society, and professional identity and coherence of purpose will continue to evolve. By shifting to a balance in the development of all of nursing's knowledge patterns, a sense of purpose grounded in the whole of knowing can develop that shapes and directs nursing practice.

CONCLUSION

This chapter has presented an overview of the five patterns of knowing, and justifies the importance of attending to all patterns of knowing when disciplinary knowledge is developed. In the next chapter we review the history of nursing knowledge development, followed by five chapters that address the particular knowledge development processes for each pattern of knowing that give rise to formal expressions of knowledge within each pattern. The last three chapters focus on authentication processes and the integration of formal expressions of knowledge in practice.

References

Adams, J. M., & Natarajan, S. (2016). Understanding influence within the context of nursing: development of the Adams influence model using practice, research, and theory. *ANS. Advances in Nursing Science, 39*(3), E40–E56. https://doi.org/10.1097/ANS.0000000000000134.

Archibald, M. M. (2012). The holism of aesthetic knowing in nursing. *Nursing Philosophy: An International Journal for Healthcare Professionals, 13*, 179–188. https://doi.org/10.1111/j.1466-769X.2012.00542.x.

Banks-Wallace, J., Despins, L., Adams-Leander, S., McBroom, L., & Tandy, L. (2008). Re/affirming and re/conceptualizing disciplinary knowledge as the foundation for doctoral education. *ANS. Advances in Nursing Science, 31*, 67–78.

Barrett, E. A. M. (2002). What is nursing science? *Nursing Science Quarterly, 15*, 51–60.

Benner, P. A. (1984). *From novice to expert: excellence and power in clinical nursing practice.* Menlo Park, CA: Addison-Wesley.

Benner, P. A. (1994). *Interpretive phenomenology: embodiment, caring and ethics in health and illness.* Thousand Oaks, CA: Sage Publications.

Benner, P. A., & Wrubel, J. (1989). *The primacy of caring: stress and coping in health and illness.* Menlo Park, CA: AddisonWesley.

Betts, C. E. (2009). Nursing and the reality of politics. *Nursing Inquiry, 16*, 261–272.

Billay, D., Myrick, F., Luhanga, F., & Yonge, O. (2007). A pragmatic view of intuitive knowledge in nursing practice. *Nursing Forum, 42*, 147–155.

Bliss, S., Baltzly, D., Bull, R., Dalton, L., & Jones, J. (2017). A role for virtue in unifying the "knowledge" and "caring" discourses in nursing theory. *Nursing Inquiry*. https://doi.org/10.1111/nin.12191.

Bonis, S. A. (2009). Knowing in nursing: a concept analysis. *Journal of Advanced Nursing, 65*, 1328–1341.

Carper, B. A. (1978). Fundamental patterns of knowing in nursing. *ANS. Advances in Nursing Science, 1*, 13–23.

Caughlin, A. (2009). *Journaling through: unleashing the power of your authentic self.* Houston, TX: Bright Sky Press.

Chinn, P. L., & Kramer, M. (2007). *Integrated theory and knowledge development in nursing* (7th ed.). St Louis, MO: Mosby.

Clements, P. T., & Averill, J. A. (2006). Finding patterns of knowing in the work of Florence Nightingale. *Nursing Outlook, 54*, 268–274.

Cloutier, J. D., Duncan, C., & Bailey, P. H. (2007). Locating Carper's aesthetic pattern of knowing within contemporary nursing evidence, praxis and theory. *International Journal of Nursing Education Scholarship, 4*, 1–11.

Copnell, B. (2008). The knowledgeable practice of critical care nurses: a poststructural inquiry. *International Journal of Nursing Studies, 45*, 588–598.

Dimitroff, L. J., Sliwoski, L., O'Brien, S., & Nichols, L. W. (2016). Change your life through journaling— The benefits of journaling for registered nurses. *Journal of Nursing Education and Practice, 7*(2), 90. https://doi.org/10.5430/jnep.v7n2p90.

Fawcett, J. (2006). Commentary: finding patterns of knowing in the work of Florence Nightingale. *Nursing Outlook, 54*, 275–277.

Fawcett, J., Watson, J., Neuman, B., Walker, P. H., & Fitzpatrick, J. J. (2001). On nursing theories and evidence. *Journal of Nursing Scholarship: An Official Publication of Sigma Theta Tau International Honor Society of Nursing / Sigma Theta Tau, 33*, 115–119.

Gallagher, A. (2013). Values for contemporary nursing practice: waving or drowning? *Nursing Ethics, 20*, 615–616. https://doi.org/10.1177/0969733013496362.

Galuska, L. A. (2012). Cultivating nursing leadership for our envisioned future. *ANS. Advances in Nursing Science, 35*(4), 333–345. https://doi.org/10.1097/ANS.0b013e318271d2cd.

Gramling, K. L. (2006). Sarah's story of nursing artistry. *Journal of Holistic Nursing: Official Journal of the American Holistic Nurses' Association, 24*, 140–142.

Hagan, K. L. (1990). *Internal affairs: a journalkeeping workbook for intimacy.* New York, NY: Harper & Row.

Hartrick Doane, G., Reimer-Kirkham, S., Antifeau, E., & Stajduhar, K. (2015). (Re)theorizing integrated knowledge translation: a heuristic for knowledge-as-action. *ANS. Advances in Nursing Science, 38*(3), 175–186. https://doi.org/10.1097/ANS.0000000000000076.

Jackson, J. R., Clements, P. T., Averill, J. B., & Zimbro, K. (2009). Patterns of knowing: proposing a theory for nursing leadership. *Nursing Economics, 27*, 149–159.

Jacobs, B. B. (2013). An innovative professional practice model: adaptation of Carper's patterns of knowing, patterns of research, and Aristotle's intellectual virtues. *ANS. Advances in Nursing Science, 36*(4), 271–288. https://doi.org/10.1097/ANS.0000000000000002.

Kangasniemi, M., Kallio, H., & Pietilä, A.-M. (2014). Towards environmentally responsible nursing: a critical interpretive synthesis. *Journal of Advanced Nursing, 70*(7), 1465–1478. https://doi.org/10.1111/jan.12347.

Lane, M. R. (2006). Arts in health care: a new paradigm for holistic nursing practice. *Journal of Holistic Nursing: Official Journal of the American Holistic Nurses' Association, 24*, 70–75.

Linderman, A., Pesut, D., & Disch, J. (2015). Sense making and knowledge transfer: capturing the knowledge and wisdom of nursing leaders. *Journal of Professional Nursing: Official Journal of the American Association of Colleges of Nursing, 31*(4), 290–297. https://doi.org/10.1016/j.profnurs.2015.02.004.

Mantzorou, M., & Mastrogiannis, D. (2011). The value and significance of knowing the patient for professional practice, according to the Carper's patterns of knowing. *Health Science Journal, 5*, 251–261.

Nelson, G. L. (2010). *Writing and being: taking back our lives through the power of language.* Novato, CA: New World Library, Kindle Edition.

Newman, M. A. (2003). A world of no boundaries. *ANS. Advances in Nursing Science, 26*, 240–245.

Pai, H.-C. (2015). The effect of a self-reflection and insight program on the nursing competence of nursing students: a longitudinal study. *Journal of Professional Nursing: Official Journal of the American Association of Colleges of Nursing, 31*(5), 424–431. https://doi.org/10.1016/j.profnurs.2015.03.003.

Paley, J., Cheyne, H., Dalgleish, L., Duncan, E. A. S., & Niven, C. A. (2007). Nursing's ways of knowing and dual process theories of cognition. *Journal of Advanced Nursing, 60*, 692–701.

Porter, S. (2010). Fundamental patterns of knowing in nursing: the challenge of evidence-based practice. *ANS. Advances in Nursing Science, 33*, 1–12.

Porter, S., & O'Halloran, P. (2009). The postmodernist war on evidence-based practice. *International Journal of Nursing Studies, 46*, 740–748.

Satterfield, J. M., Spring, B., Brownson, R. C.Mullen, E. J., Newhouse, R. P., Walker, B. B., & Whitlock, E. P., et al. (2009). Toward a transdisciplinary model of evidence-based practice. *The Milbank Quarterly, 87*, 368–390.

Terry, L., Carr, G., & Curzio, J. (2016). Expert nurses' perceptions of the relevance of Carper's patterns of knowing to junior nurses. *ANS. Advances in Nursing Science, 1*. https://doi.org/10.1097/ANS.00000000 00000142.

Thorne, S. (2014). Nursing as social justice: a case for emancipatory disciplinary theorizing. In P. Kagan, M. Smith, & P. L. Chinn (Eds.), *Philosophies and practices of emancipatory nursing: social justice as praxis* (pp. 79–90). New York, NY: Routledge.

Thorne, S., & Sawatzky, R. (2014). Particularizing the general: sustaining theoretical integrity in the context of an evidence-based practice agenda. *ANS. Advances in Nursing Science, 37*, 1–10.

Thorne, S., Stephens, J., & Truant, T. (2016). Building qualitative study design using nursing's disciplinary epistemology. *Journal of Advanced Nursing, 72*(2), 451–460. https://doi.org/10.1111/jan.12822.

Weis, D., Schank, M. J., & Matheus, R. (2006). The process of empowerment: a parish nurse perspective. *Journal of Holistic Nursing: Official Journal of the American Holistic Nurses' Association, 24*, 17–24.

Wittmann-Price, R. A., & Bhattacharya, A. (2008). Reexploring the subconcepts of the Wittmann-Price theory of emancipated decision making in women's healthcare. *ANS. Advances in Nursing Science, 31*, 225–236.

The History of Knowledge Development in Nursing

Nursing history was taught, but never accorded much importance... a casual interlude... and even more disheartening not valued. Lacking historical record, the profession is poorly informed... a void in self-awareness that affects the stature and growth of nursing as a vital, essential service.

Myra Estrin Levine (1999, p. 214)

The nursing models and frameworks that have been all too often disregarded as if they were inconvenient remnants of an immature disciplinary science can instead serve as a strong philosophical foundation for expanding our understanding of the complexity, and context within which nursing enacts [its] particular role within the health care [system].

Sally Thorne and Richard Sawatzky (2014, pp. 14–15)

Levine's quote suggests that if nurses do not know their history, they cannot value it; when nurses do not value history, they cannot learn and grow from what it teaches. Thorne and Sawatzky point out that all too often, nurses have devalued the nursing knowledge expressed in the early nursing theories and models, and that these ideas in fact form the important philosophic and value basis for our practice. As a point of reference, we have included in the Appendix our interpretive summary of a number of the broad theoretic frameworks that are foundational to defining the scope, philosophy, and general characteristics of nursing. This chapter reviews the history of nursing's knowledge development as a way to reclaim the value of nursing knowledge and to understand not only where nursing has been but also where it might go in the future.

 Discuss This...

With your colleagues, discuss your various responses to these questions:
- To what extent do the quotes from Levine, and from Thorne and Sawatzky, reflect your feelings about the study of nursing history?
- What nursing theories or models have you studied, and what do you know about the development of the ideas around which they were built?
- What do you know about Florence Nightingale and her work? Have you ever read *Notes on Nursing*? Have you read her essay "Cassandra" (1852/1979)?
- Would it surprise you to know that Florence Nightingale was widely known and respected for her statistical accomplishments during her lifetime (Beck, 2006)?
- What do you think nurses 50 years from now will say about what we are doing today?

The history of knowledge development in nursing is a vast subject indeed. In this chapter, we touch on some of the key events that are part of nursing's rich knowledge development heritage. Our purpose is to trace major historical trends that undergird serious inquiry surrounding each of nursing's patterns of knowing and spark interest in further study of the subject.

Well before the advent of modern nursing in the United States, which was marked by the beginning of the Nightingale era during the early 1900s, nursing existed in many forms that shared a common core. What the word *nursing* means and the functions of nurses have shifted to reflect the social order of the time and the demands placed on nurses. Despite shifts in their functions, nurses have played a role in the care of ill persons since the beginning of recorded history. Nursing has been fundamentally linked with a nurturing role toward the infirm, ill, and less fortunate. Much of nursing's history is tied to the history of medicine, which has dominated the accounts of changes in the care of the sick throughout time. Although much of nursing's unique history has been obscured or lost, substantial evidence supports the value and strength of nursing in the delivery of care and the promotion of health.

Early conceptions of nursing knowledge were grounded in a holistic view of health and healing. Nurses writing about nursing between the late 1800s and 1950s addressed all aspects of knowing, perhaps without recognizing it. These nurses wrote about the importance of observation and recording facts, the need to bring a sense of virtue to the care of sick people, and the characteristics of a good nurse. Early writings also addressed the art of nursing and called for responsible social action that would better the lot of the sick. With increasing interest in promoting the study of science during the 1950s in the United States, nursing shifted toward a focus on empirics as the primary concern of the discipline. Even during this period in nursing's history, however, threads of philosophic and practical commitment to holistic practices and to other patterns of knowing persisted. As the 21st century approached, nurses gave serious attention to holistic approaches in practice and in the methods used for the development of knowledge.

Current knowledge development approaches will undoubtedly continue to change with the times as societal values and resources are altered. Despite changes, strong evidence supports the claim that nurses have, throughout time, developed and used knowledge to improve practice. This chapter reviews some of the key events in nursing's knowledge development trajectory from antiquity to the present. It also addresses how societal values and resources operate to create nursing's history.

FROM ANTIQUITY TO NIGHTINGALE

There is ample evidence that, long before the work of Nightingale, nurses assisted with the routine care of the sick and, in some societies, independently provided healing care (Achterberg, 1991; Donahue, 2011; Ehrenreich & English, 1993). The care provided by these early nurses was influenced by the healing traditions within society. Pagan healers such as shamans, midwives, and other folk healers linked disease to influences that came from within a spirit world. These early healers used rituals, ceremonies, and charms to dispel perceived evil and to invoke good. Plants and herbal remedies also were used for healing. Nurses provided assistance to others who carried out healing traditions, but they were also independent providers of care.

Early Christian traditions often attributed disease to divine wrath, and punishment was meted out in the form of disease states for sinful transgressions. With the advent of early forms of scientific thought that dated from the mid-1500s to the mid-1700s, pagan and early religious views of illness were challenged. The work of scientists and philosophers such as Copernicus, Galileo, Bacon, and Newton began to lay the groundwork for a view of disease as the result of natural rather than spiritual causes. As society's understanding of the causes of disease changed, approaches such as invoking the spirits with charms and the idea of disease being a punishment for religious transgressions began to subside. It was nurses who were there to provide nurturing and assistive services consistent with the view that disease was linked to natural causes. The early religious orders offered a respectable avenue for nuns and monks to provide care to ill and infirm persons. In some societies, people who were being punished for civil offenses, people who were homeless and needed shelter, people who were addicted to drugs and alcohol, and women who were prostitutes also provided nursing care. Nurses also included women who bore the primary responsibility for the care of their ill family members.

NIGHTINGALE'S LEGACY

Although nursing as a nurturing, supportive activity appears to have always existed, it was Florence Nightingale who advocated and promoted the need for a uniformly high standard of nursing care that required both education and certain personal characteristics. The recognition of nursing as a professional endeavor distinct from medicine began with Nightingale. Her actions and writings about the subject of nursing and sanitary reforms earned her recognition as the founder of modern nursing (Dossey, 2009). For our purposes, the term *modern nursing* refers to nursing that came after the work of Nightingale. Nightingale spoke with firm conviction about the nature of nursing as a profession that could provide an avenue for women to make a meaningful contribution to society (Nightingale, 1860/1969). During the mid-1800s, women cared for the sick as daughters, wives, mothers, or maids. These socially prescribed roles influenced Nightingale's conviction that nursing should be a profession for women, but this cultural tradition was secondary to her philosophy. Her primary concern was the more pervasive plight of Victorian women. Women in her era were typically poverty stricken and forced to work at menial labor for long hours for little or no pay, or else they were—as was the case with Nightingale—idle ornaments in the households of wealthy husbands or fathers. In either case, there was no avenue for women to use their intellect, passion, and moral activity to benefit society (Nightingale, 1852/1979).

Nightingale spent the first decade of her adult life tormented by a desire to use her productive capacities in a way that would benefit society. She eventually defied the wishes of her family and broke free of the oppressive social prescriptions for her life. She obtained training as a nurse with the protestant sisters at Kaiserswerth Hospital and subsequently agreed to serve in the Crimean War (Dossey, 2009; Nightingale, 1852/1979;

Tooley, 1905; Woodham-Smith, 1983). After her service in the war, Nightingale wrote *Notes on Nursing* (1860/1969), in which she set forth the basic premises on which nursing practice should be based and articulated the proper functions of nursing. Although it was written for the lay nurses of the time, *Notes on Nursing* contains timeless wisdom that is still appropriate for today's professional nurses. In Nightingale's view, nursing required the astute observation of sick patients and their environment, the recording of these observations, and the development of knowledge about the factors that promote the reparative process (Cohen, 1984; Nightingale, 1860/1969). Nightingale's framework for nursing emphasized the use of empiric knowledge. She is recognized for using the statistics that she gathered in a way that would further the cause of health care in England and throughout the world (Dossey, 2009).

Because she was firmly committed to the idea that nursing's responsibilities were distinct from those of medicine, Nightingale maintained that the knowledge developed and used by nursing must be distinct from medical knowledge. Medicine, wrote Nightingale, focused on surgical and pharmacologic "cures," which relied heavily on empiric science. Nursing, however, was broader. Nursing was meant to assist nature with the healing of the patient. This was to be accomplished by managing the internal and external environments in an assistive way that was consistent with nature's laws. Nightingale also had a great influence on nursing education; she founded St. Thomas School in London after returning from the Crimea. She insisted that women who were trained nurses should control and staff early nursing schools and manage and control nursing practice in homes and hospitals to create a context that was supportive of nursing's art. Nightingale's influence on nursing education was felt within schools of nursing in all the British Commonwealth, in the United States, and in many other parts of the world. The first Nightingale schools were autonomous in their administration, and nurses held decision-making authority over nursing practice in institutions where students learned.

Instruction in Nightingale schools emphasized the powers of observation, the necessity of recording observations, and the potential for organizing the nursing knowledge that was gained through such observation and recording. Students also learned proper techniques of nursing. Nightingale's strong beliefs about the character and values that should be cultivated in nursing were reflected by the admissions standards and educational programs of the early schools (Dennis & Prescott, 1985). Nightingale regarded nursing as a calling and vehemently opposed registration practices of the day as a way to ensure the quality of practitioners. She argued that testing and subsequent registration might ensure a minimal knowledge base but would not guarantee the quality of the moral disposition within the individual nurse. Nightingale advocated that nursing was much more than knowledge of facts and techniques. These were important, but to her, nursing also required a certain ethical and moral disposition, a certain type of person, and an ability to act artfully. Nightingale also addressed emancipatory knowing and was concerned about the sociopolitical context within which nursing occurred. For example, in *Notes on Hospitals* as well as in other documents addressed to military administrators, she outlined the need to rectify unsanitary environmental conditions in hospitals to create a proper environment for healing (Nightingale, 1860/1969).

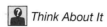 *Think About It*

> Think about what you learned, or did not learn, about Nightingale and her legacy. How did your impressions of Nightingale influence your perceptions of nursing and your nursing role?

FROM NIGHTINGALE TO SCIENCE

From the beginning of the 1900s to about 1950 was a time of great change in nursing that still continues to mold and shape knowledge development processes. Three major themes mark this period and reflect societal change patterns in the United States as they pertain to hospitals, the role of women in society, and the nature of nursing education.

Loss of the Nightingale Ideal

Despite Nightingale's insistence that nurses rather than hospital administrators or physicians control nursing care, many circumstances came together in opposition to her model for schools of nursing in the United States. The medical care system developed as a capitalist, for-profit business. This system provided the context for rapid technologic development and a complex institutionalized system to support medical interventions. Early during the 1900s, the Nightingale era was ending, and medical care was taking shape as a science. Women were viewed as incapable of practicing medicine and unqualified to be scientists. With industrialization, large populations of people moved to urban areas, and the number of hospitals increased dramatically in these areas.

Physicians and hospital administrators saw women as a source of inexpensive or free nursing labor who could further their economic goals. Many women entered nursing and provided student labor for hospitals in exchange for receiving apprenticeship training to become nurses. Many of these women came from the working class and had limited opportunities for education and meaningful work. After they were trained for nursing in hospital schools, many found themselves without employment as new student recruits filled available staff positions. Nurses were exploited both as students and as experienced workers. They were treated as submissive, obedient, and humble women who were "trained" in correct procedures and techniques. Ideally, they fulfilled their responsibilities to physicians without question. Nurses' positive desire to help people in need, coupled with their relative lack of educational preparation and social or political power, led to an extended period in history when nursing was practiced primarily under the control and direction of medicine (Ashley, 1976; Bradshaw, 2017; Evans, Pereira, & Parker, 2009; Group & Roberts, 2001; Lovell, 1980; Malka, 2007).

The Entrenchment of Apprenticeship Learning

Despite strong leaders who followed the Nightingale tradition and who viewed nursing knowledge as unique, nursing knowledge has not always been regarded as distinct from medicine. The control of nursing education and practice was transferred from the profession to hospital administrators and physicians during the early 1900s, when most of the Nightingale-modeled schools in the United States were brought under the control of hospitals (Ashley, 1976). Strong efforts to move nursing to institutions of higher learning were not enough. In a manner that was consistent with the social history of women, nursing was viewed and increasingly treated as a role that supported and supplemented medicine and certainly not as one that required a unique knowledge base (Hughes, 1980, 1990). Although training was acceptable and even necessary, true education for women and nurses was discouraged, discouraging, and limited. Indeed, education was counterproductive for women who, as nurses, were expected to follow orders and serve the needs and interests of physicians when it came to providing care (Melosh, 1982; Reverby, 1987a, 1987b).

Economic independence for women in the United States was not possible until the mid-1900s. Even a woman who earned an income was not able to have a bank account, own property, or conduct financial transactions in her own name. Normal schools were established for the training of teachers, and nursing schools were available for training nurses. To obtain long-term security, however, women were required to conform to the role of wife or daughter. Throughout the early part of the 20th century, nursing practice was based on rules, principles, and traditions that were passed along through limited apprenticeship forms of education. Nursing practice also included an ever-increasing array of delegated medical tasks that were acquired as medical knowledge expanded; these tasks were performed by nurses as extensions of physicians. Higher education for nurses was not available. What evolved as nursing knowledge was wisdom that came from years of experience.

Nursing was viewed primarily as a nurturing and technical art that required apprenticeship learning and innate personality traits that were congruent with that art (Hughes, 1990). Tradition as a basis for nursing practice was perpetuated by the nature of apprenticeship education (Ashley, 1976). Nursing students were presumed to learn at random through long hours of experience (with limited exposure to lectures or books) and to accept without question the prescriptions of practical techniques. The novice nurse acquired knowledge of what was right and wrong in practice by observing more experienced practitioners and by memorizing facts about the performance of nursing tasks. Nurse recruits also learned what sort of person a nurse should be through the imposition of rigid rules that regulated most aspects of their behavior, including sleeping, eating, socializing, and dress, both inside and outside the hospital walls. Rules were strictly enforced, with severe penalties for those who strayed outside the rules' boundaries.

PERSISTENCE OF NURSING IDEALS

Despite social impediments to the development of nursing knowledge, nursing philosophy and ideology remained committed to the idea that nursing requires a knowledge base for practice that is distinct from that of medicine (Abdellah, 1969; Hall, 1964; Henderson, 1966; Rogers, 1970). This commitment grew from the consistent recognition that, although the goals of nursing and medicine were related, the central goals and functions of nursing required knowledge not provided by medicine or by any other single discipline outside of nursing.

Although social circumstances limited the possibilities for nursing education, early nursing leaders sustained ideals that reflected Nightingale's model of education and practice. Because most nursing service was provided as free labor by students in hospitals, those who graduated secured jobs as independent practitioners who were engaged by families to assist with the care of the sick in homes and hospitals. Many nurse leaders were active in confronting a wide range of community-based social and health issues of the time, including temperance, freedom for enslaved people, the right of disenfranchised groups to vote, and the control of venereal disease. These experiences cultivated and required a broad view of nursing knowledge and a desire to change the future of nursing; technical training was not enough for these women. Despite that training, they saw nursing as independent and vital and with a firm knowledge base.

As nurses developed community-based practices, their work and writings reflected the multiple patterns of knowing in which their efforts were grounded. There is substantial evidence that graduate nurses during the early part of the 20th century had ethical and moral commitments that contributed substantively to improving health conditions in hospitals, homes, and communities. Not only did they develop health knowledge as they practiced, but they were also politically committed to finding ways to distribute this knowledge to the people who needed it (Wheeler, 1985). Consistently throughout the early 20th century, nursing leaders in the United States worked together nationally and internationally in strong connecting networks and called for a social and political ethic that would restore the control of nursing practice to nurses and promote the health and welfare of citizens.

Margaret Sanger, Lillian Wald, Lavinia Dock, Susie Walking Bear Yellowtail, Mabel Staupers, and Adah Belle Thoms are among those nurses who were challenged by specific needs in society and set about to change problematic practices that affected health care. They observed the circumstances of people in their work environment, identified health-related needs, and worked with others to meet those needs. They acted to improve health care practices by integrating ethical commitment with scientific knowledge.

For example, Sanger developed knowledge about reproduction and birth control. She fought against great odds to distribute birth control information to women who were desperate to obtain it, and she established a foundation for family-planning programs that remains viable today in the form of Planned Parenthood (Sanger, 1971). Concerned about child care and family health in the context of extremely poor sanitation in crowded immigrant tenements, Wald established the Henry Street Settlement in New York City, which is still operating today. On the basis of concepts of community health nursing and social welfare programs, Wald developed stations for distributing safe milk to families with young children and established centers for educating mothers about family care (Silverstein, 1985; Wald, 1971). Dock was an ardent suffragist and pacifist who worked for much of her professional life with Wald at the Henry Street Settlement. Dock campaigned actively for changes in labor laws that would benefit women and children. She devoted 20 years of her life to gaining the vote for women in the United States, reasoning that if women could vote, the oppressive laws that affected them could be changed (Christy, 1969).

Although much less well known, many influential nurses among minority groups also took equally significant actions to improve the health and well-being of their people.

Mary Seacole, an African-Jamaican nurse, traveled widely throughout the Caribbean, Central America, and Britain, gathering knowledge of native approaches to caring for the sick, complementing her British background. She volunteered to go to the Crimea in 1854 but was denied by the British War Office. Undaunted, she funded the journey herself and traveled to the Crimea in 1855–1856 to care for the sick in her "British Hotel" at the same time period that Florence Nightingale was in the Crimea. Her legacy, lost perhaps because of her minority identity, is now being explored anew by scholars seeking to unveil the lost history of her work (McDonald, 2012; Staring-Derks, Staring, & Anionwu, 2015).

Susie Walking Bear Yellowtail was a midwife who traveled throughout North American Indian reservations to assess the health, social, and educational problems of Native Americans, and then recommended solutions (American Nurses Association [ANA], 2007). She was instrumental in ending the abuses of women (e.g., involuntary sterilization) that were occurring within the Indian Health Care System (ANA, 2007; "Susie Walking Bear Yellowtail: 'Our Bright Morning Star,'" 2014). Mabel Staupers worked for improved access to equitable health care services for African-American citizens (ANA, 2009; Staten, n.d.). Her research into the health care needs of individuals in Harlem led to the founding of the first facility there for treating tuberculosis in African Americans. Adah Belle Thoms was among the first nursing leaders to recognize public health as a new field of nursing. In 1917, she added a course on the subject to the curriculum at New York's Lincoln School for Nurses (ANA, 2008). Thoms also founded the Blue Circle Nurses, a group of African-American nurses who worked with local communities and provided instruction regarding sanitation, diet, and appropriate clothing. She also organized a campaign to encourage members of the National Association of Colored Graduate Nurses to vote after the passage of the 19th Amendment, which gave women the right to vote (Thoms, 1929).

Similar to contemporary scholars, these and other early nursing leaders kept alive the ideals of practice as chronicled by Nightingale, and they used multiple ways of knowing to ground improvements in health care and nursing practice. They were women of strong personal character who lived their ethical convictions that nurses can and should control nursing practice. Their ethical and moral ideals of nursing practice required making observations and organizing the resulting knowledge. Art and emancipatory knowing were central to their practices as they orchestrated complex system changes that required them to interpret and maneuver through the existing social and political environments.

KNOWING PATTERNS IN THE EARLY LITERATURE

From about 1900 to 1950, nurses and others were writing about nursing and patient care in the journals of the time. These early articles reflected all the knowing patterns, although these were not named until the publication of Barbara A. Carper's doctoral research in 1978. An examination of nursing literature published before the 1950s is rich with detail about how nursing embodies, reflects, and requires multiple ways of knowing. The following sections provide some examples of how early writings addressed each pattern of knowing, including the pattern of emancipatory knowing.

Emancipatory Knowledge and Knowing

The early literature's attention to emancipatory knowing was reflected primarily by the recognition that inequities exist as well as by descriptions of situations that create inequities and injustice. The early literature also included directives about what nurses must do to change unfair social conditions. Although nurses contributed some of these early writings, other pieces were written by physicians and nonnurse educators and published in nursing journals and books or presented to nursing audiences. The following examples illustrate our heritage of emancipatory knowing.

- Effie Taylor (1934) acknowledged the existence of social inequities in a speech given at the opening session of a national nursing organization meeting. Taylor noted that the "nations of the world are sick mentally and socially and need to be enabled to live better, think better and act better" (474).
- How injustices are created is embedded in an eloquent quote from Lavinia Dock (1902) who noted the following in an early issue of *American Journal of Nursing*: "... after one has worked for a time healing wounds which should not have been inflicted, tending ailments which should not have developed, sending patients to hospitals who need not have gone if their homes were habitable, and bringing charitable aid to persons who would not have needed it if health had not been ruined by unwholesome conditions, one longs for preventive work... something that will make it less easy for so many illnesses to occur, that will bring better conditions of life" (p. 532).
- Another cause of social injustices was "anxiety over material necessities," as mentioned in a 1913 physician's address to graduates of the El Reno Sanitarium. Such anxiety "precludes living the ideal, full, free and independent effective life" (Young, 1913, p. 266).
- Marion Faber (1927) a registered nurse, noted that it is "effects of the environment that cause deformation of the personality" (p. 1048).
- Joseph Mountin, a physician and then an assistant surgeon general of the United States, stated that the "hospital hierarchy tries to provide social service according to the rules of private competitive enterprise," and this "requires a financial sleight of hand to keep the institution going" (1943, p. 34).
- According to William Kilpatrick, a doctorally prepared educator, these hierarchies resulted in a "factory system that reduces individuals to a non-entity amid the bigness of the organization" (1921, p. 791).
- Concerns about increasing levels of education led two doctorally prepared academic educators to suggest that "vested interest will preclude the development of professionalism (in nursing) as hospitals will not be able to adjust to the loss of student work hours" (Bixler & Bixler, 1945, p. 732).
- Isabel Stewart, a nurse and faculty member at Columbia University, wrote that custom and training are the great authorities and are rigid and static. Stewart further noted that "authority becomes entrenched and does not allow for change in the individual" (1921, p. 908).
- Allen Gregg, a physician and director of medical sciences at the Rockefeller Foundation, attributed injustices to "envy and malice and hate and violence" (1940, p. 738).

- Paul Johnson (1928), in an address to the Massachusetts State League of Nursing Education, stated: "[T]he first and most powerful influence upon human minds is the unconscious operation of social custom... the question of what to teach is superfluous... what is taught is the product of long experience of moral custom" (p. 1087). Johnson also suggested that, to address the conditions of social injustice, nurses must "seek by criticism and appreciation to broaden the bypath... to decrease moral provincialism which makes men blind to good beyond their own... this [moral provincialism] may be overcome by historical and cultural sympathy with others and understanding and appreciation of values that have appealed to other people" (p. 1087).
- Katherine McClure (1951), a nurse professor, noted the need to "improve the environment and conditions of the persons she nurses without remaking them to suit ourselves" (p. 221–222).
- Bixler and Bixler (1945) stated that nurses' social attitudes should reflect the conception that "every citizen is entitled to health care" (p. 733).
- Taylor (1934) wrote that nurses must have a "broad sense of justice" (p. 475), should "not know color or creed" (p. 473), and must "be for the poor as well as the rich" (p. 473).
- Kilpatrick (1921) further addressed how to undo social injustices by stating that nurses should "seek the development and expression of each in relation to all, and cause others to grow" (p. 795).
- Stewart (1921) stated that "knowledge, culture, individual development, freedom, health and expertness are used in service of the social group," emphasizing that "education has a social purpose and nursing is no exception" (p. 908).
- Noted anthropologist Margaret Mead (1956), in an address to a convention of the American Nurses Association, stated that "nursing stands between those who are vulnerable and the community that may forget them, not care for them" (p. 1002).
- Genevieve Noble (1940), a graduate nursing student, understood that nurses must notice injustice when she stated that the "nurse cannot be indifferent to the welfare and happiness of the undernourished child in the street or the maid working in her corridor" (p. 161).
- Esther Lucille Brown, a researcher for the Russell Sage Foundation who was the author of reports about nursing, recognized that "nursing must create alliances with problems outside the privileged home and hospital, and should be concerned with those who have chronic disease, are aged and physically handicapped" (Goostray & Brown, 1954, p. 720).
- Elizabeth Porter, then president of the ANA, summarized many of the social conditions that create social injustices and inequities (i.e., the focus of emancipatory knowing). Porter (1953) noted that "hunger, poverty, injustice and disease are the enemies of peace," and "when man arrogates to himself blessings that he denies others, these blessings begin to slip through his fingers"; "a chain around another's neck means there is a chain about your own"; and "passivity or acquiescence to the chains of others means you enslave yourself" (p. 948). For Porter, necessary actions included "supporting humanitarian programs on a worldwide scale," taking responsibility

to change the "conditions in which men live and the conditioning of their mind" (p. 948), and "putting the good of the world and community before the selfish interest of individuals or specialized groups" (p. 949).

- A group of nurses in Canada organized themselves as "Nurses for Social Responsibility" in 1985, and published a magazine titled *Towards Justice in Health* from 1992–1995. In their early years, they formed networks with other peace and justice groups in the community, working for peace and against war, providing education and participating in peaceful propeace (antiwar) protests. Later they also worked on behalf of abortion rights, ending violence against women, needle exchange programs, ending apartheid in South Africa and racism in Canada and other countries (Falk-Rafael & Bradley, 2014).

> **!** *Why Is This Important?*
>
> In recent years, some nurses have turned away from political action as a duty for nursing, whereas others, particularly in public health and community settings, have continued to call for nursing to take political action to improve health for all. The early nursing literature addressed the importance of emancipatory knowing by acknowledging that social injustices existed while accounting for the conditions that created them. This literature reflects the fact that nurses recognized the importance of acting in relation to the needs of others while understanding that effective change must come from a grassroots position. This literature is replete with directives for nursing actions required to rectify societal injustices and conditions that privilege one group over another. Injustices were not hidden or mystified. Rather, and perhaps concurrent with the expansion of nursing into community-based practices, the necessity to recognize social inequalities and take strong measures to rectify them was emphasized.

Ethical Knowledge and Knowing

Before the 1950s, ethics was primarily represented as virtues possessed by the nurse. Nurses were expected to be moral individuals who, it follows, do the right thing. Virtue and responsibility were paramount for nurses. Duty and responsibility included protection, truth telling, and imparting of specialized knowledge (Conrad, 1947; De Witt, 1901; Warnshius, 1926).

- An editorial in the *American Journal of Nursing* noted that "the doctor is responsible for the general conduct of the case, but the nurse is responsible for the honest performance of her own duties" (De Witt, 1901, p. 15). Further, "born qualities added to training" were critical for ethical conduct.
- According to Drake, "A good nurse will die before admitting she is even tired [for] loyal service is one of the articles of the profession's religion" (1934, pp. 134–38). Moral fitness for nursing was important, and moral examinations were recommended.
- Nurse Agnes Riddles (1928) stated that "women [nurses] should hold their position only after a moral examination as well as a technical one" (p. 29). Riddles listed a variety of moral infractions attributable to nurses of the time, including a lack of consideration for the patient, the neglecting of aseptic precautions, the disrespect for human life, and a lack of proper experience with assembling needed nursing materials.

- Charlotte Aikins (1915), presumably a nurse educator, outlined an entire curriculum for teaching ethics in *Trained Nurse and Hospital Review*. The curriculum included knowledge of "the customs and laws of the hospital world which she (student) must be admonished to accept meekly" and "personal virtues of importance such as reticence, tact, and discretion in order that she may 'do no harm'" (p. 136). "Health, carriage, voice, manner, habits and general deportment" (p. 136) also were important. During the junior year, ethics would cover "handling of supplies and appliances, avoiding accidents, use of good surgical technique, wise use of recreation and holidays, and the necessity of a good conscience" (p. 137).
- Another early nurse mentioned the need to keep preconceptions and prejudices to a minimum as a part of ethical conduct (Oettinger, 1939).
- Paul Johnson (1928), in an address to a statewide gathering of nurses, asked, "What should ethics teach?" (p. 1084). Ethics, according to Johnson, is the "science of right conduct" (p. 1085). Ethics investigates "boldly" what this is by "questioning moral tradition, examining moral facts, and searching out moral values" (p. 1085). Ethics requires "careful investigation, open-minded judgment, the practice of reasonableness and intelligent doubting" (p. 1085). Ethical sensitivity, rather than the rules approach of "laying down exact rules for conduct" (p. 1084), was important to cultivate.

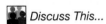 *Discuss This...*

> Discuss with your colleagues the ways you believe that ethical perspectives have changed in nursing since the early literature. The early periodical literature generally reflects a view of ethical behavior and comportment as conforming to individual virtues, although early articles also challenged virtue ethics and its position that a good person will do the right thing. Religious living, self-sacrifice, and a nearly blind duty to others' rules and prescriptions evidenced such virtues. Duty often was expressed in religious admonitions to love, live right, and have faith; duty was seen as a sacred obligation. Moral fitness for nursing was important, and moral examinations were recommended. The establishment of rules as the basis for biomedical ethics was questioned. Although most of what was considered ethical came from religious traditions and authoritative trust in others, the early writers also discussed questioning traditions and making responsible judgments, studying what one doubts, and analyzing and criticizing basic precepts. These early authors also suggested a variety of goals for ethical knowledge and knowing, including the protection of patients' privacy and rights, advocacy, and the minimization of patients' discomfort and inconvenience. Broader goals also were mentioned, such as increasing tolerance and respect by respecting the worth, autonomy, and dignity of individuals; assisting with the development of the individual; strengthening society and the self; developing economic security; and promoting peace.
>
> In your view, what, if anything, has changed?

Personal Knowledge and Knowing

The importance of the *person* of the nurse is evident in the prevailing ethics of the time, which called for a virtuous person. However, qualities of a person beyond virtue also are found in the early literature.

- Margaret Conrad (1947), writing about the nature of expert nursing care, recognized the necessity for a well-balanced, integrated personality to contribute to the care of others.
- Allen Gregg (1940), a physician, in an address given at national nurse meetings, asked nurses to "seek honestly and earnestly to find what really matters to us and what beliefs and convictions we hold" (p. 738). Gregg also redefined virtue as "the inner life as well as the outer in consistency of behavior with one's own thoughts and feelings" (p. 740) and further stated that "motives and conduct must harmonize" (p. 740). Motives must be sound, or there is "no virtue in the great sense, no independence, and no self-confidence" (p. 741). The fundamental importance of personal knowledge is acknowledged in that "only when a person is something to herself can she become anything to anybody else" (p. 741). Gregg recognized that science could not provide personal knowledge because "the social wisdom of man does not derive from chemistry and physics and mechanical skill. Decency does not visit our common dwelling place without invitation" (p. 739).
- Genevieve Noble (1940), writing as a student in "The Spirit of Nursing," emphasized the need for an inherent inner self-discipline rather than an imposed discipline for adequate nursing care.
- Katherine Oettinger (1939) gave equal importance to personal knowing and empirics by stating that "the personality of the nurse is quite as important as the distinctive facts she learns," that such a nurse is "free from conscript minds giving conscript thoughts" and is "free to change the status quo" (p. 1224).

Think About It

> In the early literature, important personal characteristics included an acceptance of the self that is grounded in self-knowledge and confidence. Personal integrity, honesty, enthusiasm, versatility, courageousness, stability, and emotional diversity were important features of personal knowledge. Such knowledge is created by engagement with life, finding out what really matters, and reflecting on it. Nursing practice requires a depth of personal knowing that acknowledges the validity of feelings, an openness to freely discussing feelings, and an examination of reciprocal emotions in dialogue and relation. A nurse of high personal character displays an inner and outer harmony and commands the respect of his or her self and of others. Nursing's historical literature suggests that a host of personal attributes that go beyond virtuous behavior, including self-discipline, knowledge of the self, and an openness to the processes of reflection to create actions with integrity are basic to good nursing care.
>
> Think about what you learned about personal knowing in your nursing education, and if this was sufficient for your practice.

Aesthetic Knowledge and Knowing

A sense that nursing has an artistic component is clearly evident in the early periodical literature.

- L. F. Simpson (1914), another physician who was speaking to nurses, stated that "real nursing is an art; and a real nurse is an artist" (p. 133).

- Conrad (1947) stated that the art of nursing included such things as "knowing what the patient wants before she is asked" (p. 162). It arises from "combining instinct, knowledge and experience" (p. 162). According to Conrad, art depends on imagination and resourcefulness and requires "true perspective" (pp. 162–163). Furthermore, art requires practice, and some nurses "never acquire it" (Simpson, 1914, p. 135).

- Austin Drake (1934), a layperson, put it the following way: "circumstances alter cases. . . the nurse adapts her roles at will according to her patient's physical state and particular mode... if he is able and desires... she talks, otherwise she is silent, intent upon her duties... the severity of the illness does not determine this" (pp. 136–137).

- Lois Mossman (1923), an assistant professor of education, acknowledged that "science cannot explain what happens when we respond to beauty of form or motion but the response is pleasurable and influences what we are doing" (p. 318). Mossman asked novice nurses to "experience beauty, to see it in the commonplace, to learn of books, poems, pictures, and music that interpret beauty and draw from them to fit the needs of those we serve" (p. 319). According to Mossman, "Life is rhythmical and lights must be set off by the shadows" (p. 319).

- Edward Garesche (1927), a Roman Catholic priest, eloquently expressed the elusiveness of assessing our art and the importance of distinguishing it from empirics: "the service of the learned professions does not bear measuring while it is being rendered" (p. 901).

- Despite the recognition of the value of empirics, the idea that science alone is an inadequate practice guide appears frequently. A physician addressing a graduating class of diploma nurses stated that "the profession of nursing is an art depending upon science. In nursing the art must always predominate though underlying science is important" (Worcester, 1902, p. 908).

≫ Consider This...

The early literature represented aesthetics as a combination of knowledge, experience, intuition, and understanding. Aesthetic knowing was creative and intuitive and consisted of exquisite judgments that were made without conscious awareness but rather were sensed intuitively by unexplained insight and hunches. Aesthetic knowledge was gained through appreciation of the arts and by subjective sensitivity to individual differences. Aesthetic knowing was also gained by personal imitation of those who possessed the art. Experience was seen as important to the development of aesthetic knowing. Aesthetic knowing required speculation, imagination, and the superimposition of impressions on facts. The practitioner who had a sincere intentionality and the ability to carry out sophisticated assessment could act artfully. It was through the interpretation of interaction that each succeeding interaction became more meaningful. Art in the more traditional sense was also recognized as important to the art/act of nursing.

How is this view of aesthetic knowing and knowledge different from what you experience now?

Empiric Knowledge and Knowing

Before the "era of science" in the mid-1950s, there was clear recognition of scientific knowledge as a source of power.

- A physician who addressed the annual meeting of the Michigan Nurses Association acknowledged that scientific knowledge had increased and asked nurses to acknowledge its power and value for producing knowledge. The physician cautioned against quackery and portrayed science as a source of legitimate criteria for the selection of information provided to patients (Warnshius, 1926). Despite the value of science, this physician also emphasized the importance of a central focus on the welfare of the patient.

- According to Margaret Conrad (1947), a baccalaureate-prepared professor of nursing, this required an understanding of the laws of nature and the principles of physics, chemistry, physiology, and psychology. In other early articles, the procedural and technical aspects of nursing were emphasized, including bed making; food tray handling and feeding; carrying out personal hygienic measures, such as bed baths and oral hygiene; and managing delegated medical procedures, such as drains, catheterizations, enemas, alcohol baths, vital signs, and medication administration (Brigh, 1944; Mountin, 1943).

- Muriel Burgess (1941), a nursing student, outlined the "facts of care," which included diagnosis; social factors such as heredity, environment, and education; and medical factors such as family history, history of the present illness, symptom onset, physical examination, and laboratory and radiography findings. Burgess further noted that the plan should include the progress of the patient and make use of graphs whenever possible. The treatments prescribed and the continuing plan for care were also important.

- Genevieve and Roy Bixler (1945), two doctorally prepared educators, addressed the development of empirics and wrote "the elements of science should be defined and organized, gathered from every science contributing to nursing and arranged in the most convenient order for thought" (p. 730). Bixler and Bixler stated that scientific compartmentalizations were artificial, arbitrary, and to be avoided by nursing science. Nursing science existed apart from practice, but its use in the service of professional practice represented a "new synthesis" (p. 731). Science, they asserted, needed to be integrated as an art.

- The 1947 editorial "Changes in Nursing Practice" in the *American Journal of Nursing* emphasized the need for nurses to develop keen observation skills because "the lack of descriptions or records of nursing care based on actual experience is appalling" (p. 655). Written observations could form the basis for a complete patient study to provide an interpretive picture of current nursing.

- In a speech at a student nurse convention, Blanche Pfefferkorn (1933), who was identified only as a registered nurse, stated that empiric knowledge came from questionnaires, detached observation, and field studies. According to Pfefferkorn, a scientific attitude was important. Scientific knowledge included "facts that were organized into a form or structure that were not dynamic and reports of field studies" (p. 260).

Regardless of the source, scientific knowledge served as a skeleton and answered questions about "what"; good science represented the "what" of nursing very well. Pfefferkorn noted that the nurse needed to know "how"—not just "what"—and stated that field studies could "enliven fact gathering by providing knowledge of how" (p. 260).

• Agnes Meade (1936), a nurse, wrote "Training the Senses in Clinical Observation" and cautioned about the following pitfall of scientific bias: "a distinguishing feature of scientific observation is that the observer knows what is being sought, and to a certain extent what is likely to be found" (p. 540).

🛈 Think About It

The early nursing literature defies a common assumption that nursing practice was based solely on tradition and habit, without due consideration of underlying empiric evidence. Early authors envisioned ways for empiric knowledge to be created and displayed. Although scientific-empiric knowledge could come from disciplines outside of nursing, there was a recognition of the unique nature of nursing science.

Empirics was typically represented as the knowledge of the underlying principles and techniques associated with nursing. Formal observation was also established as a valued technique and a skill that was critical for the development of nursing empirics. Principles, facts gleaned from observation, and procedural guides for action were important forms of empirics that were necessary for completing the routine hygienic care of patients as well as delegated medical tasks. Despite the recognition of the value of empirics, the idea that science alone is an inadequate practice guide appeared frequently. For example, a physician addressing a graduating class of diploma nurses stated that "the profession of nursing is an art depending upon science. In nursing the art must always predominate though underlying science is important" (Worcester, 1902, p. 908).

Think about the ways in which your ideas of empirics compares to the ideas expressed in the early literature.

THE EMERGENCE OF NURSING AS A SCIENCE

The shift toward a concept of nursing knowledge as predominantly scientific began in the 1950s and took a strong hold during the 1960s. This shift toward knowledge as science produced significant changes in what was considered important in nursing. Nursing gradually shifted from a perspective that emphasized technical competence, duty, and womanly virtue to a perspective that focused more on effective nursing practice (Hardy, 1978). In many ways, the shift toward science was a welcome change. However, this move was made at the sacrifice of the development of ethics for individual and collective practice, the development of a nurse's character, the artistic and aesthetic dimensions of practice, and critical attention being paid to injustices in health care practices. The development of knowledge in relation to other patterns of knowing, which was so necessary for practice and so evident in nursing's work historically, was largely neglected until the early 1990s.

The shift toward science as the basis for developing nursing knowledge was influenced by the involvement of nursing in the two world wars in the first half of the 20th century.

The wars created social circumstances that led to substantial shifts in roles for women and nurses. During the wars, with many men away from their homes, women were freed from constraints and learned to manage their responsibilities in accord with their own priorities and preferences. Many women entered the skilled or unskilled labor force while men were away in battle. Women who were nurses were needed to support the war effort by providing care for the sick and wounded. The U.S. government instituted war-related programs to make nursing preparation available to women who agreed to serve in the war (Kalisch & Kalisch, 2003; Kelly & Joel, 2001).

Partly because of the greater demand for technically skilled nurses to serve the war effort, by the decade of World War II, women had begun to enter institutions of higher learning in greater numbers. The early nursing leaders' vision of nursing education within colleges and universities began to be realized. After the end of World War II, many educational programs were established within institutions of higher learning, and graduate programs for nurses began to appear. Academic institutions required faculty to hold advanced degrees and encouraged them to meet the standards of higher education with regard to providing service to the community, teaching, and performing research. Research standards adhered to the more traditional objectivist criteria of scientific-empiric work, which limited the nature of credible scholarship among academic nurses. Nurse-scientist programs were established to enable nurses to earn doctoral degrees in other disciplines; the research skills that were learned could then be applied in nursing. As academically based nurses gained skills in the methods of science, conceptual frameworks and other types of theoretic writings began to emerge.

In 1950, *Nursing Research* was established, the first research journal for nurses (Mason, Kennedy, Schorr, & Flanagan, 2006). Books about research methodologies and explicit conceptual frameworks, often called "theories of nursing," began to appear. Early research reports often focused on describing the actions performed by nurses rather than the clinical problems of patients. Although less sophisticated with regard to method than current reports, these writings began to reflect the qualities of serious empiric scholarship and investigative skill. Various schools of thought emerged regarding the nature of nursing practice and nursing's knowledge base, providing a fresh flow of ideas that could be examined by members of the profession. These writings provided a stimulus for early efforts to develop theory and, eventually, to broaden knowledge-development efforts.

 Think About It

What nursing journals have you been reading in your educational program? Think about the content of these journals. How do the articles contribute to the ways in which you think about nursing? How do they contribute to, or influence, your practice? Which journals have been important resources for you since you first entered nursing, and why? What is missing in the journals you read?

By the 1960s, doctoral programs in nursing were being established (Carter, 2006). By the end of the 1970s, the number of doctorally prepared nurses in the United States had grown to almost 2,000. Approximately 20 doctoral programs in nursing had been established, and master's degree programs were maturing in academic stature and quality.

Master's programs began focusing on preparing advanced practitioners in nursing rather than educators and administrators, whereas doctoral programs increasingly focused on the development of nursing knowledge. Early doctoral programs were built on the ideal of the academic research degree, which was typically a doctor of philosophy (PhD). With the development of advanced educational programs, nurses could formally consider the processes for developing nursing knowledge.

Nurse scholars began to debate ideas, points of view, and methods in the light of nursing's traditions (Andrist, Nicholas, & Wolf, 2006; Group & Roberts, 2001; Hardy, 1978; Leininger, 1976; Lewenson & Hermann, 2007). These debates are reflected in the literature of the late 1960s and the early 1970s (Dickoff & James, 1968, 1971; Dickoff, James, & Wiedenbach, 1968; Ellis, 1968; Folta, 1971; Henly, 2016; Walker, 1971; Wooldridge, 1971). Fundamental differences in viewpoints on nursing science provided nurse scholars with the opportunity to learn, sharpen critical-thinking skills, and acquire knowledge about the processes and limitations of science.

As an overt and deliberative focus on knowledge development began to take shape in nursing, a prevailing view emerged of nursing as a service that required a strong base in science. Debates reflected various views of science and metatheory around the preferred methods for producing sound nursing knowledge. Despite the lively debates and substantive issues focused on scientific knowledge, the idea that nursing requires the development of a broad knowledge base that includes all patterns of knowing has never been lost. Even when this broad view was not explicitly mentioned in the debates (as was common during the 1970s), the broad conceptualizations labeled as "theories" implicitly required multiple ways of knowing. The persistent dominance of science can be attributed in part to academic nurses' need to gain legitimacy in their university communities and to nurses' need to achieve political and personal legitimacy within medicine and society in general. Regardless of the societal context, the wholistic focus of nursing has endured.

EARLY TRENDS IN THE DEVELOPMENT OF NURSING SCIENCE

Throughout the second half of the 20th century, three major trends contributed to evolving directions in the development of nursing knowledge. These trends, as would be expected, centered on the empiric pattern. However, threads of continuity reflect ethics, aesthetics, personal knowing, and emancipatory knowing, as shown in the sections that follow. Two important trends are (1) the use of theories that have been borrowed from other disciplines and (2) the development of conceptual frameworks that define nursing.

Use of Theories Borrowed from Other Disciplines

As the educational preparation of nurses expanded, theories developed in other disciplines were recognized as also being important for nursing. Problems in nursing practice with no apparent ready solution began to be viewed as resolvable, if theories and approaches to theory development from other disciplines were applied. For example, nurses recognized that young children needed the continuing love and support of their parents and families during hospitalization. The strict rules of hospitals that severely restricted visitation interrupted these primary family ties. As psychologic theories of attachment and separation developed, nurses found an explanation for the problems experienced by hospitalized children and were able to change visitation practices to provide for sustained contact between parents and children.

Although theories from other disciplines have been useful, nurses also have exercised caution rather than arbitrarily applying these theories. In some cases, the theories of other disciplines do not take into consideration significant factors that influence a nursing situation. For example, some theories of learning that are applicable to classroom learning do not adequately reflect the process of learning when an individual is faced with illness, nor do they address the ethical issues a nurse might face when disclosing sensitive information to a patient. Although borrowed theories may be useful, their usefulness cannot be assumed until they are examined from the perspective of nursing in nursing situations (Barnum, 1998; Walker & Avant, 2010). The trend of using theories from related disciplines may have been an outgrowth of predoctoral and postdoctoral fellowship funding for nurses that began in the mid-1950s. This funding nurtured a cadre of nurse scientists who studied research approaches in fields related to but outside of nursing. After these nurses were educated, they would return to nursing and conduct research, thereby contributing to nursing's knowledge base.

Development of Philosophies and Conceptual Frameworks That Define Nursing

As nurses began to reconsider the nature of nursing and the purposes for which nursing exists in the light of science, they began to question many ideas that were taken for granted in nursing and the traditional basis on which nursing was practiced. They wrote and published idealized views of nursing and of the type of knowledge, skills, and background needed for practice. As an ideal view of nursing, these frameworks and philosophies did not arise from practice per se but did reflect a reasonably attainable vision of what nursing could be. Writings of the 1960s and 1970s made significant contributions to the development of theoretic thinking in nursing. Many have been used as a basis for curricula and as guides for practice and research.

Many early nursing conceptual frameworks and philosophies include a description of the *nursing process*. This process, which is similar to both scientific methods of problem solving and research processes, is a framework for viewing nursing as a deliberate, reflective, critical, and self-correcting system. The nursing process replaced the rule-oriented and principle-oriented approaches that were grounded in a medical model in which the nurse functions as a physician's assistant. The nursing process relied heavily on what could be assessed through observation. Before there was a focus on the nursing process, unexamined rules and principles were used to guide the nurse in routine hygienic care, the performance of treatment procedures, and the administration of medications to treat disease. Because a rule-oriented approach did not encourage reflective problem solving and was not consistent with education in institutions of higher education, the shift to the nursing process as a way to approach care encouraged nurses to cultivate basic inquiry skills. *Nursing diagnosis,* which evolved from the nursing process and began to move nursing away from theoretic dependence on a medical model, was one method for organizing the domain of nursing practice. The early literature regarding nursing diagnosis included both practical and theoretic ideas about developing a taxonomy of nursing diagnoses and testing their validity.

Conceptual frameworks for nursing education and practice proliferated during the 1960s and 1970s. The then-current emphasis on systems theories is evident in the work of Callista Roy, Imogene King, Dorothy Johnson, and Betty Neuman. The movement of psychiatric care into community-based settings after the development of new drugs for the management of psychiatric illness contributed to a theoretic focus on the importance of interpersonal communication; this focus is notable in the work of Hildegard Peplau, Joyce Travelbee, and Ida Jean Orlando. The emergence of chronic disease with the control of communicable disease and a focus on wholism is reflected in Myra Levine's conservation principles framework as well as in Dorothea Orem's theoretic writings on self-care. Many nurse scientists who benefited from early funding for doctoral education received training in fields such as sociology and anthropology, in which a focus on the development of broad, grand theories was prominent; this influence is notable in the work of Madeleine Leininger. The conceptual frameworks of Martha Rogers, Rosemarie Parse, and Margaret Newman reflect theoretic perspectives linked to developments in modern physics that moved beyond earlier system concepts of equilibrium.

There was considerable debate about whether the writings of leaders such as Callista Roy, Betty Neuman, Imogene King, and Dorothea Orem and others should be called "models," "theories," or "philosophies." This debate reflected an underlying acknowledgment that empiric knowledge alone was an inadequate metatheory for practice. How to name these theorylike constructions: theories, conceptual models, theoretic frameworks, conceptual frameworks? This remains a debatable subject, and various terminologies can be found in the contemporary theoretic literature. We have chosen to refer to these broad theorylike structures as *conceptual frameworks* or *theoretic frameworks,* and their authors we call *theorists.* Regardless of labels, nursing practice consistent with these (and other) conceptual frameworks was taught in educational institutions, integrated into practice, and used to guide research. The use of conceptual frameworks cultivated a tacit recognition of the significance of multiple patterns of nursing knowledge. As nurses began to integrate these ideas into practice settings, the actual and potential relationships between nursing's conceptual frameworks and nursing practice became clearer. Practicing nurses found a new sense of purpose and direction that was consistent with the basic values of nursing, and they also achieved a sense of the increasing effectiveness as a result of systematic and thoughtful forms of nursing practice. Transferring these ideals of practice into the health care setting also served to illuminate the difficulties of finding nursing opportunities in the increasingly competitive health care system. Table 2.1 is a historical chronology of nurse theorists' work during the latter half of the 20th century.

Many of the early theorists are no longer alive, but nurses who use and continue to develop their ideas keep their work alive. Many of the theorists continued to develop their ideas and change their perspectives, but their work remains significant because their ideas have stood the test of time with regard to forming fundamental values and perspectives of the discipline (Thorne & Sawatzky, 2014). Because conceptual frameworks change as they are linked to research findings, used in education and practice, and critiqued and expanded, when you refer to another author's summary or interpretation of their work (such as our "Interpretive Summary" in the Appendix), remember that these summaries are historical in nature and may not accurately reflect the later or current thinking of the original theorist.

A wealth of information is available on the Internet about many of the nurse theorists listed in Table 2.1 and in the Appendix that can provide perspectives about more current work related to those theoretic frameworks. Even for those theorists who continue to develop their ideas, their work remains true to the essential core of the conceptual model as originally proposed. Website resources and information can be accessed with the use of key search terms or theorists' names. Applying the processes of description and critical reflection of theory as described in Chapter 8 will help to ensure your ability to evaluate appropriately the information available on theorist-related websites.

! Why Is This Important?

The conceptual frameworks developed during the 1960s and 1970s were important for broadly defining nursing and naming the phenomena central to nursing's domain of concern. These ideas were extremely valuable because they shifted nursing away from a medical model of practice that was characterized by the correct performance of routine nursing and medical procedures and the administration of medication. They broadened nursing's role in society by describing how nursing functions to achieve a socially relevant purpose and by delineating the contextual variables that were important to the practice of nursing. The philosophic values embedded in early nursing frameworks reflect central assumptions and value positions on which nursing rests. At the same time, these conceptual frameworks were characterized by a relatively functional view of nursing and health. They defined what nursing is, described the social purposes that nursing serves, detailed how nurses should function to realize these purposes, and defined the parameters and variables that influence illness and health processes.

For example, Callista Roy, Dorothea Orem, Virginia Henderson, and Hildegard Peplau focused on descriptions of illness and health: what nurses do to assist a person with moving toward health. These frameworks present explanations of how nursing actions function in practice to enhance health and well-being. The functions described are theoretic in nature in that they are conceptualized at a relatively abstract level. Nursing is viewed as a set of roles or functions rather than as concrete technical procedures. These abstract ideas about nursing functions are woven into explanations of relationships between the nurse's roles and functions and the theorist's idea of a desired nursing outcome related to health and well-being.

During the later 1970s and the 1980s, there was a noticeable qualitative shift in theoretic ideas developed for the purpose of broadly defining nursing practice. Rather than reflecting a functional perspective of the role of nursing in society, later conceptual frameworks tended to move to qualitative dimensions that characterized nursing's role not as what nurses do but as the essence of what nursing is. This shift offered the potential to move nursing from a context-dependent reactive position to a context-interactive proactive stance. These approaches combined direct observations of nurses and their

TABLE 2.1 Chronology and Key Emphases of Early Conceptual Frameworks in Nursing: 1952–1989

Year[a]	Theorist(s)	Key Emphasis
1952	Hildegard E. Peplau	The interpersonal process is a maturing force for the personality
1960	Faye G. Abdellah, Irene L. Beland, Almeda Martin, and Ruth V. Matheney	The patient's problems determine the appropriate nursing care
1961	Ida Jean Orlando	The interpersonal process alleviates distress
1964	Ernestine Wiedenbach	The helping process meets the patient's needs through the art of individualizing care
1966	Lydia E. Hall	Nursing care involves directing the patient toward self-love
	Virginia Henderson	Empathic understanding and the knowledge of the nurse help patients move toward independence
	Joyce Travelbee	The meaning found in an illness determines how people respond
1967	Myra E. Levine	Wholism is maintained by conserving integrity
1970	Martha E. Rogers	The person and the environment are energy fields that evolve negentropically
1971	Dorothea E. Orem	Self-care maintains wholeness
	Imogene M. King	Transactions provide a frame of reference for goal setting
1976	Callista Roy	Stimuli disrupt an adaptive system
	Josephine G. Paterson and Loretta T. Zderad	Nursing is an existential experience of nurturing
1978	Madeleine M. Leininger	Caring is universal and varies transculturally
1979	Jean Watson	Caring is a moral ideal that involves mind, body, and soul engagement with another
	Margaret A. Newman	Disease is a clue to preexisting life patterns
1980	Dorothy E. Johnson	Subsystems exist in dynamic stability
	Betty Neuman	Individuals, as wholistic systems, interact with environmental stressors and resist disintegration by maintaining a normal line of defense

Continued

TABLE 2.1 Chronology and Key Emphases of Early Conceptual Frameworks in Nursing: 1952–1989—cont'd

Year[a]	Theorist(s)	Key Emphasis
1981	Rosemarie Rizzo Parse	Indivisible beings and the environment co-create health
1982	Nola Pender	Health-promoting behavior is determined by individual characteristics and experiences as modulated by perceptions as well as interpersonal and situational factors
1989	Patricia Benner and Judith Wrubel	Caring is central to the essence of nursing; it sets up what matters, thus enabling connection and concern, and it creates the possibility for mutual helpfulness

(see also the Appendix, which provides more detail about these theorists' ideas)
[a]Date of first major publication.

practice with systematized insights that were guided by existing conceptual and theoretic frameworks and philosophies of nursing as well as other literature sources. For example, both Jean Watson (1979) and Patricia Benner and Judith Wrubel (1989) grounded the essence of nursing in caring. They used theoretic reasoning derived from a deliberate philosophic stance that is explicit in their writings and from the experience of the practice of nursing in many different contexts. The themes or patterns that characterize the essence of caring are those reflected in the actions, thoughts, values, and priorities of the practicing nurse.

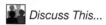 *Discuss This...*

> Discuss with a group of your colleagues the difference between what nurses do and the essence of what nursing is. Discuss the commonly repeated idea that "we still do not know what nursing is." Think about the metaphors of "nursing a drink" and "doctoring a drink" to prompt your ideas about both the functions of nursing and the essence of nursing. As you discuss these ideas, consider how you can refute the notions of uncertainty about what nursing is.

Another early formal movement defined the discipline by locating the source of nursing theory in nursing practice and calling for the systematization of practice knowledge into theory. This approach was particularly influenced by the writings of Dickoff and James and their colleagues, who were well known for theorizing about the nature of theory for a practice discipline (Dickoff & James, 1997; Dickoff et al., 1968). They proposed a radically different view for developing theory that challenged the scientific metatheory that prevailed during the 1960s. Dickoff and James described how theory is developed from the systematization of practice-based rules, guidelines, and nursing activities that are known to work. Theory was in part the systematization of practice-based variables, and it could exist at one of four levels: (1) factor isolating, (2) factor relating, (3) situation relating, or (4) situation producing.

Dickoff, James, and colleagues also recognized the value-laden nature of theory in nursing and called for an explicit recognition and naming of the values toward which theory development was proceeding; this aspect of theory they called *goal-content*. Their theory of theories proposed the formulation of prescriptions that would be used, in combination with a survey list, to reach the goal. The survey list was organized around six categories: (1) agency, (2) patiency, (3) dynamics, (4) structure, (5) terminus, and (6) procedure. The list was basically an enumeration of factors that did not qualify as prescriptions that were recognized as affecting movement toward the goal (Dickoff & James, 1968). The inclusion of values within the structure of theory and the recognition that theory was more like a flexible guide to practice (rather than a global framework to be systematically tested) provided a revolutionary view of empiric knowledge. The Dickoff and James approach to nursing metatheory, which was intensely discussed in the literature and at conferences, reflected a growing recognition that the nature and value of scientific-empiric theory for nursing was unclear. Dickoff and James asked the discipline to question the nature of theory and the value of objectivist prescriptions for practice theory and to attempt to articulate a clearer concept of nursing practice.

METALANGUAGE OF NURSING CONCEPTUAL FRAMEWORKS

Central concepts or shared images can be described when the conceptual frameworks listed in Table 2.1 are grouped around common themes. Four concepts have been widely recognized as common to nursing's conceptual frameworks: (1) nursing, (2) the person, (3) the society and environment, and (4) health. We have chosen the term *metalanguage* rather than *metaparadigm* to refer to these concepts. Although these four elements have elsewhere been considered nursing's metaparadigm (Fawcett & DeSanto-Madeya, 2012), our definition and use of the term *paradigm* is inconsistent with this terminology. The prefix *meta-* means that which is encompassing or transcending. Thus, metalanguage is language that is used to describe or analyze (include or encompass) another language or system of symbols ("Metalanguage," 1998). The following sections provide a view of these four metalanguage concepts in early conceptual frameworks. We draw on the first major publication of each of the nurse scholars in this analysis.

Nursing

In nursing's theoretic writings, nursing is generally represented as a helping process with a primary focus on interpersonal interactions between a nurse and another individual. This general idea does not clearly distinguish nursing from other helping disciplines, but it provides an important focus for deciding what type of knowledge is needed for nursing practice. In recent years, the development of caring science in nursing has refined and further focused the phenomenon of caring as the defining characteristic of inter-personal relationships in nursing (Cook & Peden, 2016; Newman, Sime, & Corcoran-Perry, 1991). The interpersonal nature of nursing practice distinguishes nursing from medicine in that medicine focuses on surgical and pharmacologic interventions, with interpersonal interactions being secondary to these interventions. Within a medical model of nursing, the nurse's primary functions relate to medical assessment, diagnosis, treatment, and medication administration as delegated medical tasks. Within a nursing framework, where interpersonal interactions are primary, technical and medical func-tions support the primary interpersonal interactions.

Although different nurse authors present conceptualizations of the nature of nurs-ing consistent with the idea of interpersonal interactions as a primary focus, important differences exist with regard to their definitions and conceptualizations. For some, the person with whom the nurse interacts largely defines the direction of the interaction and the specific actions that are taken to achieve the goals of the interaction. The nurse's role in the interaction is primarily one of facilitating. When this view of the nature of nursing is incorporated into a framework or model, nursing is viewed as enabling the will and behavior of the person who is receiving care.

Other theoretic models present a view of the interpersonal process as either shared or initiated by the nurse. In this view, nursing processes and actions rest primarily on the nurse's initiative, knowledge, and approaches. The theoretic ideas that emerge from this view focus on nursing actions to reach the goal of the interaction.

Each of these perspectives is consistent with the practice of nursing in that nurses encounter some situations in which the patient primarily directs the interaction and other situations in which the nurse is the initiator; some conceptual frameworks account for this diversity. The common significant thread is the primacy of human interaction for creating human health and wholeness.

The Person

All conceptual frameworks include ideas about the general nature of humans. The most consistent philosophic component of the idea of the person is the dimension of whole-ness or wholism. Although various conceptual frameworks may view the ill or diseased person as having problems with need fulfillment, integration, adaptation, role fulfill-ment, and so forth, the central impediment to health or healing is dealt with holistically in various senses of the word.

The nature of wholism as a concept is difficult to address from the perspective of traditional Western philosophies that are grounded in reductionism. In the reductionist view of wholism, the whole is equal to the sum of the parts; interrelationships among the parts are emphasized, and generalizations can be made about the whole from under-standing how the parts of the whole interrelate (Newman, 1979, 1999). Western culture embraces this view, and nurses, as with others in this culture, have learned to think about parts of lives, parts of bodies, and parts of human experiences.

In a purer sense that is more consistent with Eastern traditions, wholism means that the whole is greater than the sum of the parts: The whole cannot be reduced to its parts without losing something in the process. Martha Rogers, Margaret Newman, Joyce Travelbee, and Patricia Benner are among the nurse scholars whose work reflects a view that the individual is different from and greater than the sum of his or her parts. Other nursing theorists explicitly or implicitly hold to the idea that the whole is equal to the sum of the parts, assuming that the individual is a system with biologic, sociologic, and psychologic components. Although this is not consistent with wholism in its purest sense, there still is a strong commitment to the idea that all components of the individual need to be considered.

Society and Environment

The concepts of society and environment are central to the discipline of nursing and reflected across conceptual frameworks, although these concepts are not addressed as explicitly in some writings as in others. Several nursing frameworks include a concept of society or culture and present it as a critical interacting force that shapes the individual environment. Environment was central for Nightingale when she formulated her concept of nursing. Nightingale believed the primary focus for nursing was to alter the physical environment to place the human body in the best possible condition for the reparative processes of nature to occur. More recent conceptual frameworks deemphasize environment or view it as being encompassed within a concept of society; sometimes the word *society* is used to include the environment. However, the concept of environment remains a significant one (Butterfield, 2017; Jarrin, 2012; Kangasniemi, Kallio, & Pietilä, 2014; Kleffel, 1991). Martha Rogers and theorists who build on her ideas focus on a concept of environment as indistinguishable (except conceptually) from the concept of person. Most other conceptual frameworks separate the person from the environment, thus implying that boundaries separate the two. As with the concept of person, environmental concepts vary, but they appear across conceptual frameworks.

Health

The concept of health is typically identified as the goal of nursing. Nightingale (Newman, 1999; Nightingale, 1860/1969) stated that "the same laws of health or of nursing, for in reality they are the same, obtain among the well as among the sick" (p. 9), implying that health is a state of order within natural laws. Contemporary nursing models are remarkably congruent with this early conceptualization. Some frameworks are based on a conceptualization of a health–illness continuum, with the purpose of nursing being to assist the ill person with achieving the greatest possible degree of health. Other nurse authors view the concept of health as something more than or different from the absence of disease. For them, health exists independently from illness or disease. In these views, health is a dynamic process that changes with time and that varies with life circumstances. Some authors view the health process as interdependent with circumstances of the environment, whereas others view the health process as originating with the individual.

In an attempt to deal more specifically with ideas related to health, several nurse authors avoid using the terms *health* and *illness*. An example is the use of the term *conserving wholism* by Myra Levine (1967). This concept directs nurses to focus on the totality of a person's situation rather than on the typical parameters that have come to be commonly known as health. Avoiding the use of health and illness allows for the use of terms related to health that more specifically reflect nursing's concerns and that deemphasize the focus on disease or illness.

DEVELOPMENT OF MIDDLE-RANGE PRACTICE-LINKED THEORY

During the 1980s, Meleis (1987) brought into clear focus the need for nurses to develop substantive theory that provides a meaningful foundation for the development of nursing practice in relation to specific practice concepts. In accord with the observation of many practicing nurses, Meleis acknowledged the value of theories broad in scope for defining the general parameters on which nursing function is based. However, Meleis emphasized that theory of a different type was required to give more specific guidance to nursing practice; this form of theory would prove to align more closely with the empiric pattern of knowing and knowledge. Meleis's plea also reflected the need for nursing to move away from its long-term discussions and debates about the nature of theory, knowledge, and the proper functions of nursing. She called on nurses to focus on developing substance in theory and substantive, more readily observable and accessible nursing concepts grounded in a practice context.

Nursing theory of this type is developed in concert with research questions that are directly or indirectly linked to important practice issues. It avoids a focus on methodology for methodology's sake and shifts the focus to understanding nursing-related phenomena. Substantive middle-range theory can inform practice and lead to new practice approaches as well as investigate factors that influence the outcomes desired in nursing practice.

Im and Meleis (1999) introduced the idea of *situation-specific theory*, a variant of middle-range theory that underscores the importance of considering the context in which a theory will be used. Whereas middle-range theory narrows the conceptual focus of a theory and substantive middle-range theory further defines the focus as being clinically relevant concepts, situation-specific theory emphasizes the need to consider the unique context for which the theory is developed (Meleis, 2010). Situation specificity is important because of variability within particular populations, fields of practice, and subsequent approaches to clinical phenomena. Unlike substantive middle-range theory, which is presumed to be more broadly generalizable across different populations, situation-specific theory addresses the particular and unique needs of a group of people in a specific context. Situation specificity is particularly important for evidence-based practice in that best research evidence should be appropriate to the population within which the research will be used, especially when variables of importance to care have been part of the situational considerations. Substantive middle-range theory in nursing tends to cluster around a concept of interest, such as social support, uncertainty, grief, fatigue, or life transitions.

TRENDS IN KNOWLEDGE DEVELOPMENT

What counts as knowledge does not remain static. Knowledge historically reflects the social, political, and professional climate in which knowledge development occurs. The context within which knowledge is developed determines and influences what counts as knowledge and how knowledge structures are valued and evaluated. For several years after Carper (1978) published her work regarding the knowing patterns, knowledge forms and development processes other than those associated with empirics were seen as important to nursing and became more generally accepted. The adherence to a specific methodology or template for knowledge development was being replaced with a requirement for rigor and disclosure of methodology rather than following a strict formula. Although many knowledge developers in nursing remain firmly rooted in the assumptions and methodologies of empirics, knowledge structures are emerging that are not empiric in the sense that a strict interpretation of the pattern of empirics assumes. Although communicated and developed in language, these structures are not grounded in objectivist assumptions and scientific notions of reliability and validity. It is possible to conceptualize empiric knowledge broadly to include forms of interpretive work that culminate in the identification of themes (phenomenology) or detailed descriptions (ethnographies) as falling within the empiric pattern. However, some emerging knowledge forms and methods rest on different assumptions and methodologies and fall outside the realm of empirics. Several important trends in theory development and use are described in the following sections.

The Move Away from Methodolotry

A growing trend in nursing is to blend and use a variety of knowledge development processes to achieve a given research aim rather than to adhere to strict methodologic imperatives. Many scholars are moving from a focus on method and technique to a focus on problem solving or the achievement of study goals. Because the methodologic process is tailored to accomplish research objectives, various approaches to inquiry are modified and blended. The qualitative/quantitative dichotomy is being questioned as a way of categorizing methodologic approaches. There is growing recognition that qualitative data may be important to obtain in primarily experimental designs and, conversely, that quantitative data may be useful in naturalistic inquiry. Rather than combining approaches (i.e., performing both a quantitative and a qualitative study), the purpose of the research determines how findings are blended. *Critical multiplism* (Letourneau & Allen, 1999), *multivocality* (Savage, 2000), and *intersectionality* (Kelly, 2009, 2011) are examples of terms used to denote these types of methods. This trend signals maturity in nursing scholarship wherein professional research purposes take precedence over methodologic loyalties.

Interpretive and Critical Approaches

In a classic article, Allen, Benner, and Diekelman (1986) suggested three categories for the classification of research: empiric-analytic, interpretive-hermeneutic, and

critical-social. Empiric-analytic work conforms to the traditions of empirics as conceptualized by Carper, which means that the work relies on perceptually grounded and
objective replication and validation research methods. Some forms of interpretive work
remain faithful to this traditional objectivist assumption, but some forms of interpretive
work fall outside the realm of traditional objectivist empirics. Interpretive approaches,
such as grounded theory, phenomenology, analyses of language, and hermeneutic
inquiry, assess truth value (reliability and validity) by consensus between the researcher
and the participants.

The assumption of an objective reality with meaning that is independent of the
observer is not taken as a given. Grounded-theory approaches, which are now applied in
a variety of forms, are constructed out of shared understandings between the researcher
and the participants (Crotty, 1998). Methodologies grounded in the philosophy of phenomenology seek to account for the nature of the experience from the experiencer's point
of view. Although these accounts may be judged as "good" or "less than good," they
clearly do not rest on objectivist assumptions about the existence and nature of a reality
independent from the observer. As with empirics, however, their conclusions are drawn
from interpretations that are fundamentally grounded in sensory perceptions, whereas
truth value (i.e., reliability and validity) relies on a consensus of meaning that is particular
and situated. Noncritical forms of hermeneutic inquiry recognize context to be important to the shaping of knowledge. The researcher moves back and forth between what is
being interpreted and an ever-enlarging context that accounts for the researcher's unique
perspective within the situation to create a reasonable (loosely valid) understanding.

Critical approaches seek to illuminate structures of domination and in nursing are
addressing health care structures that compromise the quality of care for people on the
basis of factors such as class, economics, race, age, gender, disability, or sexual orientation
(Cowling & Chinn, 2001; Falk-Rafael & Bradley, 2014; Fontana, 2004; Kagan, Smith,
& Chinn, 2014; Kramer, 2002; Pitre, Kushner, Raine, & Hegadoren, 2013). Critical
social theory is not theory in the sense of empiric theory, which focuses on an objectivity of observation that allows for a degree of generalizable description, explanation, and
prediction. The primary purpose of critical theory is to create social and political change.
Critical theory takes the form of narrative analyses that illuminate how social practices
that are institutionalized (e.g., in political or educational institutions) enable unjust practices for the benefit of a dominant group. Critical theory may have several foci. Critical
feminist theory centers on issues of gender discrimination; critical social theory focuses
on class issues as they perpetuate unfair educational, political, and other social practices.
The "critical" focus points to a need to undo and remake oppressive social structures.

Intersectionality is a form of critical scholarship based on the premise that health disparities and social disadvantage occur in a context of many intersecting factors that have
a multiplicative effect. These intersecting factors include social identities such as gender,
race, class, ability/disability, sexual orientation, and religion. Every social group is seen
as having unique qualities, and each individual within the group is situated within the
social structure in ways that intersect with the person's unique social identities to create
social inequities. An intersectional approach yields a more comprehensive understanding of the interrelated nature of health disparities. Intersectional approaches address

two levels of analysis: the nature of structural oppression creating the disparity and the nature of the individual's intersecting identities that shape the person's experience of the situation (Kelly, 2009, 2011).

Poststructuralist Approaches

Research consistent with the analytic methodology of poststructuralism appears frequently in the nursing literature (Allen & Hardin, 2001; Arslanian-Engoren, 2002; Cloyes, 2006; Francis, 2000; Scheer, Stevens, & Mkandawire-Valhmu, 2016; Thompson, 2007; Tinley & Kinney, 2007). Poststructuralism is an outgrowth of structuralism. In linguistics, *structuralism* is the view that the meaning of words is given by context or by the linguistic frame that surrounds a word. The single word "duck," for example, has no stable referent, and whether this utterance is referring to a type of bird or is a directive to avoid hitting a low-hanging tree branch cannot be known without encountering the word in context. The poststructuralist movement moves language away from a representational view. This means that words do not stand for something that is either given objectively (as traditional forms of empirics assume) or known from a context of usage. Rather, language—or, more broadly, discourse—creates and determines possibilities. Discourses are whole systems of representations that include text, visuals, and behavioral actions that surround, are associated with, reference, or create experiences and understandings. Critical analyses that use language and systems of discourse, as data uncover how language functions to perpetuate networks of oppression and domination, add important new dimensions to nursing knowledge.

Deconstruction and Postmodernism

Deconstruction is an elusive term to define but generally refers to processes that take apart assumptions, ideologies, and frames of reference that are buried and unnoticed in text. *Text* refers to what is written as well as to other visual representations of situations and events, such as advertisements, cartoons, and film (Kress, Leite-Garcia, & van Leeuwen, 1996; van Dijk, 1997). Deconstructive work often focuses on text that is problematic in relation to sustaining inequities that create disadvantage for one group for the benefit of another. However, deconstruction is much more than even critical analysis. Deconstruction involves making explicit and coming to understand that certain features of text (e.g., implicit assumptions, ideologies, frames of reference) cannot be warranted as a basis for truths. In this way, deconstruction is useful for undermining language and social contexts that promote inequities and injustices.

Alternatively, *postmodernism* is a term with broader meaning, but as with deconstruction, it has a variety of unclear meanings and uses. In a general sense, the postmodern era is the one that followed the modern era. *Modernism,* as it relates to science, began with a move to account for natural phenomena by using scientific approaches rather than appealing to religious and metaphysical explanations. Thus, modernism signaled the end of religious authority as the basis for understanding the world. Modernism has become associated with the age of science and scientific inquiry. As discoveries in modern physics began to uncover the fallibility of scientific explanation, and the social agenda of science failed, this enabled the move toward postmodernism. Postmodernism in relation to methods of inquiry is reflected in the increasing use of nonscientific methodologies as well as the combining of multiple methods within a single research project. The reference to "anything goes" often is coupled with references to postmodernism. Although "anything goes" is reasonable in one sense, any notion of arbitrariness or relativism is unwarranted. The postmodern era has loosened the idea of what counts as legitimate knowledge, but it should not signal that sloppy approaches to knowledge development are acceptable. Although various methods may be legitimate, they must be carried out carefully and rigorously to be useful.

CLINICAL APPLICATION AND PRODUCTION OF KNOWLEDGE

Growing concern about the need to link practice and knowledge has resulted in significant trends in practice, research, and development of knowledge in nursing. These trends reflect a concern for the increased clinical relevance of theory and research, transdisciplinary relevance, and improvement in the quality of care while achieving a realistic economy in health care (Bach, Ploeg, & Black, 2009; Bliss, Baltzly, Bull, Dalton, & Jones, 2017; Hartrick Doane, Reimer-Kirkham, Antifeau, & Stajduhar, 2015; Moch et al., 2008; Ploeg, Davies, Edwards, Gifford, & Miller, 2007; Richardson-Tench, 2012; Rolfe, 2006).

Evidence-Informed Practice

During the 1990s, evidence-based nursing practice began to receive attention in the nursing literature. The idea of evidence-based practice originated in the medical literature as a way to help ensure that high-quality research was deliberately used in clinical decision making. Evidence-based medicine incorporated a variety of empiric and nonempiric knowledge forms, arranged in a hierarchy, as evidence (Mazurek-Melnyk, Stone, Fincout-Overholt, & Ackerman, 2000).

Evidence-based nursing practice also focuses on the necessity of integrating quality research into practice decisions to provide high-level nursing care. It is important to note that evidence-based nursing practice is not simply the application of single studies or using the results of metaanalyses in client care. Rather, evidence-based nursing practice requires the integration of best research evidence with such things as clinical expertise, expert opinion, health care resources, clinical state and setting, circumstances, and patient preferences (DiCenso, Guyatt, & Ciliska, 2005; Melnyk & Fineout-Overholt, 2011).

Models of research evidence generally assign the highest truth value to knowledge generated using more traditional empirics. Although case analyses and qualitative studies count as evidence, these have less credibility (Phillips et al., 2009; Schunemann, Best, Vist, & Oxman, 2003). Characterizing best research evidence as a highly empiric form of knowledge that evolves from data-based, experimental, and quasi-experimental research methodologies has received criticism that challenges the persistent predominance of empirics as a way of knowing in nursing (Fullbrook, 2003; Holmes, Perron, & O'Byrne, 2006; Mowinski-Jennings & Loan, 2001; Satterfield et al., 2009; Thorne & Sawatzky, 2014). A strictly empiric view of research evidence seems to be changing and many models of evidence-based practice acknowledge the value of such things as peer-reviewed standards and evidence-based theories although a bias for traditional research seems to prevail (Armola et al., 2009; Fineout-Overholt, Melnyk, & Schultz, 2005; Melnyk & Fineout-Overholt, 2011).

The nature of evidence-based nursing practice will likely continue to evolve. We favor an approach that views evidence-based practice as the integration of best research evidence (including less traditional knowledge development approaches) with clinical factors, expert opinion, and patient preferences and values (DiCenso et al., 2005; Melnyk & Fineout-Overholt, 2011; Salmond, 2013; Thorne & Sawatzky, 2014). The shift in terminology to *evidence-informed practice* now widely found in the literature acknowledges that although clinical decision making should consider a wide variety of credible evidence, the process must also integrate client/patient and circumstantial factors. We applaud and favor this shift in terminology and believe it more clearly represents the nature of clinical decision making. Evidence-informed nursing practice and models of evidence-based clinical decision making that acknowledge the importance of factors other than empiric research require all patterns of knowing. For example, the interpretation of patient preferences and clinical circumstances requires attending to aesthetic, ethical, and personal knowing. Understanding the politics of how health care resources affect the circumstances of care is grounded in emancipatory knowing. In short, clinical expertise requires broad knowing within all patterns.

Practice-Based Evidence and Translational Research

All health care disciplines have increasing concern for creating a closer link between what is effective in practice and evidence that is based on effective practice (Bliss et al., 2017; Hartrick Doane et al., 2015; Moch et al., 2008; Satterfield et al., 2009; Wallin, 2009). This trend is labeled by various terms, including *practice-based evidence* and *translational research*. References to practice-based evidence in the health care literature refer to the validation in practice of clinically used approaches and techniques that are known to be effective for promoting health-related goals. The call for practice-based evidence emphasizes a focus on investigating and validating what seems to be effective in practice as a way of generating research evidence for integration into evidence-based decision making (Doane & Varcoe, 2008; Fox, 2003; Hartrick Doane et al., 2015; Simons, Kushner, Jones, & James, 2003). Proponents of practice-based evidence suggest that the top-down approach (i.e., research to practice) currently valued in hierarchies of research evidence uses methodologies to generate outcomes that may not be workable in the practice arena. For example, randomized controlled clinical trials, which are taken to be highly valuable sources of empiric evidence, control for variables that are at work in the clinical environment. Proponents of practice-based evidence suggest that the stripping away of situational variables and the control necessary for many experimental studies produce a knowledge structure that is too decontextualized to be useful and thus should not be used to guide practice. Rather, evidence must be generated out of or situated within the context from which it is generated to be useful to practitioners (Simons et al., 2003).

Translational research reflects a type of "research-to-practice" approach. Simply stated, translational research is designed to take evidence a step further by validating it in the practice setting. Translational research initiatives are now part of the U.S. National Institutes of Health roadmap (Ryan et al., 2011). Interest in promoting translational research has been prominent in clinical practices where there exists an interest in moving basic research studies into practice as quickly as possible (Bakken & Jones, 2006; Hartrick Doane et al., 2015; Titler, 2004; Wallin, 2009). Thus, translational research promotes the use of research discoveries in clinical settings.

Emergence of the Practice Doctorate

Although its effect on knowledge development remains to be seen, the emergence of the doctorate of nursing science (DNS) has the potential to influence how knowledge in nursing is created and used in clinical practice and in nursing in general. The DNS, also referred to as the *practice doctorate,* was originally developed in the 1960s. However, the expansion of these early programs to prepare nurses with a practice doctorate was eclipsed by the growth of research-oriented PhD programs (Fitzpatrick & Wallace, 2009).

Recently, the DNS has begun to reemerge as a viable educational option in nursing. The American Association of Colleges of Nursing (AACN) began serious discussions about the Doctorate of Nursing Practice (DNP) in 2001 and released "The Essentials of Doctoral Education for Advanced Nursing Practice" in 2006. Currently, the AACN website lists nearly 300 schools that offer DNP programs.

In general, the DNP focuses on advanced clinical care and the application and generation of evidence that supports improved care (Acorn, Lamarche, & Edwards, 2009; AACN, 2016; Mundinger, Starck, Hathaway, Shaver, & Woods, 2009; O'Connor, 2015). According to the AACN, practice-focused doctoral programs deemphasize theory, metatheory, research methodology, and statistics that are part of research-focused programs. Foundational competencies that must be addressed by curricula in DNP programs for accreditation by the Council for Collegiate Nursing Education have been proposed. Multiple competencies within eight foundational areas are enumerated in the AACN essentials article ("The Essentials of Doctoral Education for Advanced Nursing Practice," 2006). Examples of competencies listed in the document include the following:

- Evaluate new practice approaches on the basis of nursing theories and theories from other disciplines.
- Use analytic methods to critically appraise literature and other evidence to determine and implement the best evidence for practice.
- Design and implement processes to evaluate outcomes of practice, practice patterns, and systems of care within a practice setting, health care organization, or community to determine variances in practice outcomes and population trends.
- Use research methods to collect data to generate evidence for nursing practice.
- Analyze data from practice, design evidence-based interventions, predict and analyze outcomes, and identify gaps in evidence for practice.

- Disseminate findings from evidence-based practice and research.
- Analyze epidemiological, biostatistical, environmental, and other appropriate scientific data related to individual, aggregate, and population health.
- Evaluate evidence-based care to improve patient outcomes.

In our view, these competencies can have a significant impact on the way knowledge is developed and used in nursing. The practice focus of these competencies and their basis in research and analytic clinical investigation strategies mandates that research and practice complement one another. Competencies such as these reflect the need for translational research as well as practice-based evidence. It is reasonable to assume that such competencies will require communication between academic nurses and clinical nurse researchers to achieve the goals of high-quality nursing care.

In summary, the grip of traditional empirics in nursing seems to be moderating, perhaps signaling a return to our history of wholism with regard to knowing and knowledge development. During the 1960s, a scientific metatheory dominated the literature but never really took hold. Gradually, nursing moved away from a metatheoretic focus on empirics, as expressed in objectivist research approaches that are descriptive, correlational, quasi-experimental, or experimental. Naturalistic and qualitative approaches to practice began to appear with greater frequency during the 1980s. More recently, the importance of language for determining what counts as knowledge is being recognized, and critical research that undermines unjust and inequitable social conditions is being conducted. Ongoing emphasis on evidence-based nursing practice that requires the integration of broad forms of knowledge formally acknowledges that empiric evidence is only part of what is needed for the making of good clinical decisions. A focus on practice evidence and translational research re-emphasizes moving evidence into practice in a way that benefits the patient. The foundational competencies for the practice doctorate hold the promise of creating a research agenda that more fully serves the needs and interests of people who receive nursing care.

CONTEXTS OF KNOWLEDGE DEVELOPMENT

As illustrated in this chapter, specific circumstances and contexts affect the development of knowledge. What defines knowledge, what sources identify the best knowledge, and how nurses use and construct knowledge are greatly influenced by—if not determined by—the interrelationship between values and resources at multiple levels. These levels can be categorized as individual, professional, and societal.

Values

Individual values include a specific nurse's commitment, personal philosophy, motives, beliefs, and priorities.

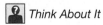 *Think About It*

Think about what sorts of research approaches you might find more valuable than others and whether you even believe that research is an important area to study. If you value research, what is your motive for learning about it? Employment in an academic setting? Making a difference in people's lives? Both? Is uncovering research evidence something you attend to because you have to or because you want to? Is it something you do after you have practiced technical skills?

Professional values are beliefs and attitudes about what is good and right that generally are held in common by members of a profession and that are used to guide professional action. These values are expressed in formal statements issued by professional groups in the form of codes, standards of practice, and ethical principles and are also reflected in themes repeated in the literature and in the collective actions taken by professional organizations. The current emphasis on the practice doctorate and the move toward evidence-based nursing practice reflect professional values that are being expressed today.

 Think About It

> How has the professional valuing of evidence-based practice influenced your learning? How has it affected the practices of nurses with whom you have come in contact? Will the profession's valuing of the professional doctorate change its research productivity for the better?

Societal values are expressed through societal choices, sanctions, and moral behavior during a given period in history. The focus on national and international security in the wake of terrorist activities and the use of monetary resources to promote security reflect its value for society.

 Think About It

> Has the valuing of national security affected the financial resources available to you as a student? How have societal values affected grant funding within academic institutions? How have they affected the topic on which you focus a research proposal for funding? Has the valuing of capitalism and corporate structures as well as the consolidation of hospital services into large entities changed your ability and others' abilities to enact evidence-informed clinical decision making?

Resources

Resources also can also be viewed as individual, professional, or societal. *Individual resources* include the natural and acquired talents that are shared among members of a discipline, including cognitive style, intellectual abilities, life circumstances, and educational preparation.

 Think About It

> How might the nature of your educational preparation (i.e., what you are exposed to and learn as a student) be a resource that you will bring to nursing. Will an ability to think in a linear fashion mean that you will bring expertise in quantitative methods to the profession? Might the gift of a nonlinear cognitive style signal your contribution to aesthetic knowing and practice? What talents will you share that evolve from those life experiences

and interests that are unique to you? Did you grow up in another country and thus can contribute a unique understanding of how to study effectively the health care needs of your country's citizens? How might the financial and other resources that you have to support additional education determine the resources that you bring to nursing?

Professional resources reflect the collective resources of the discipline for knowledge development. Examples of professional resources include a growing body of literature and practice traditions, the ability to communicate these traditions among members of the profession, the educational attainments of members of the profession, the nature of the education of the profession's members, and the methodologies and instrumentation available for knowledge development.

 Think About It

How will what you bring to nursing and develop as a practitioner, in addition to the contributions of a host of other nurses, constitute nursing's professional resources? As practitioners and students are exposed to the techniques and meanings of evidence-based practice, will knowledge resources of the discipline change? Will nurses who hold the practice doctorate change nursing's knowledge resources? Might you and others embrace critical theory or the tenets of practice-based evidence as a way to better integrate research into clinical decision making? If you are interested in knowledge development related to aesthetic knowing, are there professional resources to assist you with learning how to do this? Do available information systems ease or deter the retrieval of evidence to be integrated into clinical decision making? Has nursing made use of the Internet in such a way that it is a valuable resource for care? Are there professional practice traditions you must obey that you think are counterproductive? Will nursing pay enough for you to sustain a reasonably comfortable lifestyle? Will nursing services where you work have the political clout to advocate for improved client and patient care?

Societal resources affect the nature of the material and nonmaterial resources that are available to support knowledge development in nursing. The acquisition of societal resources depends on features of both society and the profession.

 Think About It

Political influence is required to obtain funds, materials, and space to carry out the activities of the discipline. If the political system of society reflects priorities other than those that involve nursing, societal resources are less available to nursing than to other groups who reflect those priorities. For example, how has the societal interest in national and international security affected resource allocation for nursing in your practice area? If you are a student, what trends are affecting your financial aid possibilities? Have you (or someone you know) been relocated out of your space or lost your job because of special funding initiatives? How successful will nursing be in the securing of resources to develop a broad conceptualization of knowing if scientific knowledge is still largely held to be the most valuable? Has the tax base available for health care been deflected into other arenas, thereby changing the way that you counsel an elderly person about how to obtain prescription medications?

The relationships between and among values and resources are intertwined, and, in some cases, it is difficult to determine how a given factor that affects knowledge development should be categorized. Categorization is never the goal; rather, it is important to understand how factors in a broad array of contexts interrelate to determine health care needs, how those needs are approached, and who provides care.

In addition, when individual, professional, and societal values are basically congruent, there is relative stability, and new insights tend to build on what is already established as the knowledge of the discipline. When individual, professional, or societal values change, the potential exists for creating fundamental changes in knowledge and practice. For example, political decisions that are made by government entities require value decisions about who deserves and who does not deserve to receive the resources of a society. As history shows, if female scientists are consistently provided with limited or no societal resources, this impedes the ability of women to influence value decisions about how money should be allocated.

Nursing represents a group of mostly women (a professional resource) within a societal context that devalues female scientists, which influences the profession's ability to exert influence on society to gain access to resources. The contemporary women's movement has created a stimulus for recognizing societal restrictions on nursing as a gender-segregated occupation and the effects of the systematic oppression of nurses and nursing (Group & Roberts, 2001; Malka, 2007; Roberts, 1983). Feminist theory, which shares many of the traits of nursing theory, provides a perspective for changing social values and shifting social resources. Feminism places an urgent demand on society for a values transformation that is consistent with nursing's vision of health, the health care system, and nursing (Chinn & Wheeler, 1985; Roberts & Group, 1995). As women's experience becomes increasingly valued as a resource for developing knowledge, the resulting values will conflict with traditional views, and the new values will open avenues for change.

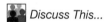 *Discuss This...*

Discuss these questions with a group of colleagues:
1. How have some of the events, trends, and issues in nursing today been grounded in or how do they depend on past events?
2. What mistakes are we making today with regard to knowledge development, and how will they affect future nursing care? What current events and trends are definitely not mistakes with regard to knowledge development, and why?
3. How would you change nursing's values and resources to promote knowledge development?

CONCLUSION

This chapter has summarized historical evidence demonstrating a steady movement to retain the early values and conceptual ideals established by early leaders in nursing, as well as movement toward change in both the functions and the essence of nursing that is responsive to the changes in culture and society. The methods that nurses use to achieve professional goals of knowledge development and practice are central to the challenges of the future.

References

Abdellah, F. G. (1969). The nature of nursing science. *Nursing Research, 18*, 390–393.

Achterberg, J. (1991). *Woman as healer.* Boston: Shambhala.

Acorn, S., Lamarche, K., & Edwards, M. (2009). Practice doctorates in nursing: developing nursing leaders. *Canadian Journal of Nursing Leadership, 22*, 85–91.

Aikins, C. A. (1915). Teaching ethics in hospital schools. *The Trained Nurse and Hospital Review, 54*, 135–137.

Allen, D., Benner, P., & Diekelman, N. (1986). Three paradigms for nursing research: methodological implications. In P. L. Chinn (Ed.), *Nursing research methodology: issues and implementation* (pp. 23–38). Rockville, MD: Aspen.

Allen, D., & Hardin, P. K. (2001). Discourse analysis and the epidemiology of meaning. *Nursing Philosophy: An International Journal for Healthcare Professionals, 2*, 163–176.

American Association of Colleges of Nursing. (2016). *The doctor of nursing practice: current issues and clarifying recommendations—report from the Task Force on the Implementation of the DNP AACN, August 2015.* http://www.aacn.nche.edu/aacn-publications/white-papers/DNP-Implementation-TF-Report-8-15.pdf.

American Nurses Association. (2007). *Susie Walking Bear Yellowtail (1903-1981) 2002 Inductee.* http://www.nursingworld.org/SusieWalkingBearYellowtail.

American Nurses Association. (2008). *Adah Belle Samuel Thoms (1870-1943) 1976 Inductee.* http://www.nursingworld.org/AdahBelleSamuelThoms.

American Nurses Association. (2009). *Mabel Keaton Staupers (1890-1989) 1996 Inductee.* http://www.nursingworld.org/MabelKeatonStaupers.

Andrist, L. C., Nicholas, P. K., & Wolf, K. (2006). *A history of nursing ideas.* Sudbury, MA: Jones & Bartlett.

Armola, R. R., Bourgault, A. M., Halm, M. A., Board, R. M., Bucher, L., … Medina, J. (2009). AACN levels of evidence: What's new? *Critical Care Nurse, 29*, 70–73.

Arslanian-Engoren, C. (2002). Feminist poststructuralism: a methodological paradigm for examining clinical decision-making. *Journal of Advanced Nursing, 37*, 512–517.

Ashley, J. (1976). *Hospitals, paternalism, and the role of the nurse.* New York, NY: Teachers College Press.

Bach, V., Ploeg, J., & Black, M. (2009). Nursing roles in end-of-life decision making in critical care settings. *Western Journal of Nursing Research, 31*, 496–512.

Bakken, S., & Jones, D. A. (2006). Contributions to translational research for quality health outcomes. *Nursing Research, 55*, S1–S2.

Barnum, B. J. S. (1998). *Nursing theory* (5th ed.). Boston, MA: Lippincott-Raven.

Beck, D.-M. (2006). Nightingale's passion for advocacy: local to global. In L. C. Andrist, P. K. Nicholas, & K. Wolf (Eds.), *A history of nursing ideas* (pp. 473–487). Sudbury, MA: Jones & Bartlett.

Benner, P. A., & Wrubel, J. (1989). *The primacy of caring: stress and coping in health and illness.* Menlo Park, CA: AddisonWesley.

Bixler, G. K., & Bixler, R. W. (1945). The professional status of nursing. *The American Journal of Nursing, 45*, 730–735.

Bliss, S., Baltzly, D., Bull, R., Dalton, L., & Jones, J. (2017). A role for virtue in unifying the "knowledge" and "caring" discourses in nursing theory. *Nursing Inquiry.* https://doi.org/10.1111/nin.12191.

Bradshaw, A. (2017). What is a nurse? The Francis report and the historic voice of nursing. *Nursing Inquiry.* https://doi.org/doi/10.1111/nin.12190/full.

Brigh, S. M. (1944). We cannot afford to hurry: training within industry applied to nursing. *The American Journal of Nursing, 44*, 223–226.

Burgess, M. E. (1941). A plan for nursing care. *The American Journal of Nursing, 41*, 215–218.

Butterfield, P. G. (2017). Thinking upstream: a 25-year retrospective and conceptual model aimed at reducing health inequities. *ANS. Advances in Nursing Science, 40*(1), 2–11. https://doi.org/10.1097/ANS.0000000000000161.

Carper, B. A. (1978). Fundamental patterns of knowing in nursing. *ANS. Advances in Nursing Science, 1*, 13–23.

Carter, M. (2006). The evolution of doctoral education in nursing. In L. C. Andrist, P. K. Nicholas, & K. Wolf (Eds.), *A history of nursing ideas* (pp. 383–392). Sudbury, MA: Jones & Bartlett.

Changes in nursing practice. (1947). *The American Journal of Nursing, 47,* 665.

Chinn, P. L., & Wheeler, C. E. (1985). Feminism and nursing. *Nursing Outlook, 33,* 74–77.

Christy, T. E. (1969). Portrait of a leader. *Nursing Outlook, 6,* 72–75.

Cloyes, K. G. (2006). An ethic of analysis: an argument for critical analysis of research interviews as an ethical practice. *ANS. Advances in Nursing Science, 29,* 84–97.

Cohen, I. B. (1984). Florence Nightingale. *Scientific American, 250,* 128–137.

Conrad, M. E. (1947). What is expert nursing care? *The American Journal of Nursing, 47,* 162–163.

Cook, L. B., & Peden, A. (2016). Finding a focus for nursing: the caring concept. *ANS. Advances in Nursing Science.* https://doi.org/10.1097/ANS.0000000000000137.

Cowling, W. R., & Chinn, P. L. (2001). Conversation across paradigms: unitary-transformative and critical feminist perspectives. *Scholarly Inquiry for Nursing Practice, 15,* 347–365.

Crotty, M. (1998). *The foundations of social research: meaning and perspective in the research process.* London: Sage.

Dennis, K. E., & Prescott, P. A. (1985). Florence Nightingale: yesterday, today, and tomorrow. *ANS. Advances in Nursing Science, 7,* 66–81.

De Witt, K. (1901). Specialities in nursing. *The American Journal of Nursing, 1,* 14–15.

DiCenso, A., Guyatt, G., & Ciliska, D. (2005). *Evidence based nursing: a guide to clinical practice.* St. Louis, MO: Mosby.

Dickoff, J., & James, P. (1968). Researching research's role in theory development. *Nursing Research, 17*(3), 204–205.

Dickoff, J., & James, P. (1971). Clarity to what end? *Nursing Research, 20,* 499–502.

Dickoff, J., & James, P. (1997). A theory of theories: a position paper. In L. H. Nicoll (Ed.), *Perspectives on nursing theory* (3rd ed.) (pp. 103–116) (Ch. 8). Philadelphia, PA: Lippincott.

Dickoff, J., James, P., & Wiedenbach, E. (1968). Theory in a practice discipline: Part II. Practice oriented research. *Nursing Research, 17*(6), 545.

Doane, G. H., & Varcoe, C. (2008). Knowledge translation in everyday nursing: from evidence-based to inquiry-based practice. *ANS. Advances in Nursing Science, 31,* 283–295.

Dock, L. L. (1902). Sanitary inspection: a new field for nurses. *The American Journal of Nursing, 3,* 529–532.

Donahue, P. M. (2011). *Nursing, the finest art: an illustrated history* (3rd ed.). St. Louis, MO: Mosby-Year Book, Inc.

Dossey, B. M. (2009). *Florence Nightingale: mystic, visionary, healer.* Philadelphia, PA: F.A. Davis.

Drake, A. (1934). How the patient judges nursing. *The Trained Nurse and Hospital Review, 93,* 135–138.

Ehrenreich, B., & English, D. (1993). *Witches, midwives and nurses: a history of women healers.* New York, NY: The Feminist Press.

Ellis, R. (1968). Characteristics of significant theories. *Nursing Research, 17,* 217–222.

Evans, A. M., Pereira, D. A., & Parker, J. M. (2009). Discourses of anxiety and transference in nursing practice: the subject of knowledge. *Nursing Inquiry, 16,* 251–260. http://search.ebscohost.com/login.aspx?direct=true&db=rzh&AN=2010378116&site=ehost-live Publisher URL: www.cinahl.com/cgi-bin/refsvc?jid=912&accno=2010378116.

Faber, M. J. (1927). The education of the self. *The American Journal of Nursing, 27,* 1047–1050.

Falk-Rafael, A., & Bradley, P. A. (2014). "Towards justice in health": an exemplar of speaking truth to power. *ANS. Advances in Nursing Science, 37*(3), 224–234. https://doi.org/10.1097/ANS.0000000000000034.

Fawcett, J., & DeSanto-Madeya, S. (2012). *Contemporary nursing knowledge: analysis and evaluation of nursing models and theories.* Philadelphia, PA: F. A. Davis Company.

Fineout-Overholt, E., Melnyk, B. M., & Schultz, A. (2005). Transforming health care from the inside out: advancing evidence-based practice in the 21st century. *Journal of Professional Nursing: Official Journal of the American Association of Colleges of Nursing, 21*(6), 335–344. https://doi.org/10.1016/j.profnurs.2005.10.005.

Fitzpatrick, J. J., & Wallace, M. (2009). *The doctor of nursing practice and clinical nurse leader: essentials of program development and implementation for clinical practice.* New York, NY: Springer Publishing.

Folta, J. R. (1971). Obfuscation or clarification: a reaction to Walker's concept of nursing theory. *Nursing Research, 20,* 196–199.

Fontana, J. S. (2004). A methodology for critical science in nursing. *ANS. Advances in Nursing Science, 27,* 93–101.

Fox, N. J. (2003). Practice-based evidence: toward collaborative and transgressive research. *Sociology, 37,* 81–102.

Francis, B. (2000). Poststructuralism and nursing: uncomfortable bedfellows? *Nursing Inquiry, 7,* 20–28.

Fullbrook, P. (2003). Developing best practice in critical care nursing: knowledge, evidence and practice. *Nursing in Critical Care, 8,* 96–102.

Garesche, E. F. (1927). Professional honor. *The American Journal of Nursing, 27,* 901–904.

Goostray, S., & Brown, E. L. (1954). American nursing: history and interpretation. *The American Journal of Nursing, 54,* 719–721.

Gregg, A. (1940). An independent estimate of nursing in our times. *The American Journal of Nursing, 40,* 735–737.

Group, Thetis M., & Roberts, J. I. (2001). *Nursing, physician control and the medical monopoly.* Westport, CT: Praeger.

Hall, L. E. (1964). Nursing: what is it? *The Canadian Nurse, 60,* 150–154.

Hardy, M. E. (1978). Perspectives on nursing theory. *ANS. Advances in Nursing Science, 1,* 37–48.

Hartrick Doane, G., Reimer-Kirkham, S., Antifeau, E., & Stajduhar, K. (2015). (Re)theorizing integrated knowledge translation: a heuristic for knowledge-as-action. *ANS. Advances in Nursing Science, 38*(3), 175–186. https://doi.org/10.1097/ANS.0000000000000076.

Henderson, V. (1966). *The nature of nursing.* New York, NY: The Macmillan Co.

Henly, S. J. (2016). Three landmark symposia on theory development in nursing: celebrating the golden anniversary of publication of the Proceedings in Nursing Research. *Nursing Research, 65*(1), 1–2. https://doi.org/10.1097/NNR.0000000000000139.

Holmes, D., Perron, A., & O'Byrne, P. (2006). Evidence, virulence, and the disappearance of nursing knowledge: a critique of the evidence based dogma. *Worldviews on Evidence-Based Nursing / Sigma Theta Tau International, Honor Society of Nursing, 3,* 95–102.

Hughes, L. (1980). The public image of the nurse. *ANS. Advances in Nursing Science, 2,* 55–72.

Hughes, L. (1990). Professionalizing domesticity: a synthesis of selected nursing historiography. *ANS. Advances in Nursing Science, 12,* 25–31.

Im, E.-O., & Meleis, A. I. (1999). Situation-specific theories: philosophical roots, properties, and approach. *ANS. Advances in Nursing Science, 22,* 11–24.

Jarrín, O. F. (2012). The integrality of situated caring in nursing and the environment. *ANS. Advances in Nursing Science, 35,* 14–24.

Johnson, P. E. (1928). What should ethics teach? *The American Journal of Nursing, 28,* 1084–1090.

Kagan, P. N., Smith, M. C., & Chinn, P. L. (2014). Introduction. In P. N. Kagan, M. C. Smith, & P. L. Chinn (Eds.), *Philosophies and practices of emancipatory nursing: social justice as praxis.* New York, NY: Routledge Taylor & Francis Group.

Kalisch, B. J., & Kalisch, P. A. (2003). *American nursing: a history* (4th ed.). Philadelphia, PA: Lippincott, Williams & Wilkins.

Kangasniemi, M., Kallio, H., & Pietilä, A.-M. (2014). Towards environmentally responsible nursing: a critical interpretive synthesis. *Journal of Advanced Nursing, 70*(7), 1465–1478. https://doi.org/10.1111/jan.12347.

Kelly, L. Y., & Joel, L. A. (2001). *The nursing experience: trends, challenges and transitions* (4th ed.). New York, NY: McGraw-Hill.

Kelly, U. A. (2009). Integrating intersectionality and biomedicine in health disparities research. *ANS. Advances in Nursing Science, 32,* E42–E56.

Kelly, U. A. (2011). Theories of intimate partner violence: from blaming the victim to acting against injustice intersectionality as an analytic framework. *ANS. Advances in Nursing Science, 34,* E29–E51.

Kilpatrick, W. H. (1921). The basis of professional ethics in nursing. *The American Journal of Nursing, 22,* 790–798.

Kleffel, D. (1991). Rethinking the environment as a domain of nursing knowledge. *ANS. Advances in Nursing Science, 14,* 40–51.

Kramer, M. (2002). Academic talk about dementia caregiving: a critical comment on language. *Research and Theory for Nursing Practice, 16*(4), 262–280.

Kress, G., Leite-Garcia, R., & van Leeuwen, T. (1996). Discourse demiotic. In G. Kress, & T. van Leeuwen (Eds.), *Reading images: the grammar of visual design* (pp. 257–291). London: Routledge.

Leininger, M. M. (1976). Doctoral programs for nurses: trends, questions, and projected plans. *Nursing Research, 25*, 201–210.

Letourneau, N., & Allen, M. (1999). Post-positivistic critical multiplism: a beginning dialogue. *Journal of Advanced Nursing, 20*, 623–630.

Levine, M. E. (1967). The four conservation principles of nursing. *Nursing Forum, 6*, 93–98.

Levine, M. E. (1999). On the humanities in nursing. *The Canadian Journal of Nursing Research = Revue Canadienne de Recherche En Sciences Infirmieres, 30*, 213–217.

Lewenson, S. B., & Hermann, E. K. (2007). *Capturing nursing history*. New York, NY: Springer Publishing.

Lovell, M. C. (1980). The politics of medical deception: challenging the trajectory of history. *ANS. Advances in Nursing Science, 2*, 73–86.

Malka, S. G. (2007). *Daring to care: American nursing and second-wave feminism*. Chicago: University of Chicago Press.

Mason, D., Kennedy, M. S., Schorr, T., & Flanagan, A. (2006). The power of the written word: the influence of nursing journals. In L. C. Andrist, P. K. Nicholas, & K. Wolf (Eds.), *A history of nursing ideas* (pp. 333–356). Sudbury, MA: Jones & Bartlett.

Mazurek-Melnyk, B., Stone, P., Fincout-Overholt, E., & Ackerman, M. (2000). Evidence-based practice: the past, the present and recommendations for the millennium. *Pediatric Nursing, 26*, 77–80.

McClure, K. (1951). Ingredients of gracious nursing. *Nursing World, 125*, 221–224.

McDonald, L. (2012). Florence Nightingale and Mary Seacole: nursing's bitter rivalry. *History Today, 62*(9), 10–16.

Meade, A. B. (1936). Training the senses in clinical observation. *The Trained Nurse and Hospital Review, 97*, 540–544.

Mead, M. (1956). Nursing—primitive and civilized. *The American Journal of Nursing, 56*, 1001–1004.

Meleis, A. I. (1987). ReVisions in knowledge development: a passion for substance. *Scholarly Inquiry for Nursing Practice, 1*, 5–19.

Meleis, A. I. (2010). *Transitions theory: middle range and situation specific theories in nursing research and practice*. New York, NY: Springer Publishing Company.

Melnyk, B. M., & Fineout-Overholt, E. (2011). *Evidence-based practice in nursing & healthcare: a guide to best practice*. Philadelphia, PA: Wolters Kluwer/Lippincott Williams & Wilkins.

Melosh, B. (1982). *The physician's hand: work culture and conflict in American nursing*. Philadelphia, PA: Temple University Press.

Metalanguage. (1998). *Britannica Encyclopedia*. https://www.britannica.com/topic/metalanguage.

Moch, S. D., Williams, C., Schmitz, S., Slaughter, J., Anderson, S. L., … Brandt, J. (2008). EBP through student-staff collaboration. *Nursing Management, 39*, 12.

Mossman, L. C. (1923). The place of beauty in life. *The Trained Nurse and Hospital Review, 81*, 318–319.

Mountin, J. W. (1943). Nursing: a critical analysis. *The American Journal of Nursing, 43*, 29–34.

Mowinski-Jennings, B., & Loan, L. A. (2001). Misconceptions among nurses about evidence based practice. *Journal of Nursing Scholarship: An Official Publication of Sigma Theta Tau International Honor Society of Nursing / Sigma Theta Tau, 33*, 121–127.

Mundinger, M. O., Starck, P., Hathaway, D., Shaver, J., & Woods, N. F. (2009). The ABCs of the doctor of nursing practice: assessing resources, building a culture of clinical scholarship, curricular models. *Journal of Professional Nursing: Official Journal of the American Association of Colleges of Nursing, 25*, 69–74.

Newman, M. A. (1979). *Theory development in nursing*. Philadelphia, PA: F.A. Davis Co.

Newman, M. A. (1999). *Health as expanding consciousness* (2nd ed.). Sudbury, MA: Jones & Bartlett.

Newman, M. A., Sime, A. M., & Corcoran-Perry, S. A. (1991). The focus of the discipline of nursing. *ANS. Advances in Nursing Science, 14*, 1–6.

Nightingale, F. (1852/1979). *Cassandra: an angry outcry against the plight of Victorian women*. New York, NY: The Feminist Press.

Nightingale, F. (1860/1969). *Notes on nursing: what it is and what it is not*. New York, NY: Dover Publications, Inc.

Noble, G. E. (1940). The spirit of nursing. *The American Journal of Nursing, 40*, 161–162.

O'Connor, B. (2015). New white paper on the doctor of nursing practice: current issues and clarifying recommendations. *Journal of Professional Nursing: Official Journal of the American Association of Colleges of Nursing, 31*(5), 378. https://doi.org/10.1016/j.profnurs.2015.08.002.

Oettinger, K. B. (1939). Toward inner freedom. *The American Journal of Nursing, 39*, 1224–1229.

Pfefferkorn, F. (1933). What of nursing field studies? *The American Journal of Nursing, 33*, 258–261.

Phillips, B., Ball, C., Sackett, D., Badenoch, D., Straus, S., … Howick, J. (2009). *Oxford Centre for Evidence-based Medicine - Levels of Evidence (March 2009)*. http://www.cebm.net/index.aspx?o=1025.

Pitre, N. Y., Kushner, K. E., Raine, K. D., & Hegadoren, K. M. (2013). Critical feminist narrative inquiry: advancing knowledge through double-hermeneutic narrative analysis. *ANS. Advances in Nursing Science, 36*, 118–132.

Ploeg, J., Davies, B., Edwards, N., Gifford, W., & Miller, P. E. (2007). Factors influencing best-practice guideline implementation: lessons learned from administrators, nursing staff, and project leaders. *Worldviews on Evidence-Based Nursing / Sigma Theta Tau International, Honor Society of Nursing, 4*, 210–219.

Porter, E. K. (1953). What it means to be a nurse. *The American Journal of Nursing, 53*, 948–950.

Reverby, S. M. (1987a). A caring dilemma: womanhood and nursing in historical perspective. *Nursing Research, 35*, 5–11.

Reverby, S. M. (1987b). *Ordered to care: the dilemma of American nursing, 1850-1945*. Cambridge, MA: Cambridge University Press.

Richardson-Tench, M. (2012). Power, discourse, subjectivity: a Foucauldian application to operating room nursing practice. *ACORN: The Journal of Perioperative Nursing in Australia, 25*, 36–37.

Riddles, A. R. (1928). The force of example. *The Trained Nurse and Hospital Review, 80*, 27–30.

Roberts, J. I., & Group, Thetis M. (1995). *Feminism and nursing: an historical perspective on power, status, and political activism in the nursing profession*. Westport, CT: Praeger.

Roberts, S. J. (1983). Oppressed group behavior: implications for nursing. *ANS. Advances in Nursing Science, 5*, 21–30.

Rogers, M. E. (1970). *An introduction to the theoretical basis of nursing*. Philadelphia, PA: F.A. Davis Co.

Rolfe, G. (2006). Judgements without rules: towards a postmodern ironist concept of research validity. *Nursing Inquiry, 13*, 7–15.

Ryan, G., Berrebi, C., Beckett, M., Taylor, S., Quiter, E., … Kahn, K. (2011). *Reengineering the clinical research enterprise to involve more community clinicians*. https://www.ncbi.nlm.nih.gov/pmc/articles/PMC3082234/.

Salmond, S. W. (2013). Finding the evidence to support evidence-based practice. *Orthopaedic Nursing / National Association of Orthopaedic Nurses, 32*, 16–22; quiz 23–24 https://doi.org/10.1097/NOR.0b013e31827d960b.

Sanger, M. (1971). *Margaret Sanger, an autobiography*. New York, NY: Dover Publications.

Satterfield, J. M., Spring, B., Brownson, R. C., Mullen, E. J., Newhouse, R. P., … Whitlock, E. P. (2009). Toward a transdisciplinary model of evidence-based practice. *The Milbank Quarterly, 87*, 368–390.

Savage, J. (2000). One voice, different tunes: issues raised by dual analysis of a segment of qualitative data. *Journal of Advanced Nursing, 31*, 1493–1500.

Scheer, V. L., Stevens, P. E., & Mkandawire-Valhmu, L. (2016). Raising questions about capitalist globalization and universalizing views on women. *ANS. Advances in Nursing Science, 39*(2), 96–107. https://doi.org/10.1097/ans.0000000000000120.

Schunemann, H. J., Best, D., Vist, G., & Oxman, A. D. (2003). Letters, numbers, symbols and words: how to communicate grades of evidence and recommendations. *Canadian Medical Association Journal, 169*, 677–680.

Silverstein, N. G. (1985). Lillian Wald at Henry Street, 1893-1895. *ANS. Advances in Nursing Science, 7*, 1–12.

Simons, H., Kushner, S., Jones, K. D., & James, D. (2003). From evidence-based practice to practice-based evidence: the idea of situated generalization. *Research Papers in Education, 18*, 347–364.

Simpson, L. F. (1914). The psychology of nursing. *The Trained Nurse and Hospital Review, 52–53*, 133–137.

Staring-Derks, C., Staring, J., & Anionwu, E. N. (2015). Mary Seacole: global nurse extraordinaire. *Journal of Advanced Nursing, 71*(3), 514–525.

Staten, C. (n.d.). *Staupers, Mabel Keaton (1890-1989)*. http://www.blackpast.org/aah/staupers-mabel-keaton-1890-1989.

Stewart, I. M. (1921). Some fundamental principles in the teaching of ethics. *The American Journal of Nursing, 21*, 906–913.

Susie Walking Bear Yellowtail: "Our Bright Morning Star." (2014). http://montanawomenshistory.org/susie-walking-bear-yellowtail-our-bright-morning-star/.

Taylor, E. J. (1934). Of what is the nature of nursing? *The American Journal of Nursing, 34*, 473–476.

The essentials of doctoral education for advanced nursing practice. (2006). http://www.aacn.nche.edu/DNP/pdf/Essentials.pdf.

Thompson, J. L. (2007). Poststructuralist feminist analysis in nursing. In C. Roy, & D. A. Jones (Eds.), *Nursing knowledge development and clinical practice* (pp. 129–143). New York, NY: Springer Publishing.

Thoms, A. B. S. (1929). *Pathfinders, a history of the progress of colored graduate nurses.* New York, NY: Garland.

Thorne, S., & Sawatzky, R. (2014). Particularizing the general: sustaining theoretical integrity in the context of an evidence-based practice agenda. *ANS. Advances in Nursing Science, 37*, 1–10.

Tinley, S. T., & Kinney, A. Y. (2007). Three philosophical approaches to the study of spirituality. *ANS. Advances in Nursing Science, 30*, 71–80.

Titler, M. G. (2004). Methods in translation science. *Worldviews on Evidence-Based Nursing / Sigma Theta Tau International, Honor Society of Nursing, 1*, 38–48.

Tooley, S. A. (1905). *The life of Florence Nightingale.* New York, NY: The Macmillan Co.

van Dijk, T. A. (1997). The study of discourse. In T. A. Dijk (Ed.), *Discourse as structure and process: discourse studies: a multidisciplinary introduction* (Vol. 1) (pp. 1–34). London: Sage Publications.

Wald, L. (1971). *The house on Henry Street.* New York, NY: Dover Publications.

Walker, L. O. (1971). Toward a clearer understanding of the concept of nursing theory. *Nursing Research, 20*, 428–435.

Walker, L. O., & Avant, K. C. (2010). *Strategies for theory construction in nursing* (5th ed.). Norwalk, CT: Appleton & Lange.

Wallin, L. (2009). Knowledge translation and implementation research in nursing. *International Journal of Nursing Studies, 46*, 576–587.

Warnshius, F. C. (1926). The future of medicine and nursing: the ideal to be sought. *The American Journal of Nursing, 26*, 123–126.

Watson, J. (1979). *Nursing: the philosophy and science of caring.* Boston, MA: Little, Brown & Co.

Wheeler, C. E. (1985). The American Journal of Nursing and the socialization of a profession. *ANS. Advances in Nursing Science, 7*, 20–33.

Woodham-Smith, C. (1983). *Florence Nightingale: 1820-1910.* New York, NY: Atheneum.

Wooldridge, P. J. (1971). Meta-theories of nursing: a commentary on Dr. Walker's article. *Nursing Research, 20*, 494–495.

Worcester, A. (1902). Is nursing really a profession. *The American Journal of Nursing, 2*, 908–917.

Young, A. D. (1913). The nurse's duty to herself. *The Trained Nurse and Hospital Review, 51*, 265–270.

Emancipatory Knowledge Development

Why have women passion, intellect, moral activity—these three—and a place in society where no one of the three can be exercised?

Florence Nightingale (1852/1979, p. 25)

Specifically, there is a need to further explore the political, economic, and social forces in communities around the country that influenced the growth of both nursing and medicine during this century. The rigidities and inflexibilities of mythical conceptions about the roles of men and women in health care and the resulting responses of community members need examination also.

Jo Ann Ashley (1976, p. X)

After one has worked for a time in healing wounds which should never have been inflicted, tending ailments which should never have developed, sending patients to hospitals who need not have gone if their homes were habitable, bringing charitable aid to persons who would not have needed charity if health had not been ruined by unwholesome conditions, one loses heart and longs for preventive work, constructive work... something that will make it less easy for so many illnesses and accidents to occur; that will help to bring better homes and workshops, better conditions of life.

Lavinia L. Dock (1902, p. 531)

The women who wrote these opening quotes represent a long tradition of emancipatory knowing in nursing. Nightingale's quote makes explicit the challenges that women of her time faced if they wanted to step outside the role that Victorian society had prescribed for them. The Ashley quote highlights the importance of examining the social processes that formed nursing and how those processes contribute to nursing's ability to deliver health care. The quote by Dock goes deeper and suggests the need to shape social processes so that they eliminate social inequities in the first place, thereby making changes that would abolish the need for emancipatory knowing and knowledge.

Nightingale stressed the importance of being aware of inequities that are created by social conditions. Ashley suggested the need to critique, to imagine a different future, and to create formal expressions that can be shared. Dock highlighted a defining dimension of praxis by suggesting the need to bring about change that creates situations of empowerment and social equity. It is the Dock quote that addresses the core reason for developing emancipatory knowledge.

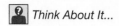 *Think About It...*

> Consider the issue of environmental pollution. To what forms of pollution does nursing contribute? To what form do you likely contribute? What options do individuals have to protect themselves, and should they pay the price for the health problems that result from exposure to pollution in the environment? Who do you think should be held accountable for the health problems that come from pollution? What is your view of nursing's duty to care for the environment?

This chapter describes the concept of emancipatory knowing and provides an overview of the foundations from which emancipatory knowing in nursing has developed. As represented in Fig. 3.1, the dimensions of emancipatory knowing surround and connect with the four fundamental patterns of knowing that are represented by the lighter center oval. In this way, emancipatory knowing places a critical lens on both nursing's knowledge development activities and the practice of nursing. The hazy indistinct outer circle that the double arrows extend beyond underscores the need for nursing to also have a critical lens that addresses the social and political contexts within which nursing functions.

This chapter includes examples of approaches that can be used to address the critical questions posed from an emancipatory perspective: "What are the barriers to freedom?" "What changes are needed?" "Who benefits?" and "What is wrong with this picture?" The creative processes of critiquing and imagining are further explained. Praxis—the process of critical reflection and action used to achieve emancipatory change—is positioned at the center of the model as well as at its outer edges. This signifies the need for an emancipatory knowing focus in the moment of practice as well as in relation to the social context in which the discipline is located.

Table 3.1 shows all of the processes related to emancipatory knowing. This chapter explains the first three rows—critical questions, creative processes, and formal expressions. The last two rows, which are shown in grey, are addressed in upcoming chapters: authentication processes in Chapter 9, and integrated expression in practice in Chapters 10 and 11.

THE CONCEPT OF EMANCIPATORY KNOWING

In 1995, Jill White (1995) proposed the addition of the knowing pattern "socio-political knowing." The concept of emancipatory knowing is related to the idea of sociopolitical knowing in that both concepts address working within a social and political system to make change (White, 2014). Both terms refer to making changes that improve patient care. We use the term *emancipatory knowing* in part because it points to the intent and hoped-for outcome of action, and because of the roots of the concept of emancipatory knowing in philosophy (Habermas, 1973, 1979).

Emancipatory knowing emphasizes action that arises from an awareness of social injustices embedded in a social and political system. Emancipatory knowing requires ongoing understanding of the network of social processes that create unjust conditions and changing them so that action to rectify injustices is no longer required. This goes

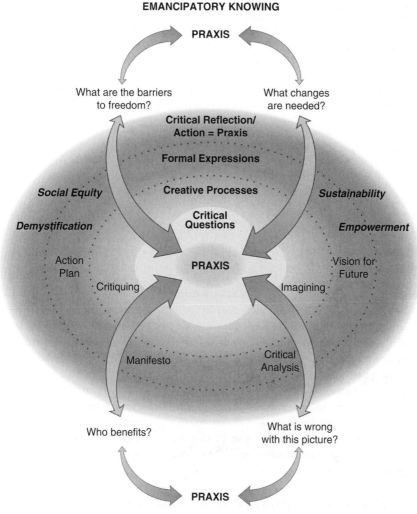

FIG. 3.1 Emancipatory Knowing.

beyond acting on recognized injustices and requires praxis—reflection and action in a continuous circle, where actions are constantly examined to ensure these are moving in the direction of social justice for all. A growing body of nursing literature affirms the essential nature of emancipatory knowing, and the vital insights that this perspective brings to all areas of nursing practice (Bickford, 2014; Butterfield, 2017; Chinn & Falk-Rafael, 2015; Kagan, Smith, & Chinn, 2014; Perry, 2015; Ray & Turkel, 2014; Scheer, Stevens, & Mkandawire-Valhmu, 2016; Thompson, 2014; Wåhlin, 2017; Walter, 2016).

Emancipatory knowing is the human ability to recognize social and political problems of injustice or inequity, to realize that things could be different, and to piece

TABLE 3.1 Dimensions of the Emancipatory Pattern of Knowing

Dimension	Emancipatory Pattern of Knowing
Critical questions	Who benefits?
	What is wrong with this picture?
	What are the barriers to freedom?
	What changes are needed?
Creative processes	Critiquing
	Imagining
Formal expressions	Action plans
	Manifestoes
	Critical analyses
	Visions for the future
Authentication processes	Social equity
	Sustainability
	Empowerment
	Demystification
Integrated expression in practice	Praxis

together complex elements of experience and context to change a situation as it is to a situation that improves people's lives. Emancipatory knowing cultivates awareness of how problematic conditions converge, reproduce, and remain in place to sustain a status quo that is unfair for some groups within society. Awareness of social injustices and inequities leads to processes that culminate in praxis, which is the integrated expression of emancipatory knowing.

Emancipatory knowing requires critical examination that aims to uncover why injustices seem to remain invisible and to identify specific social and structural changes that are required to right social and institutional wrongs. Emancipatory knowing seeks freedom from institutional and institutionalized social and political contexts that sustain injustices and that perpetuate advantages for some and disadvantages for others.

Emancipatory knowing in nursing means questioning the nature of knowledge and the ways in which knowledge itself—or what is taken to be knowledge—contributes to larger social problems. Emancipatory knowing takes into account the power dynamics that create knowledge as well as the social and political contexts that shape and influence knowledge and knowing. From an emancipatory perspective, knowledge and knowing are constructed in ways that reflect prevailing hegemony or problematic assumptions about "the way things are." *Hegemony* is the dominance of certain ideologies, beliefs, values, or views of the world over other possible viewpoints. These dominant perspectives privilege certain groups over others. Hegemonic views are often hidden and are taken for granted as "truth" or as the only possibility. Moreover, hegemony tends to recreate itself in ways that make it difficult to change.

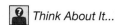 *Think About It...*

A dominant assumption or hegemonic view in nursing is that nurses practice as employees of an agency or a corporation rather than as independent practitioners. Institutionalized reimbursement practices of insurance companies and licensure laws are powerful sociopolitical structures that keep this view of how nurses can and should practice in place. Policies that govern how nurses are paid for their services make it difficult to secure reimbursement for independent nursing services. Even when reimbursement is possible, it is more difficult for nurses to receive reimbursement than it is for other health care workers, or they must be reimbursed indirectly. A few nurses have refused to accept the hegemonic assumption that they cannot or should not practice independently, and most nurses are aware that being self-employed or practicing independently is an option for others. However, the prevailing hegemonic view is that the norm is to be an employee and to work within the structures of an agency or corporation, and that it would not be feasible to practice any other way. What do you think?

Hegemonic ideologies and patterns of thinking tend to recreate themselves; in this way, they continue to seem natural and normal across time and generations. This perpetuation of hegemony happens in part when leaders and spokespersons in power speak and act in a way that is consistent with hegemony, thus reinforcing in public their ideas of how the world is and how it should function. This sort of public understanding becomes pervasive and effectively inhibits public awareness of other possibilities.

Without awareness of how things could be different, people conform to hegemonic practices and values. People are often not aware that they are trapped within a hegemonic pattern that creates disadvantages for them, and they remain unaware of alternatives. Alternatively, if they are aware, they may see the alternatives as not truly being possible.

Emancipatory knowing gives rise to the realization that there is something wrong with the way things are and that it is possible to change what is for the better. This awareness can arise when conditions become intolerable or when someone challenges or questions the hegemonic status quo. As people come to understand situations as being unjust, they can mobilize to challenge the way that things are. In so doing, these individuals exercise what may be considered *emancipatory human interest:* They clarify and define what is problematic about their situation from their point of view, and they take action to change it. They also begin to recognize that others share their experience of the situation. Together, they begin to develop actions, insights, and knowledge about the problem and about what is required to correct it or to change the situation for the better.

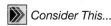 *Consider This...*

The emergence of the women's movement during the latter half of the 20th century is an example of an emancipatory process. Through the mid-1900s, the hegemonic view of women was of the ideal wife and mother who remained a subservient homemaker devoted to her family. These views of womanhood were reflected in the media, government policies, business practices, religious beliefs, and virtually every aspect of public life, as can be seen by browsing through magazines and professional journals of that time, or watching television shows aired in the 1950s and 1960s.

As women realized that this hegemonic construct of women dominated their experience, small groups of women in the United States and other countries began to examine the circumstances of their lives in consciousness-raising groups—a type of grassroots movement. Women shared experiences and feelings about their lives and formed ideas about how their lives could and should be. Many of their ideas became formalized as feminist theory. Those who spoke publicly were often derided by men and women who felt threatened by the sociocultural changes that were suggested. However, despite widespread resistance, feminist ideas began to make sense to more and more people, and many significant social and cultural changes were initiated.

One of the first changes that feminist leaders called for was a shift to gender-neutral language, and widespread changes began to occur. For example, newspapers stopped publishing their classified ads in separate "Help Wanted—Male" and "Help Wanted—Female" columns; these ads were changed to fall under a heading that simply read "Help Wanted." In this example, emancipatory knowing for women involved their shared awareness of the distress that they experienced with the restrictions that hegemonic ideals of womanhood imposed on their lives. As the outcomes of their shared awareness evolved, emancipatory knowing grew as others began to hear about and comprehend the alternatives that feminist perspectives offered.

Emancipatory Knowing and Problem Solving

Emancipatory knowing is different from but related to problem solving. It is much more than problem solving, however, because emancipatory knowing requires a deep awareness of often hidden injustices and the problematic social practices that create them. Unlike problem solving, which usually focuses on a single discrete case, emancipatory knowing requires seeing the larger picture and correcting social processes, patterns, and structures that create social inequities and injustices.

Before the social changes arising from the women's movement in Western societies, some women who wanted to perform a "man's job," such as medicine or the operation of heavy machinery, solved the problem by dressing and posing as a man. These women may have been aware that the policies and practices of their culture were unjust. Despite potential awareness of the unfairness of the practice, rather than pursuing a critical or emancipatory approach to changing societal rules and policies, they simply solved the problem by accommodating for a fundamentally unfair practice. In this example, accommodating rather than changing can be seen as a discrete, individual, and temporary solution rather than a long-term one. Asking the critical questions associated with emancipatory knowing, when you meet challenges that require this form of problem solving, is one way to initiate the corrective processes of emancipatory knowing.

Emancipatory Knowing and Critical Thinking

Emancipatory knowing differs from critical thinking in that it does not simply seek to improve one's analytic thinking ability, judgment, and problem-solving skills. Once again, the emphasis is on seeing what lies beneath issues and problems and redefining those issues and problems to reveal linkages among complex social and political contexts that create injustices. For example, a critical-thinking approach to hiring practices that are based on gender would focus on gathering the evidence and examining the rationale for restricting hiring in some jobs to women only and in others to men only. The soundness and logic of each explanation for the practice would be examined, and conclusions would be drawn about the practice. Critical-thinking approaches could reveal injustices and inequities and might result in an attempt to reduce gender-specific hiring. However, critical thinking alone would not fully examine the underlying network of social practices that keep the injustice of gender-specific hiring in place or challenge the status quo in a way that would demand long-term change.

Emancipatory Knowing and Reflective Practice

Emancipatory knowing is akin to reflective practice in that emancipatory knowing involves a constant interaction between action and reflection. This process is praxis: the integrated expression of emancipatory knowing, described in more detail later in this chapter. *Reflective practice* is a significant personal process that leads to insight about one's actions and the rationales for actions that have the potential to improve one's practice. Unlike reflective practice, however, praxis requires going beyond personal reflection to uncover deliberately what is unfair and unjust in a situation, to envision how it could be different, and to form alternate explanations and possibilities for change that come from a range of perspectives much broader than that of the individual alone (Schön, 1983).

> ### ! *Why Is This Important?*
>
> It is easy to focus on individual situations and overlook the bigger picture. The fundamental social structures that limit individuals are unevenly distributed, so that some people have advantages in overcoming individual limitations, and others do not. As an example, consider the fact that despite many changes that have opened possibilities for women in the workforce, not all women are able to pursue the options they might choose. And in addition, some women find great satisfaction and personal joy in the traditional roles of mothers and homemakers. From a reflective practice perspective, they might recognize that their experience fits a hegemonic view of ideal womanhood that could be restrictive in certain ways, but their personal experience is satisfying and rewarding, and financially feasible, and therefore requires no change. However, for many other women, this is not an option financially, and some would prefer to pursue other paths either instead of, or in addition to, the traditional roles in the home.
>
> The emancipatory knowing process of praxis would call for looking beyond personal experience alone to reflect on the broader sociocultural implications of such role prescriptions. It requires a deep sort of awareness that is not easy to cultivate, and to comprehend the circumstances that are not like your own. It also calls for considering the political, social, and economic dimensions of a situation. The personal satisfactions and rewards of homemaking for some women are not negated, but the focus shifts to broader issues and to the outcomes for women and society in general when homemaking and motherhood are prescribed as being primarily women's roles, and noticing how and why others in similar situations experience their options differently.

Emancipatory knowing does not allow us to undo hegemonic social structures by just thinking critically about injustices, solving individual or discrete problems, or reflecting on unfair social conditions. Rather, it asks, "Why do we have this problem in the first place?" For example, when approaching the situation from an emancipatory perspective, you ask, "How can we create opportunities for women in the workplace?"; you also ask, "Why are women excluded from full access to employment in the first place?" As a nurse, you ask, "How can we overcome the stigma of human immunodeficiency virus/acquired immunodeficiency syndrome?"; you also ask, "Why is this condition stigmatized in the first place?" You ask, "How do we create tolerance for transgendered persons?"; you also ask, "Why does intolerance persist?" You wonder, "How can we end the unfair policy of mandatory overtime for nurses?"; you also consider, "Why has this practice emerged, and who benefits from this policy?" As we have said many times, after these questions are asked, emancipatory knowing demands that an individual work toward the elimination of these situations.

THE REBIRTH OF EMANCIPATORY KNOWING IN NURSING

A long history of nurse activists have worked to change desperate social conditions in an effort to improve health. However, with the focus on scientific inquiry that took hold during the 1950s, an appreciation for other forms of knowing and inquiry was temporarily lost. During the 1960s and 1970s, when different forms of scholarship became more legitimate, critical perspectives began to emerge. Much of this early critical scholarship was grounded in the work of prominent critical, liberation, and poststructuralist thinkers.

Critical Theory

In the discipline of nursing, the term *critical theory* refers to a foundational perspective that grounds emancipatory knowing. This term can be confusing in that it does not reflect the usual connotation of theory in nursing. The concept of *critical* has a range of common meanings that are not relevant in the context of critical theory. In this context, *critical* implies analysis that moves beyond the surface and beyond what is usually assumed. Generally, *critical theory* is a broad term that is used to describe both the process and the product of work that takes a historically situated and sociopolitical perspective and that challenges social inequities and injustices. Such theory is critical in the sense that it analyzes the roots and consequences of social inequities and injustices that privilege one group over another (Carnegie & Kiger, 2009).

As a method, critical theory has roots in the classic sociologic traditions of Karl Marx, Max Weber, and Emile Durkheim (Morrow, 1994). These early philosophic traditions were quite unfavorable to capitalist governments such as that of the United States and were viewed in the United States as being allied with communist ideology. The extreme anticommunist sentiments that prevailed in the United States during the 20th century made it difficult for U.S. scholars to engage in discourse surrounding the emergence of critical theory and philosophy. Scholars in countries that have strong social welfare policies and values have generally been more open and accepting of critical theory. As the political structures of the world began to change and the 40-year Cold War that began in the late 1940s abated, U.S. scholars gradually became more open to critical theory. This circumstance illustrates the tremendous influence of context on people's thinking in that fears of communism created barriers to understanding critical theory and suppressed openness to the possibilities offered by critical theoretic approaches.

Critical theory began to emerge as a specific approach to the study of society through the work of scholars who were exiled from Germany by Adolf Hitler in 1932. These scholars became known as the "Frankfurt School." Within the Frankfurt School, the term *critical theory* designated a form of sociologic theory that recognized society as evolving historically and that promoted a deliberate engagement with the problems of society and the processes of social transformation. Typically (but not always), when the term *critical theory* is capitalized, it refers specifically to the work of the Frankfurt School (Morrow, 1994). We use the lowercase format throughout our discussion to indicate a perspective that encompasses a broad range of philosophies, methods, and approaches that share a common fundamental engagement with the problems of society.

During the 1960s, Jürgen Habermas assumed a prominent position in shaping new conceptions of critical theory with broad interdisciplinary connections between the human sciences and philosophy (Morrow, 1994). In his critical social theory, Habermas (1973, 1979) posited three fundamental human interests, each of which demanded its own method, as follows:

1. *Technical interest* is the human capacity to create things and processes to understand the physical world; this requires empiric methods.
2. *Practical interest* is the human capacity to communicate and to get along within a social community; this requires interpretive and philosophic methods.
3. *Emancipatory interest* is the human capacity to see that something needs to change and to take action to change it; this requires critical and reflective methods.

Each of these interests is necessary for human survival. Although critical nurse scholars have grounded their thinking in the work of a number of critical scholars and philosophers, the influence of Habermas is significant.

Liberation Theory

Paulo Freire was an important liberation theorist whose ideas have also had a significant influence among nursing scholars. Freire was a Brazilian educator who championed critical approaches to education. His work was philosophically grounded in the ideas of Karl Marx, Friedrich Engels, Georg Hegel, Gyorgy Lukacs, Herbert Marcuse, and Erich Fromm (Freire, 1970). Freire's work grew out of a project to teach peasants in rural Brazil how to read. His ideas were not only specific approaches to teaching, but they could also be used for any grassroots project of human liberation. Traditional education is based on the assumption that its primary purpose is to pass along the existing knowledge and values of the culture. Freire questioned this assumption, and in doing so, he formalized *liberation theory*, which considered education as a means of challenging the existing knowledge and values of the culture (Freire, 1970; Hooks, 1993; Weiler, 1991). Because of the broad significance of his philosophy and the practical action-oriented perspective that he articulated, Freire's ideas have had a widespread influence that has gone well beyond the scope of education.

Poststructuralism

Michel Foucault's poststructuralist philosophy has also had a major influence on nurse scholars because of his insights with regard to the power imbalances that are embedded in and sustained by verbal and symbolic social discourses. *Social discourses* are whole systems of representation—writing, images, advertisements, artwork, and everyday verbal and nonverbal language—that create perceptions of social reality. For critical poststructuralists, there is no reality in an objective sense. Rather, what seems real is created for us by dominant social discourses. Verbal and symbolic discourses are powerful because they interconnect to both enable and limit what it is socially acceptable to know (Aston, 2008; Bradbury-Jones, Sambrook, & Irvine, 2008).

 Consider This...

> Discourses of beauty for young white women suggest that a flawless face is more beautiful than a normally flawed and plainer face. Discourses also reinforce the idea that beauty of a certain type—that which is achieved by cosmetics and airbrushing—is attainable and a normal way to be. Because these messages appear everywhere, young women may only understand "beauty" as what is constructed and prescribed by these systems of discourse. Such discourses are powerful because they create barriers to societal resources for some as well as opportunities for others. Young women who cannot or choose not to achieve the popular standard of beauty may develop low self-esteem, and they risk being denied social resources, such as popularity among peers and the social interactions for which most young people yearn.
>
> This same example could be applied to young Caucasian men, for whom popular discourses prescribe what is considered a typical movie-star appearance (being handsome, having well-defined muscles, and wearing well-fashioned clothing) as opposed to that which is considered "geeky" or "nerdy" (being thin, wearing glasses, and having casual, disheveled, or mismatched clothing). It is in this way that discourses construct "realities" that create power imbalances (in our example, between young women and men who are "beautiful" or "handsome" and those who are not). As alternative discourses that counter notions of beauty begin to undermine dominant discourses, they begin to lose their power to control how young people spend their money and time (Phillips, 2006).

As a poststructuralist, Foucault viewed language and discourse, including theory, as systems of representation that are necessary in the social order in that they produce meaning or ways to comprehend the world. However, as the examples of discourses related to beauty illustrate, these systems of language and discourse also limit what is understood, known, or perceived in a way that has lasting negative consequences. According to Foucault, we can only know things as they have meaning, and it is systems of discourse that produce or construct meaning (Hall, 2001). Critical poststructuralism analyzes how discourse functions to create imbalances that disadvantage whole classes of persons, in an effort to illuminate possibilities for change (Doering, 1992; Foucault, 1980, 1984).

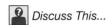 *Discuss This...*

> Read the Nursing Manifesto at http://www.nursemanifest.com/manifesto.htm. Discuss with a group of your peers ways in which critical theory, liberation theory, and post-structuralism are reflected in this document.

NURSING LITERATURE RELATED TO EMANCIPATORY KNOWING

During the latter half of the 20th century, a growing number of nurse scholars and activists began to develop disciplinary perspectives that are clearly connected to an emancipatory pattern of knowing. During the 1960s, Lydia Hall, who declared that there is no "shortage of nurses" but rather a "shortage of nursing," established the Loeb Center for Nursing and Rehabilitation at Montefiore Hospital in the Bronx, New York. Her ideas and what proceeded from them are notable examples of emancipatory knowing in nursing. Believing that nursing was the chief therapy for those recovering from chronic illness, Hall established the Loeb Center as a place where nursing (rather than medicine) could be practiced and where physicians were under the direction of nurses (Hall, 1966). Hall envisioned the Loeb Center when she noticed that nurses were taking on medical tasks and becoming what she called "physician extenders" rather than providing bodily care and nurturing the cores of individuals after medicine's curative role. Hall's model of nursing at Loeb was revolutionary because it differentiated nursing from medicine and allowed nurses to practice in an environment that did not require the performance of curative tasks associated with the growth of medical technology during the 1960s.

Early literature in nursing that reflected emancipatory knowing also grew out of feminist perspectives. As reluctant as nurses were in general to accept feminist ideas and to align themselves with the women's movement of the 1960s and 1970s in the United States, some spoke out and published ideas that challenged the status quo. One of the earliest writings that reflected an emancipatory perspective was a 1973 article in the *American Journal of Nursing* by Wilma Scott Heide (1973), who made a case for the importance of feminist ideas for nursing. In *Hospitals, Paternalism, and the Role of the Nurse,* basing her argument on historical evidence, JoAnn Ashley (1976) contended that the prevailing apprenticeship system of education in nursing situated nurses and nursing in a context that not only exploited the labor of women in hospitals, but also undermined the fundamental values of nursing related to health and health care. Her feminist analysis drew the essential connection between a misogynist (woman-hating) society and the resulting health policies and practices that constricted the role of nurses in the delivery of health care (Kagan, 2006).

Another significant publication that reflected nursing's development of emancipatory perspectives was the 1983 article "Oppressed Group Behavior: implications for Nursing" (Roberts, 1983). Drawing on Freire's work and from literature about colonized Africans, Latin Americans, African Americans, Jews, and women, Susan Jo Roberts made the case that nurses also can be viewed as an oppressed group. Emphasizing that this insight can lead to substantive action to change nursing and health care, she concluded the following:

> Nurses are an oppressed group with characteristics similar to those of [other oppressed] groups. It is hoped that with this understanding nurses can learn from the experience

of others to liberate themselves and develop an autonomous profession that can greatly contribute to the improvement of healthcare (p. 30).

Cassandra: Radical Feminist Nurses Network was founded by a group of nurses at the American Nurses Association convention in Washington, D.C., on June 30, 1982, which was the expiration date for the ratification of the Equal Rights Amendment to the U.S. Constitution. The Cassandra founders were astonished to see no acknowledgment at the convention of the political significance of the date and the major events being held throughout the District of Columbia to commemorate the death of the amendment (Chinn, 2009).

The women who formed Cassandra divided their time between various convention activities and events throughout the city to celebrate a renewal of their commitment to continue the struggle for women's full equality in U.S. society. Cassandra was formed to bring critical and feminist insights to the forefront in nursing and to use critical feminist insights as a basis for change in nursing. They named themselves after Florence Nightingale's essay titled "Cassandra," in which she asked the question that opens this chapter. The network's news journal was published until 1989, and although not widely distributed, it provided a significant source of affirmation for many practicing nurses and nurse scholars who were beginning to develop an emancipatory perspective (Chinn, 2009).

By the close of the 1980s and the beginning of the 1990s, nursing literature was beginning to reflect the strong presence of works informed by emancipatory perspectives, including critical, feminist, and poststructuralist theory (Bunting & Campbell, 1990; Campbell & Bunting, 1991; Doering, 1992; Muller & Dzurec, 1993). These early writings remain important foundations for nursing's emancipatory scholarship. These authors explained the particular critical perspectives from which they drew, and they offered critiques of nursing and nursing knowledge in addition to proposals for shifts in nursing practice and education, health care, and society that could address persistent and seemingly intractable problems in nursing.

By the mid-1990s, emancipatory perspectives appeared more frequently in nursing literature. Although remaining on the margins of dominant scholarly discourses in nursing, these perspectives gradually gained depth and quality that were increasingly recognized as noteworthy. These writings describe the nature of problems identified from an emancipatory perspective and the types of actions required to create the envisioned change. Between 1990 and 1992, a group of Canadian nurses, organized as Nurses for Social Responsibility (NSR), published the magazine *Towards Justice in Health*. Falk-Rafael and Bradley (2014) provided a critical textual analysis of the Canadian nurses' work—writings and activism that revealed an alternative and courageous voice on the political nature of health and health care, and how care was influenced by the political context of the early 1990s.

These scholarly writings challenge prevailing hegemonies and identify critical problems that typically are taken as simply "the way that the world is." These authors describe how the problems that they addressed came to be, who is advantaged and who is disadvantaged by the status quo, and how social practices intersect to keep the status quo in place; they also envision changes and the actions required to make such changes to the status quo (Falk-Rafael, 2006; MacDonnell, 2009; Messias, McDowell, & Estrada, 2009; Racine, 2009). At present, there is a strong tradition of critical analysis in nursing, as well as a conceptualization of emancipatory nursing practice that is grounded in emancipatory knowing (Bickford, 2014; Butterfield, 2017; Chinn & Falk-Rafael, 2015; Kagan et al., 2014; Perry, 2015; Ray & Turkel, 2014; Scheer et al., 2016; Thompson, 2014; Wåhlin, 2017; Walter, 2016). There is also growing evidence of nursing education initiatives that address social justice and emancipatory knowing (Snyder, 2014; Vickers, 2008; Watson & Hills, 2011).

THE DIMENSIONS OF EMANCIPATORY KNOWING

The dimensions of emancipatory knowing include critical questions; creative processes of critiquing and imagining; formal expressions; authentication processes; and the integrated practice expression of emancipatory knowing, which is praxis.

CRITICAL QUESTIONS: WHO BENEFITS? WHAT IS WRONG WITH THIS PICTURE?

The creative processes for developing emancipatory knowledge grow from the critical questions of emancipatory knowing shown in Fig. 3.1. These questions can be asked in a variety of contexts and situations, including the context of care. The questions on the model are suggestions, but any question that focuses on bringing social injustices into awareness is also a critical question. For example, critical questions can inquire about barriers to freedom, about why certain information remains invisible or hidden, or about why some people enjoy freedoms that others do not.

> **!** *Why Is This Important?*
>
> When nurses question why something seems unfair, they are operating under the assumption that all persons deserve the freedom and opportunity to develop their full potential. Such questions assume that developing and exercising one's potential is not solely a matter of individual will or desire, but that culture and society create conditions and structures within which people can thrive or fail to thrive.

When you ask the critical questions associated with emancipatory knowing, an underlying assumption is that people are not radically free to choose from among an unlimited variety of options, and that things need to change to make new options accessible to everyone. To assume that people are radically free places the responsibility for developing one's full potential totally with the individual. Critical questioning assumes that freedoms are situated, which means that the possibilities for freedom and the development of individual potential are determined by a person's situation. In other words, from a critical perspective, a person's situation is assumed to be constructed by social practices that create disadvantage for some and privilege for others. From an emancipatory perspective, any conditions that limit people from developing their full human potential can be made visible, what is imagined can become real, and humans have the innate capacity to bring about changes to improve the human condition. Asking a critical question such as "What is wrong with this picture?" requires a lens that sees beyond the obvious and beyond one's own personal experience. This makes it possible to discern problems that may exist with what people assume to be true.

Recognizing injustices and inequities can create major personal and professional dilemmas. Most people are socialized to accept an unfair status quo as the way things are (hegemony) and not to question the uncomfortable fact that some people are privileged and others are disadvantaged. To bring this kind of awareness to the surface and to act on it requires great courage, persistence, and the support of colleagues and allies who remain committed to action (Falk-Rafael & Bradley, 2014; Georges, 2013; Giddings, 2005a, 2005b). Taking action often disturbs the status quo in ways that are not only uncomfortable but also prompt harsh and swift action to keep prevailing hegemonies in place. Nonetheless, critically questioning the status quo is an initial and critical feature of emancipatory knowing that sets the stage for praxis.

 Think About It...

> Consider a nursing situation that you observed and believed to be unfair or wrong and then ask, "Who benefits from this situation?" Does your idea about how to change the situation change when you explore the answer to this question?

CREATIVE PROCESSES: CRITIQUING AND IMAGINING

The creative processes of emancipatory knowing are critiquing and imagining. Again, these dimensions of emancipatory knowing require an awareness that something is not fair or just. These two creative processes tend to happen in a circular fashion; as you realize that something is not right and needs to change, this realization brings to mind things that are wrong (critique) and how things should really be instead (imagining).

Critiquing involves analyzing the status quo from multiple points of view. For example, you deliberately examine a situation from the point of view of race, ethnicity, sexual orientation, class, gender, or any other factor that shapes human possibilities and creates inequities. The more comprehensive the critique, the more likely it is that the choices selected for action will be effective.

Imagining is the creative process that sets forth possibilities of how the world could be better, more equitable, and just. As with critiquing, the process of imagining benefits from a thorough examination of injustices from a variety of perspectives. We use the word *imagining* to describe a process of imaging and seeing possibilities and not to refer to simply dreaming about or making up scenarios without critique and examination. These dimensions of emancipatory knowing are carried out through dialogue and information sharing that lead to formal knowledge expressions of emancipatory knowing and praxis.

Within the context of emancipatory knowing, critiquing and imagining are *activist* in nature and grounded in the situation of those who experience a particular injustice.

Someone else cannot impose emancipatory processes on people who seek or need liberation. *Emancipation,* or liberation from a situation that limits one's humanity, depends on the insights, understandings, and interpretations of those who are most deeply affected, those who are disadvantaged, and those who are oppressed. Those who are disadvantaged by a situation must take steps to change the situation. Others who sense that the situation is unjust can assist and encourage those who come together to share their stories and to engage in processes of critiquing and imagining, but they cannot direct the course of action or do what needs to be done other than in a supportive way. Those most directly affected by an unjust situation are sometimes referred to as "those who are oppressed"; we refer to them simply as "people seeking liberation." Those who join with the people seeking liberation to develop insight and knowledge and ultimately to support action for change are the allies of these individuals.

Activist projects bring together those who are most directly affected by injustices and their allies so that they can discuss, identify, and define what is problematic; imagine ways to create sustainable change; and plan ways to bring about the changes that they imagine. Because the conditions of people's lives are often taken for granted as the way things are (hegemony) or assumed to be unique to the individual, the processes of critiquing and imagining occur in group settings, where individuals share with one another the conditions of their lives and come to realize that they are not alone and that their situations limit their humanity.

As mentioned previously, the people seeking liberation are the experts regarding how their particular injustice is experienced. Allies often bring skills and insights about the situation that can inform the process, but they remain fully respectful of the perspectives of the people seeking liberation. Allies can be powerful agents of change by bearing witness to the situation of those who are disadvantaged. Those who participate in the process of change may not totally fit within the roles of "people seeking liberation" or "allies." Allies often have some connection to the experience of the people seeking liberation, whereas the people seeking liberation often bring insights, understandings, and ideas that come from experiences outside the realm of the oppressive situation.

The creative processes of imagining and critiquing can occur in a variety of in-person and virtual group settings. The Nurse Manifest project involved both in-person and virtual groups; nurses shared their stories by email "to raise awareness, to inspire action, and to open discussion of issues that are vital to nursing and health care around the globe" (Jarrin, 2006; "NurseManifest Project," 2002) and also met in face-to-face groups (Jacobs, Fontana, Kehoe, Matarese, & Chinn, 2005). In the Nurse Manifest project, the people seeking liberation were the nurses actively engaged in direct patient care and employed in these roles. Some of the practicing nurses had been educators in the past and had returned to clinical practice. The allies in this project were nurse educators who had not been involved in clinical nursing for several years but who knew the experience well and who engaged with the clinical nurses to explore the experience of practicing nursing.

To be effective, the group process must provide a safe context that encourages people to discuss openly the circumstances of inequity or suffering in their lives and to talk about what would make their lives better. Members of the group share a mutual interest in changing a problematic status quo and use discussion to raise awareness of the conditions that sustain that status quo. As sharing and awareness occur, the group collectively criticizes that which limits full human potential and identifies what needs to change to create a more nurturing future.

The group process that is basic to emancipatory knowing is grounded in Freire's approach (1970), and the specifics described here were developed by Chinn (2013, 2016; 2013). These approaches to the group process are suggested as a way to assist activist groups to move effectively into the creative processes of critiquing and imagining. Groups of people seeking liberation may or may not include allies. When a group comes together out of a shared awareness that something is awry, its members are typically unclear about exactly what is wrong. They may have wrongly blamed themselves for the problem, or they may have attributed the problem to some condition that, with critique, turns out to not have contributed to the problem in a significant way. Initially, group members may not be aware that others share similar experiences. As the group process proceeds, everyone respectfully listens to each other's stories, asks questions of one another, and suggests possible reasons for their condition. This discussion creates a "background awareness" of the complexities of the situation and the differences and similarities among the members' various perspectives. It also often brings to the fore some of the most creative (and sometimes outrageous) imaginings for change that might be made.

This process begins with examining and discussing *codifications* (i.e., pictures, stories, and images) that represent what the people are experiencing. Codifications help to make visible and to bring to awareness what is problematic in a situation when it is not readily apparent. This awareness leads the group to consider possible circumstances that create and sustain the situation as it is. Through discussion in which every voice is heard, the group members come to clarify and identify in new ways what is wrong with their situation (problematization), and they begin to imagine what might occur instead. The members also begin to imagine how they might bring about various possible alternatives, discussing the merits and limitations of each action that might bring about change.

Various actions for change that are identified are seen as "untested feasibilities." Each action is "tested" by exploring its merits and limitations for action that brings about change. This emergent pattern is not orchestrated or in any way controlled or directed by any one member of the group. Rather, it is a process that emerges spontaneously in the group and emanates from the human emancipatory interest (Habermas, 1979; Hagedorn, 1995). When leadership is needed, it arises from individuals in the group who are able and willing to assume leadership for the task at hand, not from socially prescribed roles that privilege some individuals over others.

Typically, group participants come together several times over weeks or months. Because the issue of concern in groups that involve people seeking liberation is an oppressive social process and not a particular individual's experience, anyone who has experience with the oppressive social process can contribute to critiquing and imagining. Individuals may or may not attend every meeting, and new members can join the group at any time. Continuity is maintained by summarizing the critiques and imaginings that involve the oppressive social process at the end of each group meeting, and then bringing that summary forward at the beginning of the next meeting. In the case of virtual groups, the group process outcome related to critiquing and imagining is archived electronically, which gives everyone access to all contributions of all participants. All participants involved with in-person groups can make notations and personal journal entries to retain ideas and insights during the discussion and to provide a point of reference for reflection between group meetings. The process of critiquing and imagining is circular rather than linear, which means that, regardless of who is present, a constant process of reflection, reconsidering, and rethinking ideas is valued, with new critiques and imaginings coming from each circular "turn" made in the process of discussion and analysis.

As discussion progresses, participants begin to explore dominant themes that characterize the focal problem as well as the links between themes. These individuals begin to situate the themes in their historical, cultural, political, and socioeconomic contexts. From these themes, the participants also explore the circumstances that maintain the status quo: the existence of persons or circumstances that directly or indirectly benefit from the status quo and of persons or circumstances that are negated and disadvantaged by the status quo.

It is from these explorations that praxis—the integrated expression of emancipatory knowing in practice—begins to happen. Early actions are often changes that people seeking liberation begin to make in their own lives, followed by collective actions that the group pursues as a group or as individuals. Freire called this process in its entirety *conscientização,* a Portuguese term that "refers to learning to perceive social, political, and economic contradictions, and to take action against the oppressive element of reality" (1970, p. 19). Activist projects may or may not generate formal expressions of knowledge because of the primary commitment to act and to move emancipatory insights directly into actions that remove barriers to human freedom. However, formal expressions of emancipatory knowing may be formulated from the critique and imagining process, as described later.

Creative Processes and the Fundamental Patterns of Knowing

Although activist groups and their allies may have no knowledge of the fundamental knowing patterns, the creative processes of imagining and critiquing often overlap with processes within the empiric, ethical, personal, and aesthetic knowing patterns. For example, empiric methods can be used to document the extent of a problem or the nature of a structure that sustains the status quo, thereby forming a more thorough understanding of the problem. In this way, empirically based information provides data and substance that are useful for more fully critiquing and imagining possibilities for change.

For example, in a critical study seeking to understand girls' experience of menarche and create change toward a more healthy experience, a group of adolescent activists used a survey method to determine what menarche education approaches were being used in schools throughout a certain school district. The researchers also examined corporate reports to uncover the extent of profit being made by menstrual care product manufacturers who also produced the educational materials used in the schools. The participants used this information to affirm what they had suspected: that menarche education was not adequate to meet the girls' real needs but rather served the interests of powerful corporate entities. In this study, the context was a high school setting in which adolescent girls came together to explore their experiences of menarche and the meaning of those experiences, as constructed by larger sociopolitical circumstances. The study also relied on an academic ally who guided and supported their activism and published the adolescents' insights and knowledge, thereby moving it into the dimension of formal expression, where it became available to a larger professional audience (Hagedorn, 1995).

INTEGRATING CREATIVE PROCESSES AND THE FUNDAMENTAL PATTERNS OF KNOWING

The creative processes of ethical knowledge—valuing and clarifying—can be used to better understand the nature of injustices (see Chapter 4). The manifesto of the Nurse Manifest project was developed primarily from the extensive values of clarification, dialogue, and justification (Cowling, Chinn, & Hagedorn, 2009; Kagan, Smith, Cowling, & Chinn, 2009). As the members of this group critically questioned why nurses experienced so much moral distress, their discussions focused on critique that further raised awareness of a deep conflict between the values strongly held by nurses and the values enacted by the systems in which they are employed. This underlying conflict of values was identified as the problem that was fundamental to the shortage of nursing. The manifesto project led the authors to imagine ways in which nursing values could be more fully realized—or manifested—in the practice of nursing. This project began with a focused critique of the ethical dimensions of nursing's core values and the exercise of those values in practice. Subsequently, other nurses joined the project, which resulted in a more complete critique of the experiences of practicing nursing in the context of an acute nursing shortage as well as a richer set of imaginings of a desired future.

The personal knowing processes of opening and centering are vital to the emancipatory knowing dimension of critiquing and imagining (see Chapter 5). These creative processes bring to the fore the experiences of those who are most deeply affected by injustices and provide the substance required to critique the problem and imagine alternatives. For example, in a critical feminist study of the experience of nursing practice, nurses brought to their first group meeting an object or symbol (i.e., a codification) that represented their personal experience of practicing nursing. They shared the personal meanings embedded in these symbolic objects and discussed the connections that their personal experiences revealed. A food strainer brought to the group by a participant represented her feelings of a loss of control of nursing practice, which was a feeling that other nurses in the group also shared. As these nurses shared their feelings about losing control, they came to realize that this problem was not a personal failure but rather a significant injustice that came from systematic structural problems in the ways that nursing was institutionalized and practiced. Out of their sharing and critique, these nurses imagined how personal growth toward authenticity and their collective actions could change the circumstances of practicing nursing (Jacobs et al., 2005). In the Nurse Manifest project, the research team developed fictionalized stories of nursing practice from actual stories told by nurses. These fictionalized stories are an example of formal expressions of personal knowing.

The aesthetic methods of envisioning and rehearsing can be used to critique the depth of human suffering sustained by an unjust status quo and then to imagine alternatives (see Chapter 6). The items, as codifications, brought by the nurses in the study can be seen as a type of art form that illustrated their feelings and served as a basis for the creative processes of emancipatory knowing. Simple objects (e.g., a food strainer) are important in that they codify and therefore symbolize complex human experiences (Jacobs et al., 2005). Such codifications engender a rich dialogue that is useful for fully understanding the problem. In the Nurse Manifest project, Cowling created works of art as formalized expressions of aesthetic knowing that synthesized the powerful experiences reflected in the stories of nurses from around the world ("NurseManifest 2002 Research Study Report," 2002). Such artistic renderings can be used to further critique and imagine solutions to the problems of injustice represented.

 Consider This...

Consider this example: Cathy recently moved to a small southwestern community located 70 miles from a large metropolitan area in which several universities are located. Cathy has been a family nurse practitioner for many years, and she relocated to assume a full-time clinical faculty appointment to provide clinical supervision for students. The community is considered a safe environment for raising a family, but many are worried about a toxic dump that is no longer used, which is located about 3 miles outside the center of the town. As a triathlete and a survivor of thyroid cancer, she also has an interest in oncology nursing and the preventive value of exercise. After relocating, Cathy noticed that there was no health care facility in her community and that people must drive for many miles for routine or urgent care. She brought together several nurses and social workers in the community to explore her idea, and discussed the ideas with the university faculty as well. Although she was unsure whether a practice would be viable economically, the people working with her supported moving forward. Cathy and her team decided to offer care that was appropriate for a family nurse practitioner to provide, and she soon found herself seeing patients and providing care. Her patients include individuals and families from white, Native American, and Hispanic backgrounds who come to her clinic for a variety of reasons. She frequently encounters adults with diabetes and heart disease as well as children with ear infections and minor trauma. While performing physical examinations and emphasizing prevention, Cathy has also noticed a number of patients who have suspicious skin lesions, enlarged thyroid glands, or both.

What knowledge related to emancipatory knowing is required to initiate and sustain a viable practice and clinical excellence? What knowledge from within the four fundamental patterns is required to sustain the practice as viable and excellent?

FORMAL EXPRESSIONS OF EMANCIPATORY KNOWING: ACTION PLANS, MANIFESTOES, CRITICAL ANALYSES, AND VISIONS FOR THE FUTURE

Praxis may begin to occur as a direct result of critiquing and imagining processes, depending on the emancipatory interest of the activist group. However, formal expressions are often required to keep the emancipatory interest clearly in focus or to communicate to others the nature of injustices and what is needed to rectify those injustices. These formal expressions of emancipatory knowing (i.e., emancipatory knowledge) can take a number of forms. In Fig. 3.1, four formal expressions of emancipatory knowing are identified: (1) *manifestoes,* which are action-oriented and impassioned portrayals of that which is problematic, the actions required to effect change, and descriptions of the ideals that are envisioned; (2) *critical analyses,* which examine what is, how it came to be, and who is disadvantaged; (3) *vision statements,* which describe in detail an envisioned future; and (4) *action plans,* which also describe an envisioned future, as well as what is required to reach that future. Although we have identified four formal expressions of emancipatory knowing, formal expressions can take other forms. Any credible formal expression that is created expressly to assist in some way with the liberation of oppressed groups can be a formal expression of emancipatory knowing.

As stated previously, formal expressions of emancipatory knowing can arise directly from an emancipatory project. Activist groups may create various formal expressions, including action plans, manifestoes, or visions for the future, depending on the nature of their emancipatory project. In addition to formal expressions that may emerge from the work of activist groups, scholars who have a direct or indirect experience with a situation of oppression can also develop formal expressions that synthesize theoretic and empiric insights related to an unjust situation. These formal expressions can subsequently be used to raise awareness in students, mentees, and peers with regard to the source of, extent of, and remedies for social inequities. Although ideas about who can and should generate formal expressions of emancipatory knowing vary, we believe that all sources of formal expressions with an intent to correct unjust positions are valuable to the pursuit of liberation.

Fundamentally, all formal expressions of emancipatory knowing, including critical analyses, are grounded in critical social theory in a broad sense. Critical social theory in this broad sense focuses on illuminating the processes that create social injustices as well as the changes required to move toward justice and freedom for oppressed people. Within the broad perspective of critical social theory, nurse scholars generally have approached problems of social injustices with the use of the lenses of critical feminism and critical poststructuralism (Grace & Perry, 2013; Pitre, Kushner, Raine, & Hegadoren, 2013).

Critical feminism perspectives focus on social and political structures that sustain injustice and how these structures interact with gender to limit full human potential (Alex, Whitty-Rogers, & Panagopoulos, 2013; Almutairi & Rodney, 2013; Pauly, MacKinnon, & Varcoe, 2009). This approach to creating a critical analysis draws from the perspective of critical social theory as well as from any or several of the various approaches to feminism. For example, a critical feminist approach to a problem that involves economics may draw on the insights of socialist feminist thought, in which the foundation of gender inequality rests with the nature of economic structures in society.

The model of social consciousness of Giddings (2005a) is an example of a critical feminist analysis that emerged out of an activist research project (Giddings, 2005b). Giddings interviewed nurses in the United States and New Zealand who identified with the dominant Eurocentric culture, the experience of being lesbian, or the experience of being a racial minority (i.e., African American in the United States or Maori in New Zealand). The nurses were invited to participate because of their reputations as people who actively engaged in advocating for others who were disadvantaged. The purpose of the study was to explore how these nurses became aware of the plight of disadvantaged persons, how they came to speak up and act on their behalf, and what their experience of doing so in nursing had been. On the basis of the life stories of these nurses, Giddings developed a model of social consciousness that provided explanations of the challenges and barriers to nurses acting from their awareness of injustices in health care.

Similar to critical feminism, *critical poststructuralism* offers an important approach for the critical work of nursing scholars (Bradbury-Jones et al., 2008). Critical post-structuralism focuses on the role of language and discourse in the creation of oppressive conditions. Poststructuralist theory deals with how language and discourses determine or construct what is a normal and natural way to be. Discourse includes such things as representational art, advertising images, music lyrics, interview text, and written or oral accounts that reflect social processes (Georges & Benedict, 2008; Montgomery, McCauley, & Bailey, 2009; Pauly et al., 2009). When there is no language or discourse regarding alternative ways of being and acting, those alternatives simply do not exist. Analyzing what is not said, what is not represented, and how representations intersect and converge to maintain what is constructed as truth can also facilitate the emergence of ideas for changing the status quo.

For example, when the word "man" was used as a generic term to include women and other gender configurations, the subjugation of women as an outcome of this language practice was simply not recognized or perceived, and it was often denied as a possibility. In cultures in which there is no language for sexual orientation other than heterosexual and same-sex relationships, or for gender identities other than male and female, other possibilities for sexuality and gender identities are not perceived as existing. When the term *nurse* is taken to mean "female nurse," the possibility of a man who is a nurse is not perceived, and the qualifier "male" is required to bring this particular situation into awareness.

Critical postcolonialism and critical ethnography are other forms of critical scholar-ship that are used to produce formal expressions of emancipatory knowing. *Critical postcolonialism* approaches tend to focus on injustices that are created as a result of one culture taking over and subjugating another culture for its own gain. *Critical ethnography* suggests an anthropologic approach that examines structures and practices that sustain social inequities within a culture.

In critical analyses, including poststructuralist and feminist forms, multiple sources of data or materials that reflect oppressive situations can be used and combined with other sources of data to yield the most comprehensive picture of the situation (Georges & Bene-dict, 2008; Montgomery et al., 2009; Pauly et al., 2009). A scholar often begins with one data source for analysis and then turns to others in an effort to create the most complete analysis possible. Critical approaches require crossing disciplinary and academic lines that have falsely fragmented and continue to falsely fragment knowing and knowledge and that have not served the best interests of society. Academic and disciplinary lines have also sustained the academic heritage of the "ivory tower," which distances academic thinking and processes from the grassroots experiences of people in society. Without denying the valuable contributions of various disciplines to society and human welfare, the realization remains that academic disciplinary lines have tended to limit the creative process and formal expressions of emancipatory knowledge that lead to praxis, thereby resulting in limited solutions for many of the world's most persistent social problems.

Regardless of the specific methods used, critical analyses are characterized by a perspective that does the following (Fontana, 2004; Freire, 1970; Morrow, 1994):

- Trusts and remains loyal to people seeking liberation without assuming the right to speak for them
- Uncovers hidden ideologic premises (hegemony) embedded in social structures
- Examines what is assumed or presupposed in what is taken as knowledge or truth to reveal assumptions that are false
- Unveils conventions of language and symbols that limit the true representation of the situation
- Challenges current institutionalized power relations
- Projects actions and processes for changing the status quo to create equitable social relationships
- Calls forth a self-reflective attitude that constantly challenges one's own understandings
- Requires those participating in the work to disclose their personal perspectives and intentions related to their work

Taken together, these traits reveal the explicitly political and values-laden stance of critical analyses while maintaining the high standards of academic rigor. From a critical perspective, all academic processes that are used to develop knowledge are inherently laden with value, despite traditional scientific claims to the contrary. Critical analyses require that those who participate in these analyses bring to conscious awareness and disclose their own personal perspectives and share their intentions related to their work. By making these perspectives clear, the values that underpin the work are made accessible for challenge, discussion, and debate. The overriding intention is to deepen explicit ethical commitments to full human health and well-being for all and to act on those commitments (Fontana, 2004; Freire, 1970).

CONCLUSION

Emancipatory knowing makes possible the never-ending quest for improvement in nursing quality, the capacity for recognizing complex situations that shape health and well-being, and that energizes the will to act to change underlying factors that inhibit health and well-being.

References

Alex, M., Whitty-Rogers, J., & Panagopoulos, W. (2013). The language of violence in mental health: shifting the paradigm to the language of peace. *ANS. Advances in Nursing Science, 36*, 229–242.

Almutairi, A. F., & Rodney, P. (2013). Critical cultural competence for culturally diverse workforces: toward equitable and peaceful health care. *ANS. Advances in Nursing Science, 36*, 200–212.

Ashley, J. (1976). *Hospitals, paternalism, and the role of the nurse.* New York: Teachers College Press.

Aston, M. (2008). Public health nurses as social mediators navigating discourses with new mothers. *Nursing Inquiry, 15*, 280–288.

Bickford, D. (2014). Postcolonial theory, nursing knowledge, and the development of emancipatory knowing. *ANS. Advances in Nursing Science, 37*(3), 213–223. https://doi.org/10.1097/ANS.0000000000000033.

Bradbury-Jones, C., Sambrook, S., & Irvine, F. (2008). Power and empowerment in nursing: a fourth theoretical approach. *Journal of Advanced Nursing, 62*, 258–266.

Bunting, S., & Campbell, J. C. (1990). Feminism and nursing: historical perspectives. *ANS. Advances in Nursing Science, 12*, 11–24.

Butterfield, P. G. (2017). Thinking upstream: a 25-year retrospective and conceptual model aimed at reducing health inequities. *ANS. Advances in Nursing Science, 40*(1), 2–11. https://doi.org/10.1097/ANS.0000000000000161.

Campbell, J. C., & Bunting, S. (1991). Voices and paradigms: perspectives on critical and feminist theory in nursing. *ANS. Advances in Nursing Science, 13*, 1–15.

Carnegie, E., & Kiger, A. (2009). Being and doing politics: an outdated model or 21st century reality? *Journal of Advanced Nursing, 65*, 1976–1984.

Chinn, P. L. (2009, October 24). Cassandra: Radical Feminist Nurses Network: 1982-1987. http://www.peggychinn.com/cassandra.html.

Chinn, P. L. (2013). *Peace & power: new directions for building community* (8th ed.). Burlington, MA: Jones and Bartlett Learning.

Chinn, P. L. (2013, 2016). Peace & power. http://peaceandpowerblog.wordpress.com.

Chinn, P. L., & Falk-Rafael, A. (2015). Peace and power: a theory of emancipatory group process. *Journal of Nursing Scholarship: An Official Publication of Sigma Theta Tau International Honor Society of Nursing / Sigma Theta Tau, 47*(1), 62–69. https://doi.org/10.1111/jnu.12101.

Cowling, W. R., Chinn, P. L., & Hagedorn, S. (2009, April 30). *A nursing manifesto: a call to conscience and action.* http://www.nursemanifest.com/manifesto_num.htm.

Dock, L. L. (1902). Sanitary inspection: a new field for nurses. *The American Journal of Nursing, 3*, 529–532.

Doering, L. (1992). Power and knowledge in nursing: a feminist poststructuralist view. *ANS. Advances in Nursing Science, 14*, 24–33.

Falk-Rafael, A. (2006). Globalization and global health: toward nursing praxis in the global community. *ANS. Advances in Nursing Science, 29*(1), 2–14. https://www.ncbi.nlm.nih.gov/pubmed/16495684.

Falk-Rafael, A., & Bradley, P. A. (2014). "Towards justice in health": an exemplar of speaking truth to power. *ANS. Advances in Nursing Science, 37*(3), 224–234. https://doi.org/10.1097/ANS.0000000000000034.

Fontana, J. S. (2004). A methodology for critical science in nursing. *ANS. Advances in Nursing Science, 27*, 93–101.

Foucault, M. (1980). *Power/knowledge: selected interviews and other writing 1972-1977.* New York, NY: Pantheon Books.

Foucault, M. (1984). *The Foucault reader.* New York, NY: Pantheon Books.

Freire, P. (1970). *Pedagogy of the oppressed.* New York, NY: Seabury Press.

Georges, J. M. (2013). An emancipatory theory of compassion for nursing. *ANS. Advances in Nursing Science, 36*, 2–9.

Georges, J. M., & Benedict, S. (2008). Nursing gaze of the eastern front in World War II: a feminist narrative analysis. *ANS. Advances in Nursing Science, 22*, 139–152.

Giddings, L. S. (2005a). A theoretical model of social consciousness. *ANS. Advances in Nursing Science, 28*, 224–239.

Giddings, L. S. (2005b). Health disparities, social injustice, and the culture of nursing. *Nursing Research, 54*, 304–312.

Grace, P. J., & Perry, D. J. (2013). Philosophic inquiry and the goals of nursing: a critical approach for disciplinary knowledge development and action. *ANS. Advances in Nursing Science, 36*, 64–79.

Habermas, J. (1973). *Theory and practice.* Boston, MA: Beacon Press.

Habermas, J. (1979). *Communication and the evolution of society.* Boston, MA: Beacon Press.

Hagedorn, S. (1995). The politics of caring: the role of activism in primary care. *ANS. Advances in Nursing Science, 17*, 1–11.

Hall, L. E. (1966). Another view of nursing care and quality. In K. M. Straub, & K. S. Parker (Eds.), *Continuity in patient care: the role of nursing* (pp. 47–60). Washington, DC: Catholic University Press.

Hall, S. (2001). Foucault: power, knowledge and discourse. In M. Wetherell, S. Taylor, & S. J. Yates (Eds.), *Discourse theory and practice* (pp. 72–81). Thousand Oaks, CA: Sage Publications.

Heide, W. S. (1973). Nursing and women's liberation. *The American Journal of Nursing, 73*, 824–827.

Hooks, B. (1993). Bell hooks speaking about Paulo Freire—the man, his work. In P. McLaren, & P. Leonard (Eds.), *Paulo Freire: a critical encounter* (pp. 146–154). London: Routledge.

Jacobs, B. B., Fontana, J. S., Kehoe, M. H., Matarese, C., & Chinn, P. L. (2005). An emancipatory study of contemporary nursing practice. *Nursing Outlook, 53*, 6–14.

Jarrin, O. F. (2006). Results from the Nurse Manifest 2003 study: nurses' perspectives on nursing. *ANS. Advances in Nursing Science, 29*, E74–E85.

Kagan, P. N. (2006). JoAnn Ashley 30 years later: legacy for practice. *Nursing Science Quarterly, 19*, 317–327.

Kagan, P. N., Smith, M. C., & Chinn, P. L. (2014). Introduction. In P. N. Kagan, M. C. Smith, & P. L. Chinn (Eds.), *Philosophies and practices of emancipatory nursing: social justice as praxis*. New York, NY: Routledge Taylor & Francis Group.

Kagan, P. N., Smith, M. C., Cowling, W. R., & Chinn, P. L. (2009). A nursing manifesto: an emancipatory call for knowledge development, conscience, and praxis. *Nursing Philosophy: An International Journal for Healthcare Professionals, 11*, 67–84.

MacDonnell, J. A. (2009). Fostering nurses' political knowledges and practices: education and political activation in relation to lesbian health. *ANS. Advances in Nursing Science, 32*, 158–172.

Messias, D. K. H., McDowell, L., & Estrada, R. D. (2009). Language interpreting as social justice work: perspectives of formal and informal healthcare interpreters. *ANS. Advances in Nursing Science, 32*, 128–143.

Montgomery, P., McCauley, K., & Bailey, P. H. (2009). Homelessness, a state of mind?: a discourse analysis. *Issues in Mental Health Nursing, 30*, 624–630.

Morrow, R. A. (1994). *Critical theory and methodology* (vol. 3). Thousand Oaks, CA: Sage Publications.

Muller, M. E., & Dzurec, L. C. (1993). The power of the name. *ANS. Advances in Nursing Science, 15*, 15–22.

Nightingale, F. (1852/1979). *Cassandra: an angry outcry against the plight of Victorian women*. New York, NY: The Feminist Press.

NurseManifest 2002 Research Study Report. (2002). http://www.nursemanifest.com/research_reports/2002 _study/2002_study.htm.

NurseManifest Project. (2002). http://www.nursemanifest.com/.

Pauly, B., MacKinnon, K., & Varcoe, C. (2009). Revisiting "who gets care?" Access to healthcare as an arena for nursing action. *ANS. Advances in Nursing Science, 32*, 118–127.

Perry, D. J. (2015). Transcendent pluralism: A middle-range theory of nonviolent social transformation through human and ecological dignity. *ANS. Advances in Nursing Science, 38*(4), 317–329. https://doi.org /10.1097/ANS.0000000000000086.

Phillips, D. A. (2006). Masculinity, male development, gender, and identity: modern and postmodern meanings. *Issues in Mental Health Nursing, 27*, 403–423.

Pitre, N. Y., Kushner, K. E., Raine, K. D., & Hegadoren, K. M. (2013). Critical feminist narrative inquiry: advancing knowledge through double-hermeneutic narrative analysis. *ANS. Advances in Nursing Science, 36*, 118–132.

Racine, L. (2009). Applying Antonio Gramsci's philosophy to postcolonial feminist social and political activism in nursing. *Nursing Philosophy: An International Journal for Healthcare Professionals, 10*, 180–190.

Ray, M. A., & Turkel, M. C. (2014). Caring as emancipatory nursing praxis: the theory of relational caring complexity. *ANS. Advances in Nursing Science, 37*(2), 132–146. https://doi.org/10.1097/ANS.00000000 00000024.

Roberts, S. J. (1983). Oppressed group behavior: Implications for nursing. *ANS. Advances in Nursing Science, 5*, 21–30.

Scheer, V. L., Stevens, P. E., & Mkandawire-Valhmu, L. (2016). Raising questions about capitalist globalization and universalizing views on women. *ANS. Advances in Nursing Science, 39*(2), 96–107. https://doi.or g/10.1097/ans.0000000000000120.

Schön, D. (1983). *The reflective practitioner: how professionals think in action*. New York, NY: Basic Books.

Snyder, M. (2014). Emancipatory knowing: empowering nursing students toward reflection and action. *The Journal of Nursing Education, 53*(2), 65–69. https://doi.org/10.3928/01484834-20140107-01.

Thompson, J. L. (2014). Discourses of social justice: examining the ethics of democratic professionalism in nursing. *ANS. Advances in Nursing Science, 37*(3), E17–E34. https://doi.org/10.1097/ANS.0000000000 00045.

Vickers, D. A. (April, 2008). *Social justice: a concept for undergraduate nursing curricula?.* http://www.resource nter.net/images/snrs/files/sojnr_articles2/vol08num01art06.html.

Wåhlin, I. (2017). Empowerment in critical care—a concept analysis. *Scandinavian Journal of Caring Sciences, 31*(1), 164–174. https://doi.org/10.1111/scs.12331.

Walter, R. R. (2016). Emancipatory nursing praxis: a theory of social justice in nursing. *ANS. Advances in Nursing Science, 1.* https://doi.org/10.1097/ANS.0000000000000157.

Watson, J., & Hills, M. H. (2011). *Creating a caring science curriculum: an emancipatory pedagogy for nursing.* New York, NY: Springer Publishing Company. https://market.android.com/details?id=book-IsSkFAVvXdsC.

Weiler, K. (1991). Freire and a feminist pedagogy of difference. *Harvard Educational Review, 61,* 449–474.

White, J. (1995). Patterns of knowing: review, critique, and update. *ANS. Advances in Nursing Science, 17,* 73–86.

White, J. (2014). Through a socio-political lens: the relationship of practice, education, research and policy to social justice. In P. N. Kagan, P. L. Chinn, & M. C. Smith (Eds.), *Philosophies and practices of emancipatory nursing: Social justice as praxis (p. tbd).* New York, NY: Routledge, 298–308.

Ethical Knowledge Development

> *Certain fundamental ethical principles are universal and unchangeable, but the interpretation and application of truth changes and different people arrive at truth by widely different methods.... Adults who are dominated by the opinions of the herd may be morally retarded. We do not act morally unless we act from a sense of conviction and reason, guided by our own conscience.*
>
> **Isabel Stewart (1921, pp. 906, 909)**

The opening quote suggests that, although certain ethical and moral directives seem universal, when they are used in clinical settings, the ways in which to use them are not always clear. Moreover, the quote assumes that a moral truth does exist, at least in given situations, and that knowing ethical and moral truth requires not only our conscience and conviction but knowledge of moral and ethical directives. According to Stewart, moral and ethical truths are not necessarily what everyone else believes.

Ethical matters can be complicated; what to do is often not clear, and the information needed to make a sound decision may not be available. For example, consider the ethical directive "do no harm," a commonly understood ethical principle. On the surface, this may seem like a truth that is easily honored, but how is it applied in a clinical setting?

 Consider This...

Jill and Armando are expecting their first child, and they know that they may be carriers of the gene for cystic fibrosis. However, they seem to be unaware that an opportunity for genetic testing exists. You know that, in this situation, genetic testing would confirm or negate the parents' carrier status, and should they be found to be carriers, the fetus can be assessed prenatally to determine if it has inherited the genetic mutation from each parent. You also know that, if this fetus has inherited both genes, the child will most certainly develop the condition, but its severity cannot be predicted. You wonder what you should say to Jill and Armando about genetic testing. When considering this situation, you recognize that the parents are devout Catholics who likely would not want to terminate a pregnancy for any reason. Moreover, you know that there are risks to the fetus associated with prenatal diagnosis, should they choose this. In addition, you can provide no assurances about the quality of life of the child should it develop the disease, because the condition could be severe or milder. Knowing all of this, should you encourage genetic testing, and what ethical principles would guide your actions?

According to the quote from Stewart, as the nurse working with Jill and Armando, you will eventually resolve this ethical dilemma by considering the principle "do no harm" as well as other factors through your own reasoning. When making your decision, a whole host of contextual factors will be considered, including legal or policy requirements for information disclosure, what you believe the parents' response would be if genetic testing were strongly encouraged, and what you believe constitutes caring in this situation. You will make a decision, you will integrate knowledge from all of the knowing patterns in making that decision, and whatever decision is made will be the best you can do given the circumstances. What the "right" decision is may never be totally clear. You understand that, in this situation and countless others, "do no harm" becomes a complex and uncertain directive to enact.

In this chapter, we focus on methods for creating ethical knowledge. Fig. 4.1 shows the quadrant of our model that pertains to the development of this pattern of nursing knowledge. Nurses, regardless of setting, bring to practice the heritage of their own moral development and understandings, as well as knowledge of ethical and moral practice obtained through formal education. With this background, as nurses practice and reflect on their practice, they begin to ask critical questions such as "Is this right?" and "Is this responsible?" These questions set into motion the creative processes of clarifying values and exploring alternatives. As these questions are answered, knowledge that can be shared and used in practice is developed, such as ethical principles and codes. Through the collective disciplinary processes of dialogue and justification, ethical knowledge is authenticated and understood in relation to practice.

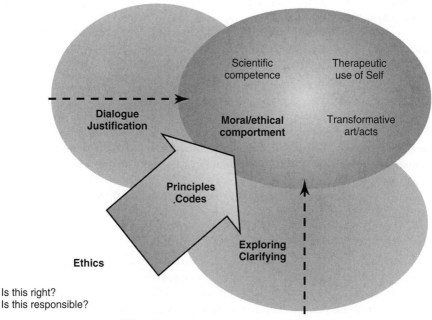

FIG. 4.1 Ethical Knowing and Knowledge.

TABLE 4.1 Dimensions of Ethical Knowledge Development

Dimension	Ethics
Critical questions	Is this right?
	Is this responsible?
Creative processes	Clarifying
	Exploring
Formal expressions	Principles and codes
Authentication processes	Dialogue
	Justification
Integrated expression in practice	Moral and ethical comportment

According to our model, nurses who make use of ethical knowledge that has been strengthened through the authentication processes of dialogue and justification can be expected to increasingly practice with *moral/ethical comportment,* the integrated expression of ethical knowing. In practice, further questioning occurs, and the stage is set for reinitiating the ongoing creative processes of clarifying values and exploring alternatives.

Table 4.1 shows the processes addressed in this chapter—the critical questions, creative processes, and formal expressions of knowledge.

ETHICS, MORALITY, AND NURSING

Clearly, nursing is a profession that requires ethical knowledge to guide practice. Whether an individual is a seasoned nurse or a beginning student, and whether a nurse working in a high-tech intensive care environment or in an isolated rural elementary school, care outcomes depend on the nurse's ethical knowing and morality. According to Levine (1989), all nursing actions are moral statements. We would add that all nursing actions also are ethical statements. But what constitutes ethical behavior? How is morality determined? These are difficult questions to answer, and even when every effort is made to address ethical issues fully and appropriately, there is no guarantee that the right decision will be made.

Whether the business of ethics really is more complex today than it was historically is questionable, but the need to make ethical decisions has *always* been part of the modern nurse's role. Ethics is now receiving renewed emphasis, and nursing organizations are deliberately focusing on the need to attend to ethical issues ("Code of Ethics for Nurses with Interpretive Statements," 2015; Numminen & Leino-Kilpi, 2009). Certainly the complexity of the current health care arena has raised questions about what is ethical behavior. Concerns about the proper care of marginalized groups, laws that regulate disclosure in health care and research practices, a focus on the rights of individuals in the health care system, and technologic advancements are among the factors that have contributed to the complexity of ethical decisions, thereby creating confusion about what is the morally right thing to do.

Ethics and *morality* are commonly interchanged terms that are sometimes used synonymously in the nursing literature. We see ethics and morality as being enmeshed, and we use both terms together in this chapter and elsewhere in this book. The distinction between ethics and morality reflects the tension between epistemology and ontology and the difficulty of separating what we know from who we are. In general, ethics relates to matters of epistemology, or knowledge, whereas morality focuses on ontology, or being. Ethics is a discipline that structures knowledge, a branch of inquiry that tries to make sense of what is right or wrong. Ethics, then, is more like "head work," the products of which include ethical principles, theories, rules, codes, and laws; lists of obligations or duties; and descriptions of moral and ethical behavior.

Ethics

Ethics may be divided into two branches: descriptive and prescriptive. *Descriptive ethics* is an empiric endeavor that systematizes what people believe ethically and how they behave in relation to those beliefs. *Prescriptive,* or normative, *ethics* is concerned with the "oughts" of behavior. With the use of cognitive reasoning processes that incorporate emotional and other nonrational sources of behavior, prescriptions for ethical behavior are put into language and set forth as theories, codes, duties, principles, and so on. In this text, our focus is on prescriptive ethics, but it is important to recognize the value of descriptive ethics for examining the nature of ethical knowledge in nursing. To understand the difference, think about the fact that there are many different beliefs about abortion; descriptive ethics provides information about what those various beliefs are, and the rationale that people offer related to their beliefs. This information can be helpful in shifting to the prescriptive challenge of what ought to be done in any circumstance, but the information alone is not sufficient to develop statements as to what ought to be done.

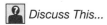 *Discuss This...*

Discuss the example of purchasing term papers over the Internet. Each person in the group probably has an opinion about this, but suppose you have been assigned to investigate whether or not your organization needs a policy about this, and if so, what that policy should be. Suppose you started by conducting a survey asking the following: (1) "Do you believe it is wrong to use purchased term papers about nurse theorists and their work to fulfill course requirements?" and (2) "Have you ever done this?" Collating and reporting their answers would be in the realm of descriptive ethics—data that documents the ethical stance of people in your organization and gives you evidence to address the question of whether or not you need a policy on this issue.

Your discussion then needs to move to the question of whether a policy is needed and what that policy might be. You might reason how and why it is not permissible to purchase term papers to meet college course requirements by invoking a rule that deception is wrong. In this example, such a practice could be understood as deceiving faculty who expect you to do your own work. It also might be understood as self-deceit, because thoroughly learning about a theorist's work is short-circuited by simply reading a paper rather than composing it. Now you are entering the realm of prescriptive ethics. Discuss what you might propose as an addition to a code of ethical behavior for students.

Morality

By contrast, morality is expressed in behavior and grounded in values. If ethics is head work, you might think of morality as "heart work" that is expressed by doing. Morality refers to our day-to-day living expressions of what we believe to be good, beliefs that are firmly embedded in our character. When people consistently behave in concert with their values, moral integrity is shown. When moral behavior is blocked by situational factors in a way that matters to persons, moral distress results. Peter and Liaschenko (2013) say moral distress results when the moral identities and responsibilities of nurses are constrained. For example, ethically you may believe that it is important to obey Provision 1 of the American Nurses Association Code of Ethics for Nurses ("Code of Ethics for Nurses with Interpretive Statements," 2015), which states that you should practice with compassion and respect for the dignity and worth of every individual. However, because time constraints imposed by a heavy patient load prohibit you from doing this in ways that really matter to you, you experience moral distress.

Morality is determined largely by situational and background experiences. Although people can appeal to ethical codes or principles to justify their actions, more often morality is shown on a less deliberative and conscious level. Daily expressions of belief about the right, the good, and the decent are filtered through lenses that are influenced by a host of factors, including family, friends, religion, gender, and developmental stage. Thus, what constitutes moral behavior varies, and what is important in one society (e.g., being on time out of respect for others) may be unimportant in another. A religious affiliation associated with one community may provide a lens that justifies war, whereas another may offer a lens that justifies pacifism.

 Think About It...

> Think of a situation you have encountered in nursing that involved decisions of "right" and "wrong." What was your own judgment about what happened, or what was done? What in your experience shapes what you think of as "right" or "wrong" in such a situation?

Interrelationship of Morality and Ethics

Morality and ethics interrelate in that ethical knowledge can provide a basis or template for judging and evaluating moral standards and behavior. Conversely, moral or immoral behavior can provide a template for judging ethical knowledge. The Nursing Code of Ethics ("Code of Ethics for Nurses with Interpretive Statements," 2015) provides specific guidelines for nurses. In addition, a number of patient bill of rights statements reflect ethical knowledge and guide moral decisions in specific situations with specific populations. For example:

- U.S. Patients' Bill of Rights in Medicare and Medicaid ("The Patients' Bill of Rights in Medicare and Medicaid," 1999) with its eight directives, summarized as follows:
  - The right to information
  - The right to choose
  - Access to emergency services
  - Being a full partner in health care decisions
  - Care without discrimination
  - The right to privacy
  - The right to speedy complaint resolution
  - Taking on new responsibilities for maintaining good health
- U.S. Affordable Care Act Patient's Bill of Rights ("ACA New Patients Bill of Rights," 2010; "Patient's Bill of Rights Under the Affordable Care Act: An Overview of the Rules on Consumer Protections," 2010) adds these rights (among others):
  - Coverage for people with preexisting conditions
  - Coverage for adult children up to age 26
- Bill of Rights for LGBTQ people and their families ("LGBT Healthcare Bill of Rights," 2016), which includes:
  - Right to visitation by anyone the patient chooses
  - Affirmation of one's gender identity
  - Designating the person who will make decisions on your behalf
- Children's Bill of Rights (Mathur, 2015) which includes rights to:
  - Receive appropriate medical treatment including therapeutic care for behavioral health
  - A voice in matters that affect them

Even with these guidelines, knowing how to act is often not so clear. Moral behavior is fluid; it occurs in the moment without time for contemplation, and it depends on situational understandings and circumstances. Legal requirements may also create moral distress and ethical conflict. Although appeals to ethical knowledge can be used to challenge and justify morality, they do not supersede the law. For example, if you have a strong moral disposition toward counseling an underage woman about her options for birth control, but such information is prohibited by state statute, an appeal to ethical knowledge (e.g., a code of rights) will not free you from legal responsibility in a court of law. In these cases, you have the choice to break the law, engage in deliberate civil disobedience to make a political statement, or work within professional organizations and local political circles to change oppressive laws.

What it is important to understand is that you, as a nurse, may act morally in relation to strong ethical precepts and end up in a court of law because your actions were illegal. Historically, changes in ethical and moral traditions have been made because people were willing to risk their lives and their personal freedom and security to ensure a broad base of human rights for others. Taking such a risk to make a political statement and to press a community to consider ethical and moral alternatives requires courage and strong moral conviction. It is also the case that ethical principles, held historically, may eventually become law. An example is the Health Insurance Portability and Accountability Act (HIPAA), which passed into law directives that protect the privacy of personal health information ("Health Information Privacy," 1996). With regard to this act, doing what was once only the "right thing to do" is now legally required.

Ideally, whatever constitutes moral behavior in nursing (elusive though that may be) needs to be in place, understood, and grounded in ethical knowledge that supports and justifies, yet challenges, that morality. Nursing, similar to other professions, has a unique set of values and a particular culture and practice that affect the ethical decision-making processes. The goal to be approached by nurses is moral and ethical coherence that is supported by laws and other societal contexts that do not prohibit but rather allow for the expression of nursing's highest moral and ethical ideals.

The following is an example of ethical directives (ethical knowledge) being used to judge behavior as ethical or not. The right-to-privacy directive in the Patients' Bill of Rights states in part that patients have the right to confidentiality. Suppose that, as you worked your shift one day in a long-term care facility, you overheard a well-meaning social worker talking with a nursing attendant in a hallway. The social worker was helping the attendant understand the nature of a resident's dementia while visitors and other residents walked by. Because the resident who is demented was identified by name in the conversation, this activity clearly constitutes a breach of confidentiality as guaranteed in the Patients' Bill of Rights. Because the right to privacy (the ethical directive) was breached, the behavior of the social worker and the attendant could be judged as immoral. Within some systems of ethical reasoning, the intent of the participants is important to ethical decision making. In this situation, the social worker had good intentions of helping the attendant better care for the resident. Might the extent that the social worker's actions would be judged immoral change if the participants knew better but just didn't care? Regardless of how an incident such as this breach of confidentiality would be judged in relation to morality, it does violate a justifiable ethical directive. Several courses of action might be appropriate, including posting the Patients' Bill of Rights in a public space as a reminder of its meaning, or approaching the social worker and the aide and bringing to their attention the inappropriateness of their behavior in reference to privacy protections.

Conversely, the following example involves behavior being used to judge the adequacy of ethical knowledge. In the Patients' Bill of Rights, another ethical directive states that patients must take more responsibility for maintaining good health. On your same shift in the long-term care facility, you notice that a newly employed nursing attendant has taken this directive to heart and is encouraging a resident with compromised cognitive function to take more responsibility for his self-care. Given the resident's cognitive state, you understand that the attendant is asking the resident to do things that are physiologically impossible, resulting in the resident's health being compromised. In this example, the attendant attempts to behave morally in light of the directive, but unknowingly is compromising other ethical principles generally accepted in health care, such as the prescription to "do no harm." In this instance, the attendant's moral expression of the ethical directive is helpful for realizing that the directive needs to be changed or clarified for persons whose cognitive function is not intact.

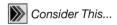 *Consider This...*

There are times when the ethical and moral judgements differ for people from different disciplines. For example, suppose you feel justified in providing information to a patient who asked you about alternative health care practices, when you know that the primary physician is unwilling to supply information about their use. When the physician discovers you have provided this information and asks to talk with you, it turns out that both she and you believe that your respective actions are morally right. You believe the patient has the right to know and thus use the precepts that surround a patient's right to information to justify your action. The physician, on the other hand, provides reasons that indicate that her intent is to do no harm. The physician states that, in the past, she had given the same information to the patient, who had not acted on the information and subsequently became extremely anxious about making treatment choices. In short, your action of providing information on the basis of the patient's right to know (autonomy) was judged as the "right thing," whereas the physician, by withholding information, was also doing the right thing by protecting the patient's vulnerabilities (doing no harm) on the basis of a reasonable knowledge of the patient's condition. In this situation, the understanding that would arise from your conversation with the physician provides you with a perspective about the right thing to do that you can draw on in the future.

Sometimes, when the moral positions of physician and nurse collide, both positions are reasonable, and both parties to the moral positions hold strong beliefs about their correctness. Differences of opinion about the best course of action in a given situation are often grounded in a preference for different ethical precepts. For example, the desire to be beneficent by ensuring that what you do results in something good for the patient or client may conflict with the equally reasonable precept of individual autonomy, or the right of patients and clients to be self-determining. Both positions may be morally justifiable but may lead to different outcomes. Moreover, the outcome of acting in relation to one or the other ethical precept cannot be known. Physicians and nurses, because of their educational experiences and health care roles, may tend to use differing and conflicting ethical precepts in approaching some care situations.

In these situations, there may be no clear answers about how to proceed, and it becomes important to identify the political processes that are operating. If the client's welfare is the concern for both parties, the nurse and physician should be successful in engaging in dialogue that questions how right and responsible any decision is. Through this process, both the physician and the nurse (and the client, when feasible) can more fully understand the nature of the decision to be made and its potential outcomes. If the nurse's or the physician's attitude reflects more of a controlling or paternalistic position in relation to the client, other strategies may be warranted. In this instance, nurse and physician should recognize the nature of power imbalances and how these are sustained, and they should seek avenues related to emancipatory knowing that fundamentally will undermine or circumvent paternalistic patterns of control.

OVERVIEW OF ETHICAL PERSPECTIVES

Within philosophic ethics, various theoretic perspectives have emerged that attempt to set forth the foundation on which to base ethical action. These approaches to ethics have been important for nursing as it attempts to create an ethical perspective on practice.

The four perspectives that often appear in nursing literature are briefly examined here: (1) teleology, (2) deontology, (3) relativism, and (4) virtue ethics.

Teleology and Deontology

Teleology and deontology are two common labels that characterize ethical systems. Most ethical codes and principles as well as systems of ethical reasoning and decision making can be broadly classified into one of these two types. In *teleology*, what is right produces good. Teleologic systems view the ends produced by a course of action as the measure that determines the action's goodness. What a right course of action yields is expressed in a familiar phrase: "the greatest good for the greatest number of people." Taken to extremes, teleologic systems could be used to justify behavior that is deemed harmful to a societal group if the harm that was done produced good for the rest of society. With the use of teleology, one could justify stripping a wealthy person of personal assets for redistribution to those who are poor and thereby producing a greater good for a greater number of people.

In *deontology*, what is right may not necessarily produce a good outcome; in other words, deontologic systems separate right from good. In deontologic systems, ethically right actions may have an undesirable outcome, as expressed by the following phrase: "the end does not justify the means." In deontologic frameworks for ethical decision making, knowledge forms such as external rules and codes determine what is right, regardless of the outcome produced. An extreme view of deontology is exemplified by someone who, because he or she is required by rule or precept to tell the truth, does the morally right thing and tells the truth, thereby causing great emotional distress to a client and that client's family (i.e., a bad outcome).

Deontologic systems suggest that the rules and the makers of the rules are in charge of ethical decision making, whereas teleologic systems assign decision-making authority to persons who make reasoned judgments about what constitutes the greatest good. Both deontologic and teleologic systems focus on the individual as a decision maker who is autonomous in action.

Relativism

Relativism exists in many varieties; it basically is the claim that what is morally and ethically correct varies across cultures and societies. In relation to ethical systems of reasoning, relativists would argue that universal generalities about what constitutes moral action cannot be made. In relativism, ethical behavior and moral viewpoints are justified by, or relative to, any one of many viewpoints or standards. What is considered moral behavior and ethical knowledge is determined by the framework used when making a judgment, and no standard or viewpoint is privileged over any other.

In relativism, any one standard of morality is as good as any other, and all ethical precepts are equally true, assuming that these can be justified with the use of an acceptable framework (Blackburn, 2005). A relativist position may argue that an ethical system grounded in deontology is just as good as one that is grounded in teleology. For relativists, ethical systems and morality depend on historical timing, the culture and language within which the justification system is embedded, and the particular group and individuals involved in decision making (Bandman & Bandman, 2001; Mappes & DeGrazia, 2006).

Relativism may be a comfortable position to take because it circumvents a responsibility to know how to behave with some degree of certainty in the face of moral and ethical dilemmas. Under the extreme relativist view, incorporating any idea of moral and ethical comportment into a knowledge development model becomes something of a nonissue; moral and ethical comportment would be relative to every possible ethical situation, and thus standards for behavior could not be generalized to all nurses. Relativist claims also preclude the advancement of ethical knowledge because no standpoint for judging behavior is taken to be better than any other.

However, some dimensions of relativism are useful and seem necessary. Nurses often face tremendous clinical complexities as part of ethical decision making that prevent knowing with much certainty the best course of action. Although moral/ethical decision making involves uncertainties with regard to taking action that cannot be solved by *a priori* knowledge of what is moral and ethical, we believe we can move toward a shared idea of what constitutes moral/ethical comportment for nursing.

Virtue Ethics

Virtue ethics introduces the character of the person as an important determiner of moral behavior/ethical decision making. Virtue or individual character is unimportant within the frame of reference provided by deontology and teleology. If ethical behavior could be reduced to the application of rules or calculations of good, character would be irrelevant. Character, however, determines how we perceive or frame situations, so a focus on the virtues of the nurse is critically important. Virtue ethics also offers a structure for moral/ethical comportment that can balance relativism by suggesting that a virtuous person will behave in a moral/ethical way. Virtue ethics allows flexibility when approaching moral/ethical situations, which deontologic and teleologic systems do not offer.

However, virtue ethics can be a particularly dangerous ethical system for a profession that is gendered in traditional female roles. Some focus on the cultivation of virtuous behavior seems important to ethical knowledge and knowing. Historically, however, for women to be virtuous meant to embrace a feminine ethic of being submissive, obedient, and self-sacrificing. It is important to question who defines what is virtuous and who benefits from the particular way in which the word *virtuous* is defined.

Our system for knowledge development includes aspects of both teleologic and deontologic perspectives. It also includes dimensions of relativism and virtue ethics. Although the knowledge forms include principles and codes, they are not taken to be infallible or to be adhered to at all costs. The creative processes of clarifying values and exploring alternatives can help to elucidate the situational contexts and decision-making frameworks that are important considerations for the modification of principles and codes. The authentication processes of dialogue and justification can function to temper rules and precepts and to sensitize them for different contexts. In addition, as the nurse acts, moral behavior and ethical knowledge are integrated with the other knowing patterns, including personal knowing, to create the best possible decision. This in turn can be further examined by questioning whether the action is right and responsible (rather than assuming that it is).

Our model of the knowing patterns incorporates a focus on virtues through the pattern of personal knowing, which grants the individual nurse the responsibility of examining what is virtuous. Emancipatory knowing suggests focusing on how and why particular virtues of nurses (e.g., caring, being on the job for patients despite heavy patient loads) may operate to maintain a problematic status quo (i.e., inadequate staffing that maximizes profits for hospital corporations to the detriment of caring nurses). The processes within the ethical knowledge quadrant help to ensure that, within the discipline, individual practitioners reflect on, discuss, and debate that which is virtuous in the context of nursing. As moral/ethical comportment is integrated in practice with other knowing patterns and subsequently examined by the critical questions ("Is this right?" and "Is this responsible?"), we expect that the growth of the discipline will evolve toward action and reflection that are consistent with praxis.

NURSING'S FOCUS ON ETHICS AND MORALITY

The virtues of a dutiful nurse were the focus of much literature about ethics during the first half of the 19th century (see Chapter 2). The historical work of Reverby (1987) underscores the nature of the nurse's duty to care while being denied the means to effect or create an environment in which caring is valued and possible. More recent nursing literature has shown increasing interest in the concept of *caring* as a centrally important focus for the development of both empiric and ethical theory. Much of the literature regarding the ethics of care centers on the relative merits of an ethic of caring compared with an ethic of justice, and how moral behavior relates to both (Barnes & Brannelly, 2008; Bell & Hulbert, 2008; Carper, 1979; Cook & Peden, 2016; Jacobs, 2013; Sander-Staudt, 2011; van Hooft, 2011; Vanlaere & Gastmans, 2011).

Nursing's focus on the caring perspective owes much to work that evolved from Carol Gilligan's critique (1982) and challenge of Kohlberg's theory of moral development (1976). Kohlberg's work staged moral development with the use of only male research participants, and Gilligan challenged its validity as a normative template for judging moral development in women. Gilligan found that women tended to care about relational concerns that focused on the needs and feelings of major players involved in the dilemma. By contrast, autonomy in decision making was a central feature of Kohlberg's theory.

Kohlberg's theory supported a morality in which actors could remain detached from the situation and appeal to rules or calculations of good as a guide to action. An approach that emphasizes detachment and objectivity in ethical decision making has been linked to traditional medical ethics approaches and critiqued as inappropriate for nursing. Fry (1989), for example, has suggested that the context of nursing practice requires a moral view of the person rather than a theory of moral action or a system of moral justification. For Fry, caring as a moral value ought to be central to any theory of ethics. Others have noted that concerns about autonomy and justice central to biomedical ethics tradition-ally have been male-gendered traits. Not only do these imply a separate-from or autono-mous stance toward ethical challenges, but they also may be inappropriate for nursing, where gendered traits are typically female (Condon, 1992).

Historically, feminists have cautioned nurses about the alignment of moral decision making in women with care perspectives because of its potential to further entrench oppressive values (Hoagland, 1990; Houston, 1990; Liaschenko, 1993; Noddings, 2003; Tong, 2008). A central criticism of care ethics for women is that it represents a type of slave morality (Sander-Staudt, 2011).

Publications about the dangers of caring theory for nurses may have waned, but we believe the previous cautions of feminist writings are still pertinent. Feminist authors have chronicled the political reality of caring and urge caution lest we embrace a femi-nine—rather than a feminist—ethic (Liaschenko, 1993; Tong, 2008). Although it can become difficult to differentiate feminine and feminist ethics, writers such as Liaschenko suggest that a *feminine ethic* reflects the uncritical acceptance and embracing, often unknowingly, of traditionally feminine values that surround caring. Embracing a femi-nine ethic of caring means promoting as ethical the enactment of the virtues associated with caring: altruism, acceptance, loving unconditionally, and other stereotypic femi-nine traits.

Although this type of caring may seem to be a perfectly good thing to do and to exemplify a very good way to be, such feminine virtues associated with caring may pre-clude nurses from understanding how this type of caring benefits the health care indus-try to the detriment of nurses' salaries, working conditions, and social value. Whereas a feminine ethic is associated with the uncritical acceptance of stereotypic female caring as a template for judging moral behavior, a *feminist ethic* is associated with critically under-standing the sociopolitical contexts that have gendered caring as feminine, and why and how this is problematic in relation to changing the situation of nurses within the health care system. In short, a feminine ethic of caring proclaims the importance of caring as being consistent with female-gendered virtues.

A feminist ethic would recognize that morality and social lives are interconnected, and that nursing's lack of power shapes our morality by determining whose ethical vision is authoritative (Tong, 2008). Feminist ethics require critical analyses that help nurses understand how to create contexts that would actually allow nurses to care. The cau-tion to embrace a feminist rather than a feminine ethic, for feminist writers such as (Liaschenko, 1993), is a plea to understand how blind adherence to the feminine virtues of caring can preclude caring by allowing for the continuance of conditions that exploit those who care. An ethics of care that does not ask who is caring for whom and whether care relationships are just is not liberatory (Sander-Staudt, 2011).

We believe that nurses must be concerned with issues of both care and justice if nurs-ing's purposes are to be realized. Walker (1993) suggested that nurses' moral expertise is not a question of mastering codes and laws but a matter of being architects of moral space within the health care setting and mediators in the conversations that are taking place. To do this requires paying attention to the vulnerabilities of both an ethic of care and an ethic of justice. As Cooper (1991) explained, we must take seriously the moral demands of care in the development of ethics. Doing so requires radical responses and moral courage as well as political astuteness. Ethical choices should be guided not only by rules and principles but also by the thoughtful analysis of feelings, intuitions, and experiences (Noddings, 1999; van Hooft, 2011).

DIMENSIONS OF ETHICAL KNOWLEDGE DEVELOPMENT

Our view of ethics is in concert with Carper's original conceptualization of the ethical pattern, which included dimensions of both morality and ethics intersecting with legally prescribed duties. Moreover, no single ethical or moral view is embraced, but nurses need to be constantly vigilant about the sociopolitical context in which they function. According to Carper, "The ethical component of nursing is focused on matters of obligation or what ought to be done. Knowledge of morality goes beyond simply knowing the norms or ethical codes of the discipline. It includes voluntary actions that can be judged as deliberately right and wrong" (1978, p. 20).

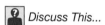 *Discuss This...*

> There are many questions that are critical for nurses to examine. Discuss these with a group of peers:
> - Toward what end should ethical knowledge be developed?
> - What ought to be done in practice to earn the label *ethical* or *moral*?
> - What values support nursing's ethics and morality?
> - Toward what clinical ends should ethical theories, reason, and ethical principles move us?
> - What sort of moral development perspective should we embrace and encourage?
> - In the context of teleology: How do we know what the greatest good is?
> - In the context of deontology: How do we know which rules are good and which are not?
> - For virtue ethics: Which virtues are worthwhile for us to cultivate?

Such questions relate to the final value from which no others can be derived and that centers our knowledge development efforts and professional activities. Although we will not answer these questions, we do provide guidelines for ways to create answers in your own situation. Because our model of knowledge development combines aspects of each of these positions, these are central questions that require thoughtful consideration.

As the dimensions of ethical knowing and knowledge development within our model are discussed in the following sections, some answers are provided, but additional questions are raised. For us, the merit of ethical knowledge will be judged based on the extent to which ethical codes and principles contribute to our collective ability to reflect and act in such a way that what we ethically know is fully consistent with what we morally do. This implies increasing the reflective awareness or consciousness on the part of nurses as nursing is practiced. It implies a move toward action that is grounded in an open awareness and choice for both the client and the nurse, in other words, a move toward health. It implies a move to reduce the moral distress that nurses face as they encounter and negotiate ethical and moral dilemmas.

The pattern of ethics focuses on nurses' day-to-day moral decision making. Ethics goes beyond what many tend to think of as ethics (i.e., the weighty, dramatic decisions that often involve end-of-life contexts or controversial political and social issues). Rather, important ethical knowing is used and created in everyday incidents and in the work of nurses (Liaschenko, Oguz, & Brunnquell, 2006). According to Thompson (2007), bioethics may be only marginally meaningful to most nurses; the language of bioethics deflects attention from the political organizations of care and the challenges of day-to-day nursing care. Ethical knowing in nursing is reflected in the decision to ignore a comment or to attend to it, in considering what to say and what not to say during everyday conversations, or in deciding whether to keep information to oneself or reveal it. Ethical decisions that are made around a conference table by an ethics committee, although important, are not our major focus or the major domain of nursing's morality and ethics. Rather, ethics arises from the work that nurses do and is about everyday uses of morality and ethical knowledge, as expressed in moral/ethical comportment in typical practice settings. Nursing's morality is largely an everyday ontology.

CRITICAL QUESTIONS: IS THIS RIGHT? IS THIS RESPONSIBLE?

In our model for knowledge development, ethical knowledge is generated with the following critical questions asked of ethical knowledge and moral behavior: "Is this right?" and "Is this responsible?" As you work as a nurse, this type of questioning is in the background whether you realize it or not. Without such questioning, you would be unable to make day-to-day moral/ethical moves.

We assume that nurses bring to their work some base set of values that guide their ethical decisions and moral behavior. As they work within the everyday world, their moral/ethical selves are challenged every day.

❗ Why This Is Important?...

Nursing's ethical and moral challenges are inherent in the ordinary things that happen, not the dramatic "hanging in the balance" kinds of challenges that are often the focus of discussions of ethics. Nonetheless being "ordinary" does not mean that these are not important challenges—they are challenges that make a significant difference in the lives of those for whom we care. Consider the kinds of situations involved in questions such as these:

- Should I reveal to an elderly woman that her well-meaning family is cleaning out her apartment and does not intend to allow her to return home because of warranted concerns for her safety?
- Should I share my views about what is responsible childbearing with a young couple who discover that they both have diabetes? Would this cause more harm than good? What would be gained? Who would gain?

If you reflect for a moment, several instances in which you have faced ordinary decisions should come to mind. You will probably notice that your decisions were made relatively quickly, without obvious reference to ethical codes or principles, and that you did wonder what was right and responsible. As you consider these questions in the moment of practice, you act in relation to your knowledge about what is ethical with consideration for other patterns of knowing. You will also reflect on the principles, codes, and other ethical knowledge forms that guided your actions apart from actual practice, in an attempt to understand more fully what was done and what should have been done in the situation.

CREATIVE PROCESSES: CLARIFYING VALUES AND EXPLORING ALTERNATIVES

As you or others inquire about how right and responsible your decisions are within your particular context, different perspectives on ethical decision making will become apparent. Clarifying values and exploring alternatives are the creative processes that begin to answer these questions. Simply stated, as you consider whether your moral/ethical behavior (as guided by disciplinary ethical knowledge) is right and responsible, you clarify the values that come into play as the situation unfolds, particularly those that create a dilemma. During this process, you are drawn to consider and explore various actions and options that flow from each value, which leads to the further clarification of the values themselves. Moreover, you and others can revisit and revise ethical knowledge forms to make them better guides for moral/ethical comportment.

Values Clarification

Values clarification processes deliberatively question and raise awareness of the personal values that undergird action. In this way, these processes have the potential to improve the moral/ethical correctness or "rightness" of a decision and subsequent behavior. The specific values that give rise to a nurse's moral/ethical decisions and actions (and subsequently ethical knowledge expressions) are often hidden. Values can be viewed as the background information or assumptions that create moral and ethical questions and actions. Values provide a lens that brings into focus certain aspects of a moral problem while at the same time distancing or blurring others. Values vary among individuals and reflect the contexts of our experiences with family members, friends, social institutions, gender boundaries, and age. The questioning of values with the use of formal techniques of clarification assumes that values may not always be "good." It also assumes that a disjunction exists between the values that we believe are important for influencing our actions and those that actually do influence what we do and say.

There are various techniques for values clarification (Bandman & Bandman, 2001; Catalano, 2008; Simon, Howe, & Kirschenbaum, 1995). Fundamentally, these processes involve the use of rational thought and emotional awareness to understand and examine the values that guide your actions. Approaches can involve the use of real or contrived dilemmas, group or individual work, self-analyses, interviews, or any number of other methods that free individuals to examine and embrace their values. The clarification of values is often an emotionally charged activity that involves deeply held personal beliefs. Individuals or groups who engage in values-clarification processes need an environment that allows for the freedom of value choices and for the affirmation of the values clarified. Regardless of the techniques used, values clarification is an individual process that seeks to unveil values that are often taken for granted. Values clarification is important because it emphasizes affective thinking and behavior-motivated choice and allows you to question how responsible your moral/ethical decisions are.

Various approaches for values clarification generally follow some basic general guidelines. First, it is important to select or create a moral/ethical dilemma that you and those working with you will emotionally relate to and that you will not see as fictitious to your practice. Although common approaches (e.g., Which person would you throw from the sinking boat?) may suffice, we believe that it is more beneficial if the situations relate to actual or potential nursing practice. Second, it is important to focus on clarifying individual values that emerge from the process, regardless of the process used for clarification. When engaging in values clarification, there may be a tendency to avoid what is difficult. Lively discussions about what should be done are not a substitute for a deliberative focus on one's personal values. A third guideline emphasizes writing about or listing personal values that emerge. *Journaling* about your values helps you make values explicit and clarify what the values are, and it provides a forum for examining how and why values change. Because it is difficult to provide a public forum in which nurses can freely examine their values, journaling is a particularly important tool, especially when the moral/ethical dilemmas that are the focus for deliberation are derived from practice situations that you are likely to encounter.

Exploration of Alternatives

The exploration of alternatives is an important process for understanding the moral/ethical correctness of a decision. Unlike values clarification (i.e., an attempt to understand emotionally, clarify, embrace, and perhaps change individually held values), an exploration of alternatives seeks to more objectively understand and analyze the values inherent in a certain situation and the various actions that flow from those values. During the process of exploring alternatives, you examine how different courses of action might flow from or challenge your values. As you explore what is or what could be happening morally and ethically in a situation, you begin to see alternative actions and even alternatives to your personal values. In addition, you begin to recognize the merits and pitfalls of different approaches to moral and ethical decision making. You strive to set aside your own values as much as possible and to view value structures—both your own and those of others—from different perspectives. During the process of exploring alternatives, you strive to gain clarity on an issue and examine various points of view, both factually and logically, as well as different approaches to resolving a dilemma.

As with values clarification, the situations that you choose for the exploration of alternatives arise from your practice. You explore the values that are important to the situation and the various actions that flow from those values. If factual evidence for one point of view is provided, that evidence is examined for accuracy. An ethical decision that is arrived at logically is then tested in some manner (e.g., by looking at its consistency with a principle or code for ethical behavior). However, when you are exploring alternatives, you are concerned not only with factual evidence but also with the preferences and beliefs of those who are involved in the situation. For example, when people are involved in end-of-life care, each individual will have personal beliefs and preferences about how best to care for the person who is dying. Each person's personal beliefs and values regarding death and life influence how he or she approaches the situation. The facts about the dying person's physical condition, physiologic indicators that the end of life is near, and observable behaviors are all factors that influence the situation. However, many alternative actions can be taken, even when all the facts remain constant. As you explore all the alternative actions that arise from the various values of those involved and the dilemmas that arise from competing ethical values, you gain insight and understanding of the situation, ultimately with increased clarity about those actions that are right, good, just, and responsible.

Values Clarification and Exploration of Alternatives Using Ethical Decision Trees

A number of sources suggest the use of decision trees as an approach to ethical decision making (Burkhardt & Nathaniel, 2007; Ellis & Hartley, 2004; Frame & Williams, 2005). Although the elements that constitute ethical decision-making trees vary somewhat, fundamentally they are depicted as flowcharts or a series of ordered questions that begin with the identification of the ethical issue or problem. After the problem is identified, the user is guided linearly through a number of steps that, when followed, suggest an ethically correct decision.

Ethical decision trees call for the gathering of facts about the situation in relation to the ethical framework that is being used. Options are considered, situational factors are identified, and an evaluation of various courses of action is required before a decision is proposed. Some decision trees prescribe, at least in part, the ethical framework to be used, whereas others expect the user to designate or choose the framework that is relevant to the situation.

Ethical decision trees are particularly useful when there is enough time for effective consideration and clarification of the requisite details within the elements of the tree before a decision is made. Ethical decision-making trees reflect what Liaschenko and Peter (2004) identify as a *disciplinary* type of ethics that suggests the professional activities of nurses that are understood in a certain way are inherently moral. They propose that approaches that limit what counts as a moral or ethical concern and that authorize how these concerns are resolved—as decision trees often do—incompletely reflect the complexity of contemporary health care.

However, decision trees can be useful as a learning tool. As with the nursing process, ethical decision trees offer a system that, once learned, helps nurses more quickly integrate the details involved in ethical situations and make an appropriate decision. The trees also make the factors and processes involved in ethical decisions less opaque and help learners understand what is and what is not ethically justifiable.

Completing decision trees can be useful for values clarification and the exploration of alternatives. Case studies of ethical problems can be organized into decision trees rather than being discussed directly. Decision trees can be completed by individual participants and then examined with the use of questions for values clarification. In addition, as participants individually complete decision trees, details that are important to consider within various elements required by the tree (e.g., the consequences of an action) will not be self-evident. When placing details of an ethical situation within a decision tree, it is important to notice which details require deliberation before making a choice and which can go unquestioned.

During this process, individual values tend to be clarified. As different members of the group suggest what must be included as relevant, the validity of various views within the group is likely to be challenged. Some members may notice that certain details were omitted that, in their view, should have been included. Others may not have even considered certain details as being relevant, whereas still others may offer reasons for omission as well as for inclusion. As discussions and disagreements occur, underlying values are made more visible to individual participants within the group. In addition, when individuals separately or groups collectively reflect on the extent and conditions of their agreement with a completed decision tree, values are clarified and alternatives explored.

Finally, changing the details that are entered in the elements of a decision tree and noticing how it affects both the processes and the outcomes of decision making is a useful clarification technique. Similar processes can assist in exploring alternatives using completed decision trees. Elements required within the trees as well as the details in completed trees can be questioned for underlying assumptions and conditions of context that have precluded the possibility of making some decisions. As participants notice the details within various elements as well as the elements themselves, the underlying values and how these are operating come to light.

Both values clarification and the exploration of alternatives are important processes for understanding the nature of right and responsible moral/ethical decisions in relation to the knowledge form that is generated. The juxtaposition of personally cherished but problematic values (from values clarification) and possible alternative values (from the exploration of alternatives) deepens an individual's understanding of what is possible and what is necessary for nursing practice. When problematic value positions are challenged by a person who sees that alternative positions are possible in certain situations, personal values can change.

The creative processes of clarifying and exploring include (whether recognized or not) references to justice and care perspectives that involve ethical decision making, as well as to ethical principles and codes that are consistent with the deontologic and teleologic perspectives. Within our model, therefore, exploring and clarifying processes occur when questions are raised about what is right behavior and what is responsible behavior. From these creative processes, formal expressions of ethical knowledge are created and recreated, and the integrated expression of ethical knowledge in practice as moral/ethical comportment is promoted.

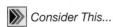 Consider This...

Penny Thompson, a geriatric nurse, works in a small community hospital in upstate Wisconsin. The hospital serves several small communities near Lake Michigan. As she goes about her routine work one afternoon, she is paged to the emergency department and asked to report quickly because "Charlie and Agnes are back." Charlie and Agnes Miller are in their mid-80s, and they have been permanent residents of the area for more than 40 years. Their children have married and moved away, but they have strong ties to their lakefront property and they hope to live out the remainder of their lives there. Lately, Charlie has been acting strangely and, as Agnes says, generally "getting into trouble." Several incidents have brought Charlie and Agnes to the emergency department, and this is their fourth visit in less than a month. This time, Agnes called an ambulance: Charlie could not get up from his shower chair, he seemed incoherent, and he was in danger of falling. Until recently, Charlie has generally been able to manage himself. However, for the past year, he has had increasing trouble with balance and walking, and he has also begun to swear and talk loudly as he relates stories of his past work on the railroad. This is unusual, because swearing used to be something that he would never do. Most troublingly for Agnes has been his tendency to drive their pickup truck irresponsibly. During the past 6 months, he has had several incidents of overturning mailboxes, he drove off the road into a ditch a few times, and once he ran into the neighbor's garage wall and caused significant damage. After one winter's day incident of driving into the ditch, Charlie, cold and confused, was picked up by a passerby; however, Charlie was unable to remember his address, so he was taken to the local police station. Neighbors, who are concerned for their safety and their property, have been calling the police when they see Charlie driving, and, on multiple occasions, officers have escorted him home. Charlie has been generally healthy throughout his life, but he does have a history of hypertension as well as a permanent colostomy as a result of colon cancer surgery 5 years ago. Although Penny has tried on several occasions to refer Charlie for a diagnostic workup, this would require travel to a health sciences center located several hours away, and Charlie refuses to go, declaring, "There's nothing wrong with me!" Agnes feels powerless to manage Charlie, and she is reluctant to trouble the children because "they have their own lives." However, Agnes is increasingly unable to continue with the situation as it is. What knowledge related to ethical knowing is required to manage this situation? What knowledge from within the other patterns of knowing is required to manage this situation?

FORMAL EXPRESSIONS OF ETHICAL KNOWING: PRINCIPLES AND CODES

The formal expressions of ethical knowledge that we have identified are principles and codes, which are common in nursing (Numminen & Leino-Kilpi, 2009; Salmela, Koskinen, & Eriksson, 2017; Schmidt, MacWilliams, & Neal-Boylan, 2017). However, other forms do exist. Ethical knowledge may be sets of rules; statements of duties, rights, or obligations; theory; or laws. The Nightingale Pledge (which, we would like to add, was not created by Florence Nightingale) and the Hippocratic Oath also are forms of ethical knowledge. An individual nurse or a group of nurses setting forth an ethical position for disciplinary use could put that position in the form of an article, a case analysis, or even a poem (Bliss, Baltzly, Bull, Dalton, & Jones, 2017; Jacobs, 2013; Kangasniemi, Pakkanen, & Korhonen, 2015; Norlyk, Haahr, Dreyer, & Martinsen, 2017; Salmela et al., 2017; Sanner-Stiehr & Ward-Smith, 2017; Schmidt et al., 2017; Van Der Zande, Baart, & Vosman, 2014).

We choose principles and codes as generic forms of ethical knowledge because they are attainable and common forms of ethical knowledge in nursing. For example, the American Nurses Association has created a Code of Ethics for Nurses ("Code of Ethics for Nurses with Interpretive Statements," 2015). Nurses are also taught to operate within common forms of ethical knowledge, such as principles of autonomy and beneficence. We prefer to avoid associating ethical knowledge forms with theory to prevent confusion about the differences between ethical and empiric theories. Regardless of its form, we believe that, eventually, ethical knowledge can be reduced to principles and codes, which are shorthand ways of expressing ethical knowing.

CONCLUSION

This chapter focused on the development of ethics in nursing. Ethical perspectives common in nursing were reviewed and the nature of ethics in nursing explored. Critical questions and creative processes of values clarification and exploration of alternatives lead to formal expressions of ethical knowledge.

References

ACA New Patients Bill of Rights. (2010, June 22). https://www.cms.gov/CCIIO/Resources/Fact-Sheets-and-FAQs/aca-new-patients-bill-of-rights.html.

Bandman, E. L., & Bandman, B. (2001). *Nursing ethics through the life span* (4th ed.). Upper Saddle River, NJ: Prentice Hall.

Barnes, M., & Brannelly, T. (2008). Achieving care and social justice for people with dementia. *Nursing Ethics, 15,* 384–395.

Bell, S. E., & Hulbert, J. R. (2008). Translating social justice into clinical nurse specialist practice. *Clinical Nurse Specialist: The Journal for Advanced Nursing Practice, 22,* 293–301.

Blackburn, S. (2005). *Truth: a guide.* New York, NY: Oxford University Press.

Bliss, S., Baltzly, D., Bull, R., Dalton, L., & Jones, J. (2017). A role for virtue in unifying the "knowledge" and "caring" discourses in nursing theory. *Nursing Inquiry.* https://doi.org/10.1111/nin.12191.

Burkhardt, M. A., & Nathaniel, A. K. (2007). *Ethics and issues in contemporary nursing* (3rd ed.). New York, NY: Delmar Publishers.

Carper, B. A. (1978). Fundamental patterns of knowing in nursing. *ANS. Advances in Nursing Science, 1,* 13–23.

Carper, B. A. (1979). The ethics of caring. *ANS. Advances in Nursing Science, 1,* 11–19.

Catalano, J. T. (2008). *Nursing now: today's issues, tomorrow's trends* (5th ed.). Philadelphia, PA: F.A. Davis.

Code of Ethics for Nurses with Interpretive Statements. (2015). http://www.nursingworld.org/MainMenu Categories/EthicsStandards/CodeofEthicsforNurses/Code-of-Ethics-For-Nurses.html.

Condon, E. H. (1992). Nursing and the caring metaphor: gender and political influences on an ethics of care. *Nursing Outlook, 40,* 14–19.

Cook, L. B., & Peden, A. (2016). Finding a focus for nursing: the caring concept. *ANS. Advances in Nursing Science.* https://doi.org/10.1097/ANS.0000000000000137.

Cooper, M. C. (1991). Principle-oriented ethics and the ethic of care: a creative tension. *ANS. Advances in Nursing Science, 14,* 22–31.

Ellis, J. R., & Hartley, C. L. (2004). *Nursing in today's world: trends, issues and management* (8th ed.). Philadelphia, PA: Lippincott, Williams & Wilkins.

Frame, M. W., & Williams, C. B. (2005). A model of ethical decision-making from a multicultural perspective. *Counseling and Values, 49,* 165–179.

Fry, S. T. (1989). Toward a theory of nursing ethics. *ANS. Advances in Nursing Science, 11,* 9–22.

Gilligan, C. (1982). *In a different voice: psychological theory and women's development.* Boston, MA: Harvard University Press.

Health Information Privacy. (1996). http://www.hhs.gov/ocr/privacy/.

Hoagland, S. L. (1990). Some concerns about Nel Noddings' caring. *Hypatia, 5,* 109–114.

Houston, B. (1990). Caring and exploitation. *Hypatia, 5,* 115–119.

Jacobs, B. B. (2013). An innovative professional practice model: Adaptation of Carper's patterns of knowing, patterns of research, and Aristotle's intellectual virtues. *ANS. Advances in Nursing Science, 36*(4), 271–288. https://doi.org/10.1097/ANS.0000000000000002.

Kangasniemi, M., Pakkanen, P., & Korhonen, A. (2015). Professional ethics in nursing: an integrative review. *Journal of Advanced Nursing, 71*(8), 1744–1757. https://doi.org/10.1111/jan.12619.

Kohlberg, L. (1976). Moral stages and moralization: the cognitive-developmental approach. In T. Lickona (Ed.), *Moral development and behavior: theory, research, and social issues.* New York, NY: Holt, Rinhart & Winston.

Levine, M. E. (1989). The ethics of nursing rhetoric. *Image - The Journal of Nursing Scholarship, 21,* 4–6.

LGBT Healthcare Bill of Rights. (2016). http://healthcarebillofrights.org/Read-The-Bill.

Liaschenko, J. (1993). Feminist ethics and cultural ethos: revisiting a nursing debate. *ANS. Advances in Nursing Science, 15,* 71–81.

Liaschenko, J., & Peter, E. (2004). Nursing ethics and conceptualizations of nursing: profession, practice, work. *Journal of Advanced Nursing, 46,* 488–495.

Liaschenko, J., Oguz, N. Y., & Brunnquell, D. (2006). Critique of the "tragic case" method in ethics education. *Journal of Medical Ethics, 32,* 672–677.

Mappes, R. A., & DeGrazia, D. (2006). *Biomedical ethics* (5th ed.). New York, NY: McGraw-Hill.

Mathur, R. (2015, October). Children's bill of rights. https://campaignforchildren.org/wp-content/uploads/sites/2/2015/10/Childrens-Bill-of-Rights.pdf.

Noddings, N. (1999). Care, justice, and equity. In M. S. Katz, N. Noddings, & K. A. Strike (Eds.), *Justice and caring: the search for common ground in education* (pp. 7–20). New York, NY: Teachers College Press.

Noddings, N. (2003). *Caring: a feminine approach to ethics & moral education* (2nd ed.). Berkeley, CA: University of California Press.

Norlyk, A., Haahr, A., Dreyer, P., & Martinsen, B. (2017). Lost in transformation? Reviving ethics of care in hospital cultures of evidence-based healthcare. *Nursing Inquiry.* https://doi.org/10.1111/nin.12187.

Numminen, O., & Leino-Kilpi, H. (2009). Nurses' codes of ethics in practice and education: a review of the literature. *Scandinavian Journal of Caring Sciences, 23,* 380–394.

Patient's Bill of Rights Under the Affordable Care Act: An Overview of the Rules on Consumer Protections. (2010). http://www.phlp.org/wp-content/uploads/2010/08/Catalyst-Patients_Bill_of_Rights_Fact_Sheet_8.20.10.pdf.

Peter, E., & Liaschenko, J. (2013). Moral distress reexamined: a feminist interpretation of nurses' identities, relationships, and responsibilities. *Journal of Bioethical Inquiry, 10*(3), 337–345. https://doi.org/10.1007/s11673-013-9456-5.

Reverby, S. M. (1987). *Ordered to care: the dilemma of American nursing.* Cambridge, MA: Cambridge University Press, 1850–1945.

Salmela, S., Koskinen, C., & Eriksson, K. (2017). Nurse leaders as managers of ethically sustainable caring cultures. *Journal of Advanced Nursing, 73*(4), 871–882. https://doi.org/10.1111/jan.13184.

Sander-Staudt, M. (2011). Care ethics. http://www.iep.utm.edu/care-eth/.

Sanner-Stiehr, E., & Ward-Smith, P. (2017). Lateral violence in nursing: implications and strategies for nurse educators. *Journal of Professional Nursing: Official Journal of the American Association of Colleges of Nursing, 33*(2), 113–118. https://doi.org/10.1016/j.profnurs.2016.08.007.

Schmidt, B. J., MacWilliams, B. R., & Neal-Boylan, L. (2017). Becoming inclusive: a code of conduct for inclusion and diversity. *Journal of Professional Nursing: Official Journal of the American Association of Colleges of Nursing, 33*(2), 102–107. https://doi.org/10.1016/j.profnurs.2016.08.014.

Simon, S., Howe, L., & Kirschenbaum, H. (1995). *Values clarification: a handbook of practical strategies for teachers and students (Revised).* New York, NY: Hart Publishing Co.

Stewart, I. M. (1921). Some fundamental principles in the teaching of ethics. *The American Journal of Nursing,* *21,* 906–913.

The Patients' Bill of Rights in Medicare and Medicaid. (1999). http://archive.hhs.gov/news/press/1999pres/990412.html.

Thompson, J. L. (2007). Poststructuralist feminist analysis in nursing. In C. Roy, & D. A. Jones (Eds.), *Nursing knowledge development and clinical practice* (pp. 129–143). New York, NY: Springer Publishing.

Tong, R. (2008). *Feminist thought: a more comprehensive introduction* (3rd ed.). Boulder, CO: Westview Press.

Van Der Zande, M., Baart, A., & Vosman, F. (2014). Ethical sensitivity in practice: Finding tacit moral knowing. *Journal of Advanced Nursing, 70*(1), 68–76. https://doi.org/10.1111/jan.12154.

van Hooft, S. (2011). Caring, objectivity and justice: an integrative view. *Nursing Ethics, 18*(2), 149–160. https://doi.org/10.1177/0969733010388927.

Vanlaere, L., & Gastmans, C. (2011). A personalist approach to care ethics. *Nursing Ethics, 18*(2), 161–173. https://doi.org/10.1177/0969733010388924.

Walker, M. U. (1993). Keeping moral space open. *The Hastings Center Report, 23,* 33–40.

Personal Knowledge Development

Self is a dynamic concept, ever deepening as we expand and broaden our relationships with others. The Self is created in relation to others.

Beverly Hall and Janet Allan (1994, p. 112)

T he opening quote for this chapter suggests that people know who they are through their relationships with others, and that who a person is changes over time. In this context, the idea of relationships does not imply only close or intimate relationships, as with a partner or spouse. Rather, relationships include contacts and interactions with the people you relate to from day to day. These relationships can be close in varying degrees, casual, and even so subtle as to go unnoticed. In addition, in the context of personal knowing for this text, you can also have a relationship with your Self that reflects who you really are compared with the Self you project or you want others to see.

 Consider This...

A young woman named Alia might be characterized a "jet-setter." Alia has much wealth at her disposal and has not had to work or become educated to maintain her standard of living. She is hospitalized because she was driving while alcohol impaired and sustained multiple injuries when her sports car ran off a cliff.

Christie is assigned to care for Alia. Christie has come to know her own personal Self as a hardworking person who is responsible. Christie knows this largely because her parents and teachers have reflected to her and her brothers the importance of "making something of themselves." Her parents taught their children to work hard, to get a good education, and to contribute meaningfully to society. Christie did this, although it was not easy. Her parents also reflected to the children that those who have wealth and do nothing productive are undeserving if not contemptible. As a result, as a nurse she has a deeply held value that worthiness is a byproduct of being responsible and socially productive. At the same time, Christie was also taught in her nursing program that each person deserves to be respected and cared for as an individual, despite who they may be, and that each person is inherently valuable. Because of who Christie is, as a personal Self, if she did become aware that her nursing care for Alia was lacking in any way, she would be distressed.

As Christie cares for Alia, it is inevitable that who Christie is as a person—her core Self—will affect her nursing care. Without fully realizing it, because of her background, experiences, and values, Christie might hold resentments or stereotypes about people who are wealthy and privileged. She might become slightly punitive and withhold comfort measures just a little while longer than she otherwise would, or she might conveniently forget to call the kitchen when a special menu request is made, explaining to Alia that she became busy with another patient. She might not make an effort to understand anything about Alia as a human being, but rather focus on her care as just another situation to tolerate and get through. In this example, the Self of Christie and her care would benefit by a focus on personal knowing.

Personal knowing is the basis for the expression of an authentic or genuine Self. It is also essential for a healing relationship and fundamental to the essence of what it means to be human (Green, 2009; Zolnierek, 2014). In the "Consider this" example of the nurse caring for Alia, assume that Christie was able to tolerate Alia despite her feelings toward wealthy people and thus was able to provide acceptable care. Tolerance alone does not engender the growth of personal knowing. If Christie began to reflect on how she truly felt about Alia, she could then begin to recognize the basis of her feelings and how those feelings affect her nursing care. As Christie reflects on her background and how it influences who she is, she can make a conscious choice about the person that she wants to be as a nurse. Through this process, the nurse becomes more genuine and authentic. Her actions grow to be more in harmony with what she would choose them to be: compassionate and caring toward Alia, just as they would be toward any other person.

In this chapter we examine various meanings of personal knowing, and various ideas that are related to, or influence the development of, personal knowing. In a sense, all knowing is personal, because people can only know their own understandings, mental images, perceptions, experiences, memories, and thoughts (Bonis, 2009). However, for the purposes of this text and for the construct of patterns of knowing in nursing, we use the concept of *personal knowing* to refer to a process of Self-knowing that is conscious; it is developed deliberately to know fully who you are and to understand your actions and relationships. Personal knowing is shaped by your relationships with others, and it also shapes your relationships when caring for others. As such, personal knowing is a conscious process that cultivates your wholeness and the wholeness of others.

Fig. 5.1 provides an overview of the personal knowing pattern of our model for knowledge development in nursing. Nurses bring to their practice the Self they are. As they care for others and reflect on their caring practices, knowing arises as they ask critical questions: "Do I know what I do?" and "Do I do what I know?" The creative processes of opening and centering flow from these questions, and these creative processes foster the development of formal expressions of personal knowing. As seen in Fig. 5.1, the integrated expression of personal knowing in practice is the therapeutic use of the Self.

Table 5.1 lists the processes of creating personal knowing, showing the dimensions that we explore in this chapter—the processes of opening and centering, and the formal expressions of personal knowing—the genuine Self and the stories that reflect the genuine Self in written form. This chapter opens with an exploration of the conceptual meanings of personal knowing in nursing and then

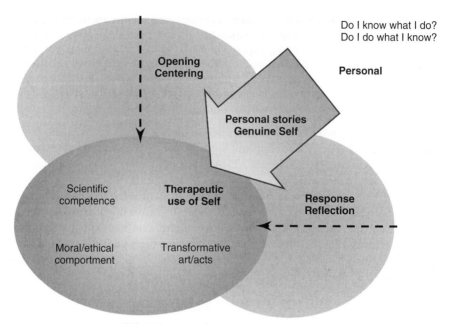

FIG. 5.1 Personal Knowing and Knowledge.

TABLE 5.1 Dimensions of Personal Knowing

Dimension	Personal
Critical questions	Do I know what I do? Do I do what I know?
Creative processes	Opening Centering
Formal expressions	Personal stories Genuine self
Authentication processes	Response Reflection
Integrated expression in practice	Therapeutic use of self

details the critical questions, creative processes, and formal expressions of personal knowing.

Personal knowing requires that you be in touch with who you are and understand that who you are as a person affects your behavior, attitudes, and values both positively and negatively. Personal knowing involves much more than simply knowing basic characteristics that define who you are—your weight, birthdate, certain personality characteristics, tendencies, preferences, biases etc. Rather, knowing the Self—personal knowing—involves awareness of your inner experience in each situation, recognition of the ways you are interacting in the moment and bringing together in the moment your understanding and insights. Through personal knowing, you live your life with deliberate intent; your actions come to be in harmony with your deepest intentions. In short, personal knowing is the dynamic process of becoming a whole, aware Self and of knowing the other as being valued and whole. It brings you to a place of knowing what you do and doing what you know.

 Think About It...

- What is the difference, for you, between "knowing about the self" and "knowing the Self"?
- How has your Self-knowing benefited or compromised your nursing care?
- Have you ever cared for someone who you simply cannot relate to or who represents something you cannot accept? How was care affected?
- Is there anything about your Self that you know you would like to shift in order to be a better nurse?
- How difficult or easy would it be for you to change some aspect of your Self? What would it require?

PERSONAL KNOWING IN NURSING

Personal knowing as knowledge of the Self is perhaps the most difficult pattern to understand, because the nature of the Self and knowing the Self are elusive concepts. The ideal of personal knowing is to become a more whole and authentic Self. To know who you are, you need to embrace, internalize, and reflect on the responses that you receive from others as a clue to the Self that you are. As you more fully understand your Self, you realize possibilities for who you might become in the future as you grow and develop.

Personal knowing is expressed as the Self: the person you are. In other words, you are known to others because of who you are. Initially, people recognize you because you have a certain appearance; your face and other features of your physical self are recognizable. People begin to know you by name. As they come to really know you as a person, people recognize not only your physical appearance but qualities of your Self that are expressed through your actions and the daily choices that you make. You might be known as someone who has a great sense of humor, who likes beans but not carrots, who loves to dance, or who is afraid of heights. All these things and many more constitute the "you" that others come to know, and these make you distinctly recognizable as you and not someone else. Others experience and know you as unique by virtue of your personal qualities that are conveyed through being in the world within the context of the culture.

You know your Self as the person you are in part because of how others perceive you. You may not appreciate your sense of humor, for example, unless other people come to recognize this in you and give you feedback. You might not be aware that your food likes and dislikes are so obvious to others, and once you sense how they react to your being a certain kind of eater, you might decide to learn to change how you approach your food choices. At a deeper level, you may begin to see yourself as somewhat selfish or insensitive. Regardless, as you reflect not only on the reactions of others but also on how it feels to you *to be* you, you begin to make deliberate choices about the type of person you really want to be in the world. This process is what we refer to as *personal knowing*. It is an ongoing process that leads to change and growth toward wholeness, authenticity, mind-body-spirit congruence, and genuineness.

One formal expression of personal knowing is the *genuine* Self. The genuine Self conveys directly, without words, who one is. Personal or autobiographic stories are also formal expressions of personal knowing but are less direct than the actual Self (i.e., the person you are in the world). Personal stories are limited in their capacity to convey the fullness of the person, but they provide a means of communication with a wide audience and illuminate various paths to the creation of a more genuine Self.

Response and *reflection* are the authentication processes within the personal knowing pattern. Response and reflection in relation to personal knowledge expressions are necessary for us to know who we are as individuals, and they are the basis for continued growth. According to our model, nurses who practice using personal knowledge that has been strengthened through the authentication processes of reflection and response will increasingly improve with regard to the ability to use the Self therapeutically.

CONCEPTUAL MEANINGS OF PERSONAL KNOWING

Carper's early description of personal knowing points directly to transcendent interpersonal encounters as central, defining qualities of personal knowing:

> One does not know about the self; one simply strives to know the self. This knowing is a process of symbolically standing in relation to another human being and confronting that human being as a person. This "I-Thou" encounter is unmediated by conceptual categories or particulars abstracted from complex organic wholes. The relation is one of reciprocity, a state of being that cannot be described or even experienced—it only can be actualized (1978, p. 18).

For Carper, personal knowing is connected to an "I-Thou" encounter that actualizes the Self in a way that is instantaneous and transcendent. If you have ever had an experience, most likely a powerful and memorable one, during which you "just knew" or "understood" something about another and your Self without contemplating or thinking about the person, you most likely have experienced what Carper conceptualized personal knowing to be. This sort of personal knowing happens in a compelling human-to-human moment, and it is both transcendent and immediate. For Carper, personal knowing actualizes the wholeness and integrity in each encounter and immediately knows and affirms the Self of the person.

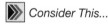 *Consider This...*

> Examples are difficult because personal knowing as conceptualized by Carper is not explained or recounted, it is only experienced. However, an encounter described by a young nurse, Rebecca, serves as an example. A young man she was caring for was slowly dying from an abdominal gunshot wound sustained while committing a petty

crime. One day, during the course of care, this young man motioned for Rebecca to come to his bedside. As she approached, he held out his arms, pulled her in close to his face, and whispered, "You are the best nurse I ever had." In that moment, this young man was fully known not as a criminal or a dying man but simply as a person. It was an unmediated and unexpected knowing of Self and other that just was. To this day, the recollection of this moment that occurred more than 40 years ago is still vivid and powerful for Rebecca. We believe that this type of in-the-moment knowing of another is the "I-Thou" experience that Carper associated with personal knowing.

PERSONAL KNOWING AS SPIRITUAL IN NATURE

Personal knowing has been linked with spirit and to what is sometimes referred to as *spiritual understanding* (Barnum, 2010; Bishop & Scudder, 1990; Pesut, 2008; Pesut, Fowler, Taylor, Reimer-Kirkham, & Sawatzky, 2008; Register & Herman, 2010). *Spirit* is a term derived from the Latin word for "breath" and "breathing," which are basic to sustaining life and being (Huebner, 1985).

The term *spiritual* is often associated with religion, a tradition that Hall (1997) identified as deriving from the fact that Western culture limits the expression of what is known either to science or to religion. Because of this, alternative conceptualizations of the spiritual have not been as visible as those that associate spirituality with religion. Many people do connect their spirituality with religious beliefs; however, that which is spiritual does not of necessity link with religiosity (Campesino & Schwartz, 2006; McSherry & Cash, 2004; Pesut, 2016; Pesut et al., 2008; Tinley & Kinney, 2007). Rather, the spiritual is a complex combination of values, attitudes, and hopes that is linked to the transcendent and that guides and directs a person's life. It is particularly associated with life experiences that bring one to the brink of uncertainty: the "existential boundary issues" of life and death, good and evil, hopes and dreams, and despair and suffering. Personal knowing, when viewed as being spiritual in nature, provides a way for people to understand and shape their lives as they confront difficult challenges. This form of spirituality helps people to face the inevitable realities of life that create vulnerabilities and that cannot be overcome. Spirituality nurtures a personal agency for relating to such vulnerabilities (Hart, 1997).

Hall (1997) presented a conception of human spirit and spirituality as reaching within to learn to accept, love, and value what you find there and learning to be yourself authentically and with confidence. What you find may not be what you want to find, but you either change or come to live with, accept, and love what is within. This spirituality is not a process of self-centered exploration, nor is it linear. Rather, it is an unfolding process that is grounded in the context of everyday experience in relationship with others.

Think About It...

- Would you describe the experience of Rebecca who was told she was the best ever to be a spiritual one?
- Have you had what you would describe as spiritual experiences during the course of caring for others?
- What characteristics make such experiences spiritual?

PERSONAL KNOWING AS SELF-IN-RELATION

Hall and Allan (1994) explained the vital link between personal knowing and relationships with others in their concept of Self-in-relation. Personal knowing and wholistic nursing practice are possible through Self-in-relation, which is the core of caring and healing. These authors' ideas are grounded in traditional Chinese medicine, which philosophically views the mind, body, spirit, and environment as an integrated whole. The embodied Self is an open system that belongs to a social world. The caring relationships that nurses enter into can reflect four dynamics that nurture Self-in-relation, as follows:

Caring by giving requires being present and involved in relation with others. In this process, mutual sharing develops the Self and the other by giving to one another and by affirming the value and purpose of each life.

Empowerment develops a sense of the Self as being responsible for one's own health and involves the context in which health is possible for everyone. Empowerment in relationship gives rise to the ability to influence one's own health outcomes. When the self is fully in relation with the other, both are empowered, and unconditional love occurs. Both learn the joy of reciprocity, which occurs when what each brings to the interaction is deeply valued.

Knowing the value of a human life comes from a mutual quest to find meaning in life. In a healing relationship, questions of living and dying come to the surface, thus inviting an openness to explore what is possible in a particular time and space. Openness while fully engaging with another person in this quest develops the self in each.

Sense of community is the most important and yet the most elusive concept. Basically, this dynamic means that a supportive and caring community is required for the development of Self-in-relation.

PERSONAL KNOWING AS DISCOVERY OF THE SELF AND THE OTHER

Moch (1990) defined personal knowing as the discovery of the Self and other that is arrived at through reflection, the synthesis of perceptions, and connecting with what is known. She identified three overlapping components of personal knowing: (1) experiential knowing, (2) interpersonal knowing, and (3) intuitive knowing.

Experiential knowing is the understanding and knowledge that comes from participating in the events of daily living; it is deepened by attending to the experience, studying the process of the experience, and connecting the experience to previous understandings. Attending to the experience involves being aware of what one is feeling and sensing, and observing the Self and others. For Moch, both cognitive and spiritual processes contribute to deriving meaning from experience. *Interpersonal knowing* is increased awareness as a result of interaction or being with another. It emerges from intense attending to the moment, opening the Self to the other, and conveying feelings to one another. *Intuitive knowing* is the immediate knowing of something without the conscious use of reason.

Moch (1990) identified the following attributes of personal knowing:

- Personal knowing can be viewed only in the context of wholeness; there is no knowing apart from the knower.

- Personal knowing includes a process of encountering. The ideal encounter is one of mutual respect that affirms those involved in the encounter.
- Personal knowing involves passion, commitment, and integrity. Passion affirms something as valuable, commitment motivates the search for personal meaning, and integrity brings thought and action together as an authentic whole.
- Personal knowing is the instantaneous "aha" experience during which one's perspective shifts, either consciously or unconsciously.

PERSONAL KNOWING AS UNKNOWING

Munhall (1993) reflected Carper's point that knowing the other sets aside personal assumptions and generalizations. She stressed the nature of a genuinely authentic encounter by conceptualizing a pattern of "unknowing" to signify the openness to the other that must occur during such an encounter. Unknowing creates a stance that is completely open to the experiences and perceptions of others as they experience them and not filtered by the nurse's own structures of understanding. Unknowing means setting aside all that is assumed to be known about the other, as well as previously held organizing structures that make sense of the world. This requires a "decentering" from the perspective of the Self and a movement toward considering the perspective of the other. This occurs when the nurse takes a deliberate stance of complete openness and receptivity to the unique subjectivity of the other and remains open to a deep knowledge of the other, to different meanings and interpretations, and to varying perceptions of the world. Unknowing is similar to the phenomenologic process of "bracketing" but specifically refers to a type of personal openness that is more than intellectual; it is a full mind-body-spirit openness that creates existential availability to know another deeply.

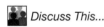 *Discuss This...*

> Ask a trusted friend or colleague to share with you his or her impressions of who you are as a nurse. Let the person know that you are not seeking compliments or praise but that you want an honest reflection of how you come across to others in your practice. Reflect on the perceptions that this person shares with you. Are there aspects of his or her perceptions that you feel are not fully consistent with who you are? Did he or she describe traits that you would like to develop in different ways?

SUMMARY: COMMON MEANINGS FOR PERSONAL KNOWING

Despite certain distinctions in each of these conceptualizations of the meaning of personal knowing, important threads are common to all. These threads form the conceptual understandings on which our approaches to developing personal knowing are based, as follows:

- Personal knowing grows out of relationships and interactions with others and out of deep reflection on experiences with others.
- Personal knowing goes beyond cognitive reasoning; it depends on reflection that brings about an awareness of meaning and direction in one's life.

- Personal knowing brings about congruence between one's actions and one's values.
- Personal knowing brings about a wholeness that embraces the entirety of existence and experience.

DIMENSIONS OF PERSONAL KNOWING

Personal knowing is fundamental to nursing because interpersonal relationships are inherent in nursing practice. Meaningful interpersonal connections do not occur in a vacuum and are not happenstance. Well-developed personal knowing is a requirement for being fully present with another. Personal knowing can be nurtured and encouraged as an important dimension of competent, quality care (Pai, 2015).

The label "personal knowing" can be misleading in that it can imply a solitary and individual process that involves only the unique perceptions of the individual. However, as shown by our overview of the conceptualizations of personal knowing, relatedness is essential for the development of personal knowing. Personal knowing does require deep inner reflection that is sometimes solitary and that comes from within the individual; in other words, it involves a form of the Self in relation with the Self. However, personal knowing also requires openness to experience the world and to have mutual meaningful interactions with others. Contemporary popular notions of self-actualization and individuation reinforce images of the individual on a lone, often self-indulgent journey of discovery. Moreover, contemporary cultures that primarily value empiric knowing reinforce the limited and mistaken notion that people are essentially rational egos who seek individual autonomy, rights, and freedoms (Hart, 1997). Despite these dominant cultural contexts, personal knowing is not a quest of a rational, autonomous ego. Rather, personal knowing as we view it is intimately connected to relationships with others. In the following section, we focus on the epistemological aspects of how we come to know and express the whole, genuine Self and enhance the authentic being of the other.

CRITICAL QUESTIONS: DO I KNOW WHAT I DO? DO I DO WHAT I KNOW?

In our model of knowledge development in nursing, the pattern of personal knowing requires asking two critical questions: "Do I know what I do?" and "Do I do what I know?" These questions, as with the other patterns, can be asked apart from the context of practice or in the moment of practice. These questions assess the character of the Self and the extent of the therapeutic use of the Self in care situations, and they initiate the ongoing process of personal knowing.

 Think About It...

Think about caring for a person whom you typically view in a negative light. We use the examples of an older person with dementia, a morbidly obese woman with diabetes, and a homosexual man with acquired immunodeficiency syndrome. The care provided for people with traits that are often stigmatized is often jeopardized and influenced by the typical stereotypes associated with who they are and what they are experiencing. You may not want to face some of your own inner thoughts and feelings, but facing your inner Self honestly is a necessary part of knowing the Self.

All nurses bring to their work an understanding of the Self that guides how they use that Self therapeutically. Asking the critical question "Do I do what I know?" creates an awareness of the values of the good nursing care that you believe in and reflection on the extent to which you are providing that form of care in this situation. The critical question "Do I know what I do?" brings about reflection on what you know to be the care you are providing and the realization that perhaps your practice is falling short because of the stigma and stereotyping that prevail with regard to particular individuals.

Each of the critical questions points to important aspects of the experience and processes involved in developing personal knowing. As you honestly ask and answer these questions, you will uncover areas for growth of the Self toward authenticity so that you will move toward doing what you know and knowing what you do.

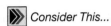 *Consider This...*

You are supervising nursing students and Sally has been assigned to care for 54-year-old John. John was born with a genetic condition that resulted in severe body disfigurement. Although mobile with a walker and persistent, his legs are twisted and it is a struggle for him to move about. His chest is enlarged and he has severe scoliosis. Other significant abnormalities of the head and chest area are also apparent as a result of his genetic makeup. As you make your rounds to see how the students are progressing you find Sally standing outside John's room looking at his electronic record. Sally has not been in to speak to John yet and you are somewhat surprised when Sally says, "I just don't know what to do."

Is Sally's personal knowing deficient, or is she doing what she knows?

- What, for Sally, might need to change in order for her to productively care for John?
- Might fear to approach another who is different suggest a need to work on personal knowing?
- How might getting to know John as a person add to personal knowing for Sally?

CREATIVE PROCESSES: OPENING AND CENTERING

As you or others ask the critical questions, the extent to which your "knowing Self" and your "doing Self" are congruent becomes clearer, and creative processes that acknowledge and develop your personal knowing can be initiated. The creative processes involved in developing personal knowing evolve in unique and individual patterns throughout a person's life, but there are ways to develop personal knowing that can be described and carried out.

The ability to grow toward becoming a more genuine and authentic Self requires deliberate preparation and intent. Fig. 5.2 depicts the creative processes of opening and centering. Over time, these processes ground the individual in the center of the Self (represented by the heart in the figure) so that the Self is known, valued, affirmed, and loved for what it is. Specific opening and centering practices that can be used are journaling,

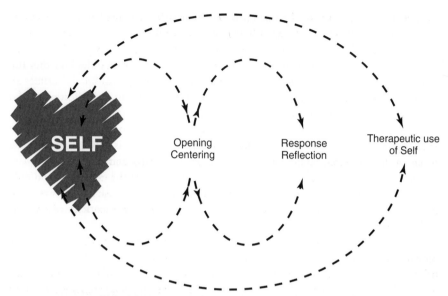

FIG. 5.2 Creative Processes of Opening and Centering.

meditation, and various body-mind-spirit practices such as yoga, tai chi, labyrinth walking, drumming, and chanting. These types of meditations bring mind-body-spirit into wholeness, create a time-space of inner calm and peace, and bring personal intentions and meanings to realization at a deep level that transcends consciousness. Such practices also make it possible to bring deeper meanings to conscious awareness to shape your actions in harmony with your inner intentions.

From time to time, realizations that come from private opening and centering processes enter into shared experiences with others, thus providing the opportunity to exchange responses and to integrate new perceptions and reflections. As you return to your private time-space of opening and centering, responses that you have received from others deepen and enrich your experience of your Self. In the figure, the inner dotted loops represent reflection as it moves through opening and centering, back and forth between the heart center of the Self and the interactive responses of others, to depict the circular movement among the aspects of opening and centering. Opening and centering provide the core strength and character that are necessary to enter into an authentic encounter in which the heart center or the Self of the person opens to be fully present with and for the other. The larger dotted oval represents how private opening and centering processes that are shared with others to create a more genuine and authentic Self in turn foster increasingly authentic encounters with others and support the therapeutic use of the Self.

The processes of opening and centering to grow in personal knowing are different from therapy or counseling. Therapy can assist a person with his or her quest for personal knowing, but therapy involves other purposes that focus on returning one's Self from a troubled or disturbed situation to one that is less troubled and more able to cope with life's difficulties. Therapy often involves an unequal relationship in which one person provides therapeutic guidance and the other receives it. Many practices that are used for opening and centering (e.g., meditation, journaling, labyrinth walking, tai chi) can also be used for therapeutic purposes. However, opening and centering are vital processes that are required to fully know the Self and to constantly deepen inner knowing and self-wisdom, regardless of therapeutic or healing needs.

For some, opening and centering can be closely linked to the concept or experience of prayer. Prayer is often thought of as a process of communing with a higher power, a divine being, or the universe. Meditative opening and centering are ways of listening to your own heart, your own Self, and your own inner wisdom (Hall, 2008). For those who have a spiritual view of the divine or universal essence as residing within, or part of the Self, this experience is very close to our concept of opening and centering

The creative processes of personal knowing can be integrated into daily life and can provide a focus on knowing the Self as a whole, authentic being. These processes contribute to self-healing and focus the energy of the Self without interference from outside sources. Opening and centering can be facilitated by others or enhanced by joining with others to share in a particular self-healing practice. However, opening and centering require one's own deepest intentions and attention. When opening and centering to nurture Self-knowing, the individual reaches into an attentive mind-body-spirit center to come to know and love what resides within.

Opening and centering are interrelated and occur in many different ways and in many different contexts. The processes of opening and centering focus on your lived experience and the meaning of that experience. These processes can be engaged spontaneously or can be deliberately scheduled as individual, solitary processes that contribute to self-knowing (Beckerman, 1994).

In the following section we discuss two specific practices that you can use for opening and centering: journaling and meditation. These practices nurture Self-knowing and prepare the Self for authentic encounters. Although we focus here on journaling and meditation, you may find and use many other approaches to the creative processes of opening and centering.

OPENING AND CENTERING PRACTICES: JOURNALING AND MEDITATION

Journaling is an avenue for opening and centering that nurtures Self-knowing. It is a private encounter with the inner Self. Through journaling, you can be your Self without fear of judgment by others. You can acknowledge those things about your Self that might otherwise be hidden. Journaling provides a platform for understanding the Self, for growth, and for change (Banks-Wallace, 2008).

Meditation often goes hand in hand with journaling. Meditation requires clearing the mind and inviting a deep inner awareness to emerge. Both journaling and meditation benefit from consistent and regular practice, time devoted to the practice, and solitude away from other people and things. There are many different reasons for journaling. In the context of developing personal knowing, what you write is never to be shared with others unless you choose to do so. To be a useful practice for full discovery and knowledge of the Self, your journal should be something that you write with the intention of keeping it private to maintain your sense of safety for the expression of whatever feelings and perceptions emerge from deep within. In your journaling, you can let fears, anxieties, anger, and fantasies surface without even your own censoring. There are no critics peering into the inner Self; even your own critical judgment is withheld as you seek to know and understand your deepest Self.

We reserve the term *journal* for the type of private opening and centering process writing that is not to be shared with others. If you do decide to share something from your journal but you are not comfortable sharing it in the form in which it appears in your journal, you can extract and revise segments from your journal with the intent of sharing with others for response. Alternatively, you might be required to write what someone refers to as a "journal" as an assignment that must be shared with one or more other people. When you write something that you are required to share or that you plan to share, consider starting with the kind of private writing that we describe here, to gain the deepest insights so that your inner knowing can flourish. You can then revise your private journal into a document that can be shared, and you can include only what you are willing to share with others (Nelson, 2010).

As you settle into a time for journaling, begin with meditation: Sit still and quietly, turn your focus to your breath, and take several deep breaths. Let the sense of your being settle into a centered space. You can repeat a sound, a mantra, or an affirmation that brings your focus closer to your center and to your deepest intentions, hopes, and desires. Affirmations should begin with "I" and be stated in the present tense. In addition, they should be positive, reflect your personal way of talking, and be stated as if what you want to become has already happened. For example, you might repeat an affirmation such as "I am a loving and accepting person" or "I am at peace with the path of my life" (Chinn, 2013).

When you feel ready, move to your journal to begin to bring your inner perceptions to the page. Journaling can include recounting facts and events, but it should move beyond these to explore how you feel and what is going on inside of you. As other people enter your reflections, you can move back to your own center and explore your sense of being in the situation and the relationship. When journaling as an approach to personal knowing, it is important to let your innermost thoughts come to the surface, however difficult it may be. Acknowledging the nature of our deepest Self is critical to realizing our full, genuine, and authentic Self.

Journaling is a process of working from both the conscious and the subconscious and of engaging in an inner experience with the Self. The inner experience sensitizes your perceptions of events, people, and situations and brings you to a place of harmony and wholeness with who you are in relation to your world (Beckerman, 1994).

As you journal, abandon rules about written expression to express your feelings and perceptions fully. You can doodle, draw, and let nonverbal images find expression on the page. Let the unexpected emerge without censorship or judgment. Imagine what you hope and dream for and what your deepest desires are. If you feel drawn to analyze and judge what is coming forth, move back to nonverbal meditation, focus on your breath, and turn your attention once again to being open and feeling unconditional love and value for who you are. Insights will come from your journaling that enhance your ability to analyze and rationally think through problems, so you can let go of anything that is drawing your attention toward the rational processes of problem solving while you are journaling. Use journaling to deepen your own inner sense of worth and self-love, which will grant you greater clarity and strength to address the issues that you face day to day. While you are meditating and journaling, always treat yourself as if you totally love yourself (Nelson, 2010).

You can enter into journaling with a specific intent, or you can enter the time-space with no particular intent other than to let your perceptions of your inner being come to the surface. If you are new to journaling, or if you have had an experience or are involved in a situation that is saturating your consciousness, you can use a specific intent to focus your journaling and meditation. Again, the intent is not to solve problems but rather to explore a particular aspect of your inner Self. Images can also be used to focus your journaling and to draw you into your inner Self. Beckerman (1994) used works of art that depicted caring and focused her journaling on her perceptions of caring within the works of art. You can create an intention around your hopes and dreams, around memories, or around experiences. For example, you could write a prayer to express your deepest hopes and dreams. You could spend time journaling about different "selves" you have been throughout your life, such as your child Self, your afraid Self, and your confident Self. Typically, starting with a focus simply opens doors and begins the journey to deep reflection; the path of the reflection then moves in directions of personal change and growth.

The creative processes of opening and centering assist with the knowing of the genuine, authentic Self and with coming to understand and love who and what we are. It is this self-knowing and self-love that subsequently mobilize and allow us to continue to grow and change in ways that continue to heal and create wholeness in the Self and in others and to create a Self that is therapeutic in the context of care.

 Think About It...

Think back about Sally who is assigned to care for John (see p. 123).
- What sorts of things do you imagine Sally would journal about?
- How might the meditative exploration of her feelings about John lead to personal knowing and mitigate her fear?
- What factors about Sally might be revealed in her journal that account for her fear?
- Was there ever a patient or family you feared? How did you deal with it? What did you learn about your Self in this situation? Would meditative journaling been useful?
- Have you left a nursing care situation feeling regret or sadness at how you behaved? What would you say in your journal about it?

FORMAL EXPRESSIONS OF PERSONAL KNOWING: PERSONAL STORIES AND THE GENUINE SELF

Personal stories and the genuine Self are the formal expressions of personal knowing that emerge from the creative processes of opening and centering. The genuine Self, as Carper (1978) initially proposed, is the active, acted-in-the-world form of expression of personal knowing.

Personal stories provide a written form of expression of personal knowledge (Banks, 2014). Formally developed stories written in the first-person voice of the nurse provide a means of conveying personal knowing in a form that can be widely communicated within the discipline. Personal stories can recount an instance that occurred in practice that conveys to others something about the experience of the therapeutic use of the Self.

Personal stories developed from your journal are a way of sharing insights that come to you from journaling while keeping your journal a protected and private document. You may have journaled about feelings and emotions surrounding a situation without writing the story of the situation. As you identify what you want to share, you might not include anything from your very personal journaling, but rather use your journal to bring you back to the experience as a way to develop the story for sharing. Your journal will also draw you into deeper reflection regarding the meaning of the situation, which you can weave into your story in language, metaphors, analogies, or symbols. In some instances, you may find excerpts that you do want to extract and share or to integrate into a written or verbal story (Nelson, 2010).

Personal stories provide a glimpse of who you are in a form that is not confined to the time and space of the moment. Personal stories are limited in their capacity to convey the fullness of the Self but provide a means of communication about who you are with a wide audience. Personal stories convey essences of experience that are not communicated in theories or clinical histories. Personal stories are not trivial pastimes or entertainment; they are vital within a discipline that depends on meaningful interpersonal connections. In addition, personal stories are important to the discipline to create a shared understanding of what it means to know and develop the Self. The written expression of personal knowing opens opportunities for responses from others as well as for possibilities for deeper reflection.

Personal stories are distinct from other types of stories in that they are personal accounts of your own experiences. They reveal the thoughts, feelings, insights, and values that come from your own inner Self. Other characters and players may enter into your story, but it is your own thoughts, words, and feelings that are the focus of the story. For example, if you compose a story about your encounter with a person who is dying, the story provides a window into your experience, not into the experience of the dying person. Your story might include dialogue with the person you cared for or may recount what you observed about that person, but the main content of the story is how you felt and what you experienced as you cared for this person.

As formally developed personal stories are created and shared within the discipline, the insights conveyed in the stories give others in the discipline an opportunity for reflection and response that involves their potential for conveying the nature of the therapeutic use of the Self. When made available to others, these stories have the potential to enrich and deepen personal knowing as they inspire others to change the nature of the Self. Although written stories are in one sense limited in their capacity to convey the essence of a person, they are rich in that they convey inner processes and meanings that are not easily perceived as part of the interpersonal experience. These personal stories provide vicarious experiences that enrich those experiences provided by response and reflection in relation to the Self alone.

In addition to personal stories as a form of expression of personal knowing, personal knowing is expressed as the genuine Self. In other words, who you are as a person and your being in the world is an ongoing and living expression of your personal knowing.

 Think About It...

Have you encountered a story about nursing that has stayed with you, a story that you cannot forget? Why is this story so powerful for you, and what does it reflect about the nature of nursing? What insights about the nature of nursing does this story reveal?

Has there been a nurse you know who you feel is fully authentic and genuine. How might you approach a personal story about this nurse as a way to help your classmates understand the nature of a genuine Self?

CONCLUSION

In this chapter we have explored various conceptualizations of personal knowing in the nursing literature. For us, personal knowing is seen as knowledge of Self that is examined by asking the critical questions: "Do I know what I do?" and "Do I do what I know?" Journaling and meditation facilitate the creative processes of opening and centering that are central to the ongoing development of personal knowing. The formal expressions include the embodied Self or the human person, as well as stories that reflect personal knowing.

References

Banks, J. (2014). And that's going to help black women how? Storytelling and striving to stay true to the task of liberation in the academy. In P. Kagan, M. Smith, & P. Chinn (Eds.), *Philosophies and practices of emancipatory nursing: Social justice as praxis* (pp. 188–204). New York, NY: Routledge Taylor & Francis Group.

Banks-Wallace, J. (2008). Eureka! I finally get IT: Journaling as a tool for promoting praxis in research. *The ABNF Journal: Official Journal of the Association of Black Nursing Faculty in Higher Education, Inc, 19,* 24–27.

Barnum, B. S. (2010). *Spirituality in nursing: The challenges of complexity* (3rd ed.). New York: Springer Publishing Company.

Beckerman, A. (1994). A personal journal of caring through esthetic knowing. ANS. *Advances in Nursing Science, 17,* 71–79.

Bishop, A., & Scudder, J. (1990). *The practice, moral and personal sense of nursing.* New York, NY: National League for Nursing.

Bonis, S. A. (2009). Knowing in nursing: A concept analysis. *Journal of Advanced Nursing, 65,* 1328–1341.

Campesino, M., & Schwartz, G. E. (2006). Spirituality among Latinas/os: Implications of culture in conceptualization and measurement. ANS. *Advances in Nursing Science, 29,* 69–81.

Carper, B. A. (1978). Fundamental patterns of knowing in nursing. ANS. *Advances in Nursing Science, 1*, 13–23.

Chinn, P. L. (2013). *Peace & power: New directions for building community* (8th ed.). Burlington, MA: Jones and Bartlett Learning.

Green, C. (2009). A comprehensive theory of the human person from philosophy and nursing. Nursing Philosophy: *An International Journal for Healthcare Professionals, 10*, 263–274.

Hall, B. A. (1997). Spirituality in terminal illness: An alternative view of theory. *Journal of Holistic Nursing: Official Journal of the American Holistic Nurses' Association, 15*, 82–96.

Hall, B. A. (2008). *Surviving and thriving after a life-threatening diagnosis* (2nd ed.). Bloomington, IN: AuthorHouse.

Hall, B. A., & Allan, J. D. (1994). Self in relation: A prolegomenon for holistic nursing. *Nursing Outlook, 42*, 110–166.

Hart, H. (1997). Conceptual understanding and knowing other-wise: Reflections on rationality and spirituality in philosophy. In J. H. Olthuis (Ed.), *Knowing other-wise* (pp. 19–53). New York, NY: Fordham University Press.

Huebner, D. E. (1985). Spirituality and knowing. In E. Eisner (Ed.), *Learning and teaching the ways of knowing* (pp. 159–173). Chicago, IL: University of Chicago Press.

McSherry, W., & Cash, K. (2004). The language of spirituality: An emerging taxonomy. *International Journal of Nursing Studies, 41*, 151–161.

Moch, S. D. (1990). Personal knowing: Evolving research and practice. *Scholarly Inquiry for Nursing Practice, 4*, 155–165.

Munhall, P. L. (1993). "Unknowing": Toward another pattern of knowing in nursing. *Nursing Outlook, 41*, 125–128.

Nelson, G. L. (2010). *Writing and being: Taking back our lives through the power of language*. Novato, CA: New World Library, Kindle Edition.

Pai, H.-C. (2015). The effect of a self-reflection and insight program on the nursing competence of nursing students: A longitudinal study. Journal of Professional Nursing:. *Official Journal of the American Association of Colleges of Nursing, 31*(5), 424–431. https://doi.org/10.1016/j.profnurs.2015.03.003.

Pesut, B. (2008). A conversation on diverse perspectives of spirituality in nursing literature. Nursing Philosophy: *An International Journal for Healthcare Professionals, 9*, 98–109.

Pesut, B. (2016). There be dragons: Effects of unexplored religion on nurses' competence in spiritual care. *Nursing Inquiry, 23*(3), 191–199. https://doi.org/10.1111/nin.12135.

Pesut, B., Fowler, M., Taylor, E. J., Reimer-Kirkham, S., & Sawatzky, R. (2008). Conceptualising spirituality and religion for healthcare. *Journal of Clinical Nursing, 17*, 2803–2810.

Register, M. E., & Herman, J. (2010). Quality of life revisited: The concept of connectedness in older adults. ANS. *Advances in Nursing Science, 33*, 53–63. https://doi.org/10.1097/ANS.0b013e3181c9e1aa.

Tinley, S. T., & Kinney, A. Y. (2007). Three philosophical approaches to the study of spirituality. *ANS. Advances in Nursing Science, 30*, 71–80.

Zolnierek, C. D. (2014). An integrative review of knowing the patient. *Journal of Nursing Scholarship: An Official Publication of Sigma Theta Tau International Honor Society of Nursing / Sigma Theta Tau, 46*(1), 3–10. https://doi.org/10.1111/jnu.12049.

Aesthetic Knowledge Development

Chapter

6

The first requisite [of nursing] is the practical belief that the greatest likeness among humans is their difference. The unspoken lesson of anatomy, the autopsy room, chemistry lab builds up the insidious biological impression of the body as a predictable entity—no wonder normal and alike become confused!

Katherine Brownell Oettinger (1939, pp. 1224–1225)

Nursing is an art: and if it is to be made an art, it requires an exclusive devotion as hard a preparation as any painter's or sculptor's work; for what is the having to do with dead canvas or dead marble, compared with having to do with the living body, the temple of God's spirit? It is one of the Fine Arts: I had almost said, the finest of Fine Arts.

Florence Nightingale . . .

The opening Oettinger quote penned 75 years ago remains timeless. Oettinger acknowledged the core premise of aesthetic knowing: That situations and humans, while alike in general and predictable ways, remain unique and different. Aesthetics focuses on knowing how to understand and act in relation to those individual differences to create a positive outcome. Oettinger understood that those aspects of humanness that make people alike fall within the realm of empirics, and she cautioned that "alike" is not necessarily the same as "normal." Oettinger implied that, although humans do generally share things in common (e.g., certain features of anatomy and physiology), they are more alike in their uniqueness.

The well-known quote of Nightingale underscores the importance of art in nursing. As we shall see from this chapter the art/act of nursing is nursing's finest art; and is the formalized expression of the pattern of aesthetics. Although empirics addresses what is common and predictable, it is aesthetic knowing that helps us deal with circumstances that are unique to the situation—changing, ongoing circumstances that require our finest art.

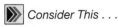 Consider This . . .

You are working with a certified nurse practitioner in an outpatient clinic when a scantily dressed 13-year-old girl we'll call Niki arrives and, after the usual preliminaries, is escorted to an examination room accompanied by her mother. As you and the nurse practitioner review Niki's intake questionnaire, you notice that she is complaining of urinary frequency and burning and that her urinalysis showed results typical of a uri-nary tract infection. A pregnancy screen also reveals that Niki is pregnant, although this is not acknowledged on her questionnaire. You discuss your approach to care with the nurse practitioner, recognizing the probable diagnosis and pregnancy.

In this situation, you will consider the *empiric data:* the urinary dipstick results, the pregnancy test, the reported symptoms, and the indicated treatments. You might also consider the *ethics* of questioning Niki about sexual activity or abuse given her young age and the presence of her mother. You acknowledge your *personal knowing* as someone who is somewhat intolerant of parents who would let a young girl dress so provocatively, and you tell yourself to keep those attitudes in check and try to understand what that means; you also are aware of a deep compassion for this child, who may be in a very precarious situation. You understand through *emancipatory knowing* that this type of dress is socially acceptable for young women despite its culturally constructed provoca-tive meaning.

Before going into the examination room, you and the nurse practitioner briefly discuss your plan. The plan includes, in part, that you expect to work with Niki and her mother from a place of compassion for Niki's plight. You will do an assessment to uncover any other problems or issues that might require attention, and you will explore more about the situation in the home and at school. After you get a clearer picture of the situation, you will discuss a possible plan of care with Niki and her mother and finish with some preventive teaching about her pregnancy and urinary tract infection prevention. You have thought about the *aesthetics* of your encounter, and you plan to try to create the best outcome by gaining Niki's trust before broaching the subject of her sexual behavior or possible abuse when her mother is asked to go to another room, where she will talk with the nurse practitioner. You do not know whether Niki's mother knows that her daughter is pregnant, and you are not sure how best to reveal it, but you do know that knowledge of her pregnancy must come out during this visit. This type of planning integrates all the knowing patterns, whether they are consciously recognized or not, and it considers what, in general, seems reasonable for this situation.

As you open the door and enter the room, you notice immediately that something is terribly wrong and that the situation is not what you expected. Your eyes immediately go to Niki, who has obviously been crying. The clothes she was wearing are awry, and she is huddled on the examination table as far away from her mother as possible. Her mother is looking very angry. The look on your face and your hesitation registers your surprise at what you see, and, before you can say anything, Niki's mother angrily de-clares, "This little slut just told me she's pregnant."

You immediately move to deal creatively with the situation. The anger of the mother may be the first thing you attend to, but then you immediately consider other elements of the situation: how Niki looks; the fact that her clothes are awry, which suggests a minor physical confrontation; and the body language that indicates estrangement. You notice these as well as countless other details all at once. Your assessment is not linear or conscious, and you say and do something immediately to assuage the mother's anger. On the basis of the unique response that you receive after this action, you make other moves that include verbalizations and movements. You continue this sort of "artful dance," balancing and tempering your ongoing responses according to the responses received from Niki and her mother. Eventually, the situation calms down.

Recounting the how, what, and why of your actions in a particular situation is not possible, because actions that arise from aesthetic knowing occur immediately in the moment, with consideration of elements that are present but typically not consciously and deliberatively recognized. Your aesthetic knowing gives rise to nursing actions that move the situation to a desired outcome—that transform the situation from what is, to another possibility. This is the nature of aesthetics; it is artful, balanced, and in a sense beautiful, rather than clumsy or uncertain. You complete a transformative art/act and transform a situation that is uncomfortable or undesirable into a situation of calm where healing can occur. You do this rather quickly by noticing and responding to the whole situation all at once. Each situation is totally unique and will never be duplicated exactly, and it can only be understood and managed in the moment. Moreover, although you know when you act artfully, you can never fully explain what you did. You can recount the situation in a story and describe how you felt, what you thought, and generally what happened, but it is not possible to describe fully the details of how you knew what you knew in the moment, that is, the fullness of aesthetic knowing that is essential to creating your actions in the moment.

 Discuss This . . .

> Share with your peers what comes to mind when you hear the phrase "the art of nursing." Keep notes about all of the ideas that are mentioned, then read the rest of this chapter. When you have completed the chapter, come back to your discussion and discuss your original ideas and how these ideas influence your nursing practice.

This chapter details the pattern of aesthetics. Aesthetic knowing in nursing is the aspect of knowing that requires an understanding of deep meanings in a situation and that, on the basis of those meanings, calls forth the creative resources of the nurse that transform experience into what is not yet real but envisioned as possible. It is the dimension of knowing that understands how human experiences that are common (e.g., grief, joy, anxiety, fear, love) are expressed and experienced uniquely. In practice, aesthetic knowing is expressed by means of *transformative art/acts*.

Fig. 6.1 depicts the dimensions of aesthetic knowing. In our model, the aesthetic pattern of knowing in nursing requires asking the questions, "What does this mean?" and "How is it significant?" From these questions, the creative processes of envisioning and rehearsing nurture the artistic expression of aesthetic knowing. Aesthetic knowing can be shared to some extent through its formal expressions of aesthetic criticism and works of art. Poetry, stories, and photographs are also artful forms of expression for aesthetic knowing. These formal expressions provide for the discipline a source of appreciation and inspiration that further nurtures aesthetic knowing. In practice, aesthetic knowing is expressed in transformative art/acts, in which the nurse moves experience from what is to a new realm that would not otherwise be possible. Table 6.1 summarizes the dimensions of aesthetic knowledge development. In this chapter we address the dimensions of critical questions, creative processes, and formal expressions (shown in bold in Table 6.1).

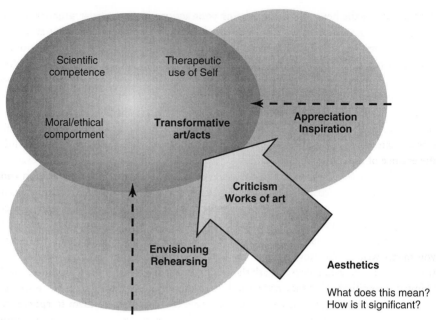

FIG. 6.1 Aesthetic Knowing and Knowledge.

TABLE 6.1 Dimensions of the Development of Aesthetic Knowing

Dimension	Aesthetics
Critical questions	What does this mean? How is this significant?
Creative processes	Envisioning Rehearsing
Formal expressions	Aesthetic criticism Works of art
Authentication processes	Appreciation Inspiration
Integrated expression in practice	Transformative art/acts

As nurses move into caring encounters, they have some idea of situational factors that might be present based on prior experiences with similar situations. The critical questions of aesthetics are "What does this (situation) mean?" and "How is it significant?" In the example of you as the nurse practitioner, seeing Niki, you made a plan based on your past experiences with similar situations. However, as soon as you entered the room, those same questions were asked again, all at once in the moment, although not deliberatively or with conscious intent. After the meaning became apparent that the mother was angry, you sensed (envisioned) what was required to calm the situation and, in the moment, selected a response. Various responses were stored up in your background of experience both in practice and from deliberate rehearsal of different kinds of responses that you could call forth in an unexpected situation that required a calming influence. Because you had practiced through role playing how to calm a situation and knew it could be effective when doing so, you acted in this situation with skill and confidence. You continued to ask questions about meaning and significance (critical questions) and to envision a desired outcome, and select from various rehearsed possibilities all at once. This is the essence of the transformative art/act.

As you reflect on this situation, you could write about it to describe the situation and your own internal experience of the scenario as it unfolded. As you begin to explore what it all meant or could mean and how your education and experience inform your reflection of the situation, you create an aesthetic criticism. Such a written account will never be as rich as the actual situation, but certain elements can be expressed. Alternatively, you might write a poem or create a drawing that represents the situation. After such a work has been created, others can ask the critical questions, "What does this mean?" and "How is it significant?" as they review and study the formal expressions of your aesthetic knowing. They could ask themselves if your representations helped them to appreciate the meaning and significance of the situation, and if its meaning and significance inspire them in a way that would be helpful in their own practices. As a preceptor, mentor, or teacher, you might guide your students to rehearse and envision what they might do in a similar setting as a way to help them to cultivate aesthetic knowing. In these ways, others learn how to create transformative art/acts more effectively.

We begin this chapter with a discussion of the meaning of art and aesthetics as the background for our conceptualization of aesthetics in nursing. Next, we present a conceptual definition of the art of nursing and discuss our definition in the light of other conceptualizations of the art of nursing that have appeared in nursing literature.

ART AND AESTHETICS

Aesthetics is a noun that derives from the Latin and Greek words that refer to perception. It has evolved to refer specifically to the study of and ideas about *artistically valid* forms. The adjective *aesthetic,* as in an aesthetic work of art, identifies an object or experience as being artistically valid. That which is artistically valid is coherent in form and substance and thus conveys a meaning of a whole beyond the formative elements; the artistically valid also evokes a response. In the following sections, the terms *aesthetic* and *artistically valid* are used interchangeably.

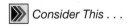 Consider This . . .

Consider the famous painting *Mona Lisa.* Aesthetics would address theoretic and philosophic views about its artistic validity. If an art critic declared the painting to be artistically valid, it would mean, in the critic's view, that it had a coherence about it that conveyed some meaning that was understood across multiple critics. Coherence may be proposed because of color contrast and proportion within the painting that emphasize the subject's large figure and face. The response that is evoked is one of interest or mystique—the painting engages the viewer—and lingers in the viewer's memory.

THE NATURE OF AESTHETICS

The aesthetic as we use it does not equate to that which is commonly viewed as beautiful or lovely. The standards by which something is taken to be appealing or beautiful vary widely in different disciplines and within different contexts and cultures. Individuals, given their unique perceptions and tastes, respond differently to an art object or experience. In the philosophy of aesthetics, beauty is not taken as a matter of taste. Rather, it takes a form that brings forth a response that draws a person in, so that you notice what is expressed. The substance of what is aesthetic (perhaps even addressed as beauty) in philosophy, may, in fact, represent something like shame, grief, or death. However, the expressive form is considered beautiful in that it satisfies aesthetic criteria and thus is considered to be artistically valid.

General traits distinguish what is artistically valid or aesthetic in form from what is not. That which is artistically valid places various elements into a pattern to form a whole that symbolizes meaning beyond the elements themselves. The form evokes a response, a feeling, an insight, or a sense of connection with the experience portrayed in the art. The response that art evokes is very often strong or even transformative, which means that the experience of the art is unforgettable, it leaves a strong impression, or it provides insight into the human condition.

The meanings conveyed and the responses evoked are connected to the cultural heritage from which the art form arises. Those outside the culture may not fully recognize the meanings that are derived from the culture, but they can still recognize the work as artistically valid. They will recognize the wholeness of the form and see there is meaning in the work, although the meaning may differ from that in the culture of origin. The cultural heritage of nursing points to the primacy of interpersonal interactions, and thus nurses will tend to be drawn to works that evoke a sense of caring and meaningful interpersonal connection.

THE NATURE OF ART

Art is both the process of creating an aesthetic object or experience and the product that is created. The process of creating and what is produced must display characteristics that are artistically valid to properly be called "art." Art is not limited to the fine arts or to what is often labeled as art. Rather, art is present in all human activities that involve forming elements into a whole. In our example of Niki, the transformative art/act was art in action, and it was artful because the nurse's actions and being were in synchrony with all that unfolded as part of the situation. The nurse was an integrated part of a whole and created an unfolding of possibilities that would not otherwise have been possible.

Art is not defined by taste or by what someone likes. Matters of taste or preference, such as "I like that painting (or what that nurse did)" or "I do not like that painting (or what that nurse did)" do not define something as being art. Neither is art in the traditional sense considered art because it can be sold for profit. For example, a local "art show" might sell out of its posters of a popular rock band, but this does not mean the poster was in fact a work of art. Rather, the extent to which art as process is satisfying and the extent to which art the product assumes coherence as a whole and elicits a feeling response determines the extent to which the experience can be called "art".

Art as a process requires skill in the technical and mechanical aspects of working with the elements from which the product is formed. It also requires an ability to imagine the whole before it is expressed and creatively integrate elements of form into a whole. This process can be readily illustrated in the fine arts; for example, a musician acquires technical and mechanical skills with an instrument and learns to bring the elements of sound together into a musical performance that generates a response from the listener. Art as a product creates a response that can transform experience. This transformation of experience occurs when a person—whether an observer or a participant—is drawn into a realm that would not otherwise be accessible, such as the realm of chaos that a performance of Wagner's *Ride of the Valkyries* might engender.

In summary, art is the process and product of bringing diverse elements together into a whole that evokes a response and that moves one's experience or perception into a realm that is not otherwise possible. Aesthetics concerns the nature and characteristics of art as process and product. It seeks to determine the extent to which what is said to be art is in fact artistically valid in form.

ART AND AESTHETICS IN NURSING

Nurses have a notable history of appreciating art and creating aesthetically pleasing environments to enhance healing and well-being. Familiar examples include the use of music to create a sense of calm, visual arts to convey health and illness experiences, dance or free-form movement to enhance physical coordination and strength, and drawing as a therapeutic modality. Works of art have also been used to illustrate and interpret meanings of health and illness experiences in education and research (Archibald et al., 2017; Bender & Elias, 2016; Chinn & Watson, 1994; Darbyshire, 1994; Dean, 2013; Honan et al., 2016; Lamb, 2009; Liehr et al., 2013; Pellico & Chinn, 2007). Although we acknowledge and encourage these therapeutic uses of artistic processes, this is not the focus that concerns aesthetic knowledge development, and this is different from what we are addressing as "the art of nursing." Rather, aesthetic knowledge development is directed toward those aspects of knowing that are essential to the "doing" of nursing itself, which is what we consider "the art of nursing."

Aesthetics is typically associated with what is generally referred to as *art*. Perhaps because of this, aesthetics has had little emphasis in nursing. However, aesthetics has always been integral to nursing practice. Aesthetic qualities can be seen as art in all aspects of nursing practice, from notes written in a chart to theoretic formulations, from a single brief interaction with an individual to sustained interactions with groups and communities, and from an unexpected encounter to a thoughtfully planned design for a system of care. In all these wide-ranging nursing experiences, nurses artfully draw on and use emancipatory, empiric, ethical, personal, and aesthetic knowing. It is the dimension of aesthetic knowing that endows nursing experiences with aesthetic qualities and that differentiates excellent and skilled nursing from the impersonal or mechanical-like performance of technical acts and routinized procedures.

Moreover, things that ordinarily would not be labeled as "art" do have aesthetic characteristics. For example, an empiric theory is formed from conceptual ideas linked in a pattern having a meaning that the concepts alone could not convey. The appeal (i.e., a subtle feeling response) of a theory often derives from the *aesthetic shape* of the theory. Without this quality, the theory lacks a certain attractiveness or appeal to the community of scientists.

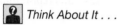 *Think About It . . .*

> Reflect on your personal experiences with "the arts"—learning to play an instrument, participating in a play, dancing, singing. What has this experience meant to you? What have these experiences contributed to your health, your physical or mental well-being? Your experience with nursing?

AESTHETIC KNOWING

Aesthetic knowing requires knowledge of the experience toward which the art form is directed as well as knowledge of the art form itself. For example, a poet requires knowledge of a life experience that is reflected in the poem, as well as knowledge of the art form itself—the techniques and methods used to create something that can be considered poetry. The visual artist requires knowledge of the experience or situation that will be visually presented as a painting or sculpture, as well as knowledge of the technical aspects of painting or sculpting required to achieve the desired visual representations.

In nursing, aesthetic knowing requires knowledge of the following:
- The experience of nursing (the art form)
- The experience of health and illness (that which nursing art/act transforms)

These two aspects of knowledge grow as nurses are educated, as they have experiences in practice, and as they learn about the experiences of other nurses. For example, nurses learn about the experience of dying by studying theories of death and dying, by reading or hearing stories about dying, and by caring for people who are dying and experiencing their feelings and those of their loved ones. Nurses learn about caring for someone who is dying as they are guided through this type of clinical experience in school, as they hear the stories of other nurses who have cared for people who are dying, and as they experience working with people who are dying.

Background knowledge of the experience of nursing and of the experiences of health and illness are essential, but they are not sufficient for aesthetic practice. For example, to bring an aesthetic quality into the experience of caring for someone who is dying, you also need to cultivate the ability to enact nursing's art form itself—the art of nursing.

CONCEPTUAL DEFINITIONS OF THE ART OF NURSING

As demonstrated, the idea of the art of nursing has had several different meanings reflected in the nursing literature since the time of Florence Nightingale. Although no single clear definition of the art of nursing prevails, nurse scholars have consistently recognized the art of nursing and emphasized how vital this aspect of nursing is in relation to who nurses are and what they do. Although historically nursing art referred largely to technical skills that were often learned in the "nursing arts laboratory," the art of nursing has taken on a meaning that is more closely related to art as aesthetic practice.

The art of nursing as aesthetic practice can be a difficult concept to understand. One difficulty is that the nurse's art is expressed in the knowing-being of the nurse. Briefly, nursing art does not simply reflect what and how the nurse knows (epistemology); it also refers to the nurse's being and doing (ontology). The embodied nature of "the art of nursing" is part of what makes it difficult to understand. The term *embodied* means that nursing art requires mind-body-spirit involvement in a creative experience that is transformative. The body moves through the nursing situation, the mind understands meaning, and the spirit feels—all at once—and artfully acts to transform experience. In this sense, nursing art is a form of performance art that involves the nurse and the person for whom the nurse is providing care. Like a theatrical production or an orchestral concert, the nurse's performance art can have various degrees of artistic validity. As with all art forms, artistic skill can be taught and learned. Even for those who are most talented in the art form, artistic competence requires discipline and practice; it does not come naturally.

Recognizing the challenges inherent in defining the art of nursing, we propose a definition that was derived from an aesthetic inquiry project that began as the result of conversations with practicing nurses who, without exception, recognized meaning in the phrase "the art of nursing." Conversations and storytelling among nurses focused on their experiences of the art of nursing, the various meanings that they saw in photographs, or in rehearsals or the role playing of various alternative approaches to nursing practice. The conversations with nurses were supplemented with introspection and more formalized aesthetic inquiry techniques carried out by project leaders. Chinn, Maeve, and Bostick (1997) observed nurses as they practiced nursing, reviewed photographs of nurses as they practiced, and used journaling to explore deeper symbolic and personal meanings of the practices observed.

The following definition emerged from this aesthetic inquiry project and is used in this text:

The nurse's synchronous arrangement of narrative and movement into a form that transforms experiences into a realm that would not otherwise be possible. The arrangement is spontaneous, in-the-moment, and intuitive. The ability to make the moves that are transformative is grounded in a deep understanding of nursing, including relevant theory, facts, technical skill, personal knowing, and ethical understanding; and this ability requires rehearsal in deliberative application of these understandings, p. 90).

This definition identifies synchronous narrative and movement as the elements that form the aesthetics of nursing, which is what in this textbook we refer to as the *transformative art/act. Narrative* includes words, gestures, and intonations of speech. *Synchrony* refers to the coordination and rhythm of the experience. Synchrony of intention and action is also implied. Synchrony and narrative must come together to form an integral whole. In the example of Niki at the opening of this chapter, narrative would include elements such as what you said, the somewhat surprised look on your face when you entered the room, and the loudness or softness with which you spoke at different times when trying to restore calm. Synchrony refers to how you moved your embodied Self within the situation; who you approached and when; how and where you touched Niki or her mother with the intent to calm; as well as how you were synchronizing your words with what you were doing. Synchronous narrative and movement, as the elements that form the aesthetic in nursing, can be taught and conveyed.

Johnson (1994) identified the following five conceptualizations for the art of nursing:
- The ability to grasp meaning during patient encounters
- The ability to establish a meaningful connection with the person being cared for
- The ability to skillfully perform nursing activities
- The ability to rationally determine an appropriate course of nursing action
- The ability to morally conduct one's nursing practice

All of these are relevant to our conceptualization of the art of nursing. The following sections explain these connections.

Grasping Meaning During Patient Encounters

In our definition of the art of nursing, the ability to grasp meaning during a patient encounter is required if the nurse is to transform an experience from what is to what is possible. Our explicit reference to the intuitive, in-the-moment arrangement of movement and narrative refers to the intuitive element as it unfolds within the transformative art/act, not to intuitive elements that inform or point to a specific outcome or problem. In other words, as a nurse in the moment of care, you may not have an immediate grasp of what the moment means to a person or family and what to do about it. Rather, your intuitive sense detects all that is going on and calls forth a response, and you act spontaneously to care for the person or family in the moment.

The focus from which your nursing art form emerges is the intuitive use of your creative resources to form experience. You are open to making moves within an experience that you have not anticipated and planned, and you have not necessarily confirmed the patient's or family's perceptions of the situation. Rather, your moves come from a perceptual grasp of the various possibilities for forming the situation that resides within the experience. Your own creative energy moves the encounter forward as a work of art in process.

 Consider This . . .

As a way to better understand what is meant by "grasping meaning in the situation," think about how you cannot really know how to be in a situation until you are actually in it. As an experienced practitioner, as you move into clinically complex care situations, you comprehend—all at once—what a situation is calling forth, and you respond wholly. As you respond, your being and your behavior call forth in the other or others a response that they in turn wholly understand and to which they respond. These sorts of all-at-once, instantaneous, and simultaneous response patterns, which transform the experience in the moment, constitute the *art/act.*

The intuitive aspect of creating form is what is referred to as *creativity.* It is a knowing in the moment of creating that enables the artist to express unique possibilities that fit together, make sense for the situation, and come together in the right relationship. It then follows that the intuitive perception of a right relationship within a nursing encounter depends on a deep grasp of the meaning embedded in the situation.

Although our definition is clearly applicable to patient encounters, it also applies to nursing actions that do not involve a direct patient encounter. The ability to design a system of care is grounded in a grasp of meaning in the experience of people for whom the system is designed. Here, spontaneous and intuitive aspects of the process of creating the design are part of the formative process. The nurse-designer does not intuit an end point or set about to design it. Rather, the nurse-designer is immersed in the experience of creating the design and remains open to a stream of possibilities that can only emerge as the design takes shape.

Establishing a Meaningful Connection with the Person Being Cared For

Our definition of the art of nursing assumes a deep and meaningful connection with the other. A transformative move requires presence with the other. To be transformative and artful, an art/act must be grounded in a profound level of connection between the nurse and the other. In the context of such a connection, there is a synchronicity or rhythmicity between the nurse and the other. The "synchronous arrangement of narrative and movement" in an interaction refers to the timing and flow among all elements in the situation and reflects a deep level of connection between the nurse and the person for whom care is being provided.

Skillfully Performing Nursing Activities

The performance of nursing skills is one of the earliest conceptualizations of nursing art, and it is an element of meaning often expressed by nurses in Chinn's aesthetic inquiry. Nurses first pointed to tasks and procedures that are required in the "doing" of nursing, noting that it is *how* they do what they do that characterizes their art. However, in our definition, skills alone do not constitute the art of nursing. Rather, skillful performance is expressed in the nurse's movement and narrative, which may or may not involve tasks and procedures. Skillful performance is developed over time from a background of practice (rehearsal) that makes possible what Heidegger (1962) identified as "ready-to-hand" knowing. Artful nursing includes and indeed often requires skilled technical performance. However, our definition implies an integration of skill with relevant theory, facts, and personal knowing as well as with emancipatory and ethical understanding.

Rationally Determining an Appropriate Course of Action

Research regarding clinical judgment and rational reasoning suggests that intuitive and aesthetic components are necessary for sound practice. In our conceptualization of the art of nursing, rational reasoning is not a defining element. Rather, as with technical skills, rational thinking ability and clinical judgment processes create the background necessary for aesthetic capability. Nursing art as synchronous movement to transform experience is an art form; it is not rationally formed, and there is no "outcome" that is defined in advance. As in other art forms, the nurse has a vision or an idea of what improved health and well-being would be like for a person in a particular situation. However, the exact outcome of a particular situation is not projected in the moment of the transformative art/act. Rather, the direction of health and well-being is intuitively shaped and formed as it occurs. In this sense, the creation of health and well-being is a "work in progress."

 Why Is This Important?

>The role of rationality in aesthetics is similar to, but different from, rationality in empirics. Consider the example of composing a musical score—it is essential that a composer makes use of accepted theories of rhythm when constructing a musical score and has an idea about what the music might be like in the end. However, during the process, she is inspired to integrate rhythmic variations that may defy common conventions, and the exact form of the music shifts as it unfolds. In the process, the composer places a unique signature on the work that gives it artistic character. The final score generally reflects what the composer envisioned, but it is not exactly what might have been predicted at the outset. Likewise, as a nurse, you call on your theoretic understanding of a particular type of illness experience when developing a rational plan of care for appropriate nursing action. Although you do plan, you remain open to spontaneous events that create opportunities to change the plan as the caring process unfolds in synchrony with the person and family involved in a particular experience. It is this spontaneous unfolding of the process, when integrated with your prior rational understanding, that creates artistic form. The particular ways in which the nurse shifts or moves through the experience is the artistic signature that endows the experience with a particular and unique quality.

Morally Conducting One's Nursing Practice

Our definition of the art of nursing points to ethical understanding as background that is essential for aesthetic practice. A significant ethical dimension is inherent in transformative art/acts that are basic to the art of nursing. Nurses who participated in the aesthetic inquiry from which our definition was derived told many stories of their practices that involved ethical dilemmas and elicited actions that they associated with the art of nursing. There is a value component in the idea of transformative art/acts that implies a significant ethical dimension

Inherent in the art of nursing is that transforming creates a change in what something is to what it otherwise would not be. In the context of nursing, the change is, by definition, one toward a higher level of health and well-being. A transformative art/act could not be recognized as artistically valid if it violated ethical sensibilities. However, transformative art/acts alone do not convey ethical understanding. Rather, transformative moves can come out of significant ethical and moral dilemmas and contribute to the development of ethical sensibilities.

THE DIMENSIONS OF AESTHETIC KNOWING

As seen in Fig. 6.1 at the beginning of this chapter, the dimensions of aesthetic knowing include the critical questions, "What does this mean?" and "How is it significant?" These critical questions engage the creative processes of envisioning and rehearsing possibilities. From these creative processes, aesthetic criticism can be constructed as a form of knowledge of the artistry of nursing that can be shared with others. Works of art also emerge as representations of what is known, and they are also a form of aesthetic knowledge that can be made available to the broader audience within and outside the discipline. Art forms that can be created in nursing to represent the meaning and significance of nursing and health experiences include poetry, photography and other visual art forms, story, drama, and dance. The authentication processes of appreciation and inspiration examine the extent to which formal expressions of aesthetic knowing are aesthetic in nature and thus can be used to cultivate aesthetic knowing in nursing. Transformative art/acts are the integrated expressions of aesthetic knowing in practice. Synchronous movement and narrative that transform the health–illness experience, from what is into a realm that would not otherwise be possible, characterize these art/acts.

Critical Questions: What Does This Mean? How Is It Significant?

The critical questions for aesthetic knowing ("What does this mean?" and "How is it significant?") can be asked of formal expressions of knowing or in the context of practice to create a transformative art/act. As a nurse engages in transformative art/acts, various possibilities emerge instantaneously in the moment, without conscious thought. Outside of practice, these questions initiate an envisioning and rehearsing process that is conscious and deliberative and that can be used to cultivate aesthetic knowing.

Creative Processes: Envisioning and Rehearsing

Envisioning and rehearsing are two interrelated processes from which creative products of aesthetic knowing emerge. Typically, envisioning and rehearsing have not been deliberately taught, nor do nurses identify these processes as something that they do. However, many of the practices that Chinn, Maeve, and Bostick (1997) came to view as envisioning and rehearsing were activities in which nurses engaged. Often these activities were hidden from view, engaged in during nurses' time away from their job responsibilities, and assumed to be insignificant and trivial yet often necessary to cope with difficult situations. As the nurses participating in the study described situations that represented their art, they related how they shared stories about the situations in phone conversations after work, over a meal, or in a secluded area during a downtime. Their storytelling episodes always included an account of the response of the listener and the ways in which their interactive talk formed and re-formed how they saw similar situations and how they came to trust their own intuitive senses. When the nurses associated these and similar activities as being necessary and important aspects of developing an aesthetic knowing of their art form, the importance of these activities was immediately grasped.

Envisioning involves imagining a typical end point scenario or a response that one hopes to elicit by the performance or display of the art form. For a comedian, the envisioned obvious end point is the audience's laughter; a less obvious but hoped-for end point is that the audience will catch subtle meanings conveyed in the comedy (i.e., "get" the point of the joke). For a musician, the envisioned end point for a particular piece of music might be to convey a sense of longing, a sense of joy, or a sense of excitement. For a novelist, the envisioned end point is transporting the reader into a realm outside that reader's own experience and into the realm of the characters and situations depicted in the novel. For a nurse, envisioned end points are those that represent health and well-being, such as calm, relaxation, comfort, and the ability to navigate health-related situations.

Rehearsing is either a physical or a mental walk-through of the skills required for the performance or display of the art form, ultimately involving the presence of a coach, teacher, or critic. The writer presents excerpts or pieces of writing to reviewers for critique and feedback. The comedian engages small audiences to listen and respond to segments of a routine. The musician performs for a teacher or mentor.

 Consider This . . .

A useful analogy for understanding the processes of envisioning and rehearsing in nursing is *improvisation*. In an improvisational art the display (or performance) is possible because the performer is skilled in the various moves and sequences that improvisation requires. The skills are developed through repeated practice, thus making it possible for the performer to call these skills forth in a unique situation. Repeated and intense rehearsal and the development of a wide range of finely tuned skills makes the skills fully embodied. Over time, the artist must also rehearse imagined improvisational scenarios before a coach or critic to receive direction that allows the artist to refine his or her ability so that intended meanings are conveyed.

In improvisational drama, the actor (nursing student) practices sequences of movements (techniques), postural and facial expressions (body language), and voice intonations (soft and soothing or loud urgent speech) that convey wide ranges of emotion (from calm to immediacy). They also practice and narrate lines ("Shh, it's OK" or "Hurry with that crash cart!") that give verbal expression to a possible experience (this is going to be frightening for the patient or the patient is going to arrest). The director (critic, coach, or teacher) gives the actor (nursing student) feedback and guidance that lead the actor into new territory. The director (teacher) may also guide the actor (nursing student) to repeat and perfect the sequence of movements to bring them to a refined, embodied level. Eventually, the actor's skills are so finely tuned that the actor's focus remains on the process that is emerging in the improvised situation rather than on the technical skills required for the process of improvisation.

In the following sections, we describe three practices for envisioning and rehearsing narrative and movement as elements that are basic to nursing's art: (1) creating and recreating storylines, (2) creating and developing embodied synchronous movement, and (3) rehearsing and engaging a connoisseur-critic. The practices that we describe are not linear or sequential; they are interwoven and integral to aesthetic knowing. They are presented separately here to describe in some detail what they are and how they function to contribute to aesthetic knowing. Each of these practices fosters both envisioning and rehearsing.

Creating and Recreating Storylines

When nurses tell stories to one another, they move into a realm created from the imagination and not bound by the constraints of the workaday world. Even when the story begins with the intention of conveying an accurate account of a real experience, in the telling of the story, the narrator creates emotion, stresses points of emphasis, exaggerates or downplays selected elements of the story, and selects certain features to include or exclude. Often the desires of the storyteller come into the story in ways that surprise even the storyteller. For example, the storyteller may unexpectedly give an account of what he or she wishes had been done in the situation as if it actually happened, rather than accounting for what did happen. In this way, the storyteller forms various types of meanings and significances for the story, providing multiple possible responses to the critical questions of "What does this mean?" and "How is it significant?" If viewed through the lens of empirics, the story would have little or no worth. When viewed through the lens of aesthetics, however, the story has exquisite value as a frame from which to explore possible meanings and to create visions and possibilities for the future.

To develop aesthetic knowing with the use of the creative envisioning and rehearsing processes, we recommend that the story be told in the voice of the person who receives nursing care. Stories that are told in the voice of the nurse are more often reflective of personal knowing and explore the nurse's personal meanings. Stories that are told in the voice of the person receiving nursing care inspire empathy as well as a deeper understanding of the experience that is the story's focus. Stories told from the perspective of the other also help to develop an embodied knowing of the other's experience. We recommend stories that illuminate some health or illness experience toward which nursing's art form is directed.

The story can come from actual experience, but aesthetic storytelling does not require adhering to the factual truth of a situation as does an empiric case study or anecdotal account. Rather, the storyteller purposely exaggerates, fictionalizes, emphasizes, and reshapes the actual experience to enhance listeners' perceptions of certain meanings that the storyteller intends to convey in the story. In this way, the story comes from the imagination more than from the actual experience, although the imagination is inspired by the actual experience. The well-developed story will reveal possibilities in human experience that often are not perceived empirically or understood rationally.

The storyline is the *plot* of the story. A plot requires that the essential characters of a story be placed in a situation that suggests a tension that builds toward an uncertain ending, thereby moving the story toward any one of several possible endings. The storyteller knows which of the uncertain endings will eventually emerge, but the listener or reader can only be drawn into the story if the ending remains uncertain. The listener or reader senses any number of possible endings, some dreaded and others hoped for. In the best of stories, the worst possible ending and the best possible ending both remain viable to the listener or reader until the very end, thus keeping the reader engaged. Characters other than the essential characters can shift and move in and out of the story, but the main characters play essential roles throughout to maintain the tension of uncertainty. This tension of uncertainty is appealing in part because this is exactly the way one's own real-life story is emerging from day to day and even from moment to moment. Nurses move in and out of people's real-life stories, often playing essential roles that can and do influence movement toward a hoped-for future.

During the initial creation of a storyline, you typically begin by recounting an experience very much the way it actually happened in practice, with creative license to embellish along the way. Then, you recreate the situation by telling the story as you might have wished it to unfold. You retell the story and describe your actions (movements and narrative) as you might have acted in the situation, perhaps describing what you wish you had done instead of what you actually did. You continue to create different storylines that involve the same situation, inserting different imagined possibilities for what you might have done and said in ways that you can imagine would lead to a different possible ending.

⟫ Consider This . . .

In our opening example, when recounting the story of Niki, you might insert a different approach to your initial encounter with Niki and her mother, when you knew that the pregnancy test was positive but did not know if Niki or her mother knew this. You could create a storyline in which you candidly tell them about the results of the pregnancy test; you could then imagine how Niki and her mother would react at this point in the unfolding story and how you would handle such a scenario. You might create a storyline in which Niki did not know she was pregnant, one in which her mother was overjoyed, one in which the mother became very frightened, and one in which both immediately revealed incest occurring in the home and expressed despair regarding how to stop it. Each of these scenarios leads to mentally rehearsing possible creative possibilities that can be used in actual practice.

Stories serve several purposes that are related to aesthetic knowing. Most important, from the perspective of aesthetics, each storyline brings forth new perceptions of meaning that could be possible in the situation. For example, the storylines in the case of Niki provide the opportunity to explore various nursing approaches to the situation and to imagine different responses from Niki and her mother and how you, or those with whom you share the story, would respond to each of the possible scenarios. The different storylines bring to awareness various meanings that could be present in a care situation. As various meanings come into awareness, new possibilities for creative engagement with each meaning can emerge. Stories elicit profound reflection on meaning that involves both personal meaning and the meaning for others in the story. In this way, the story brings to awareness the aesthetic knowledge that is embedded in experiences and that contributes to aesthetic practice.

Creating and recreating storylines also provide a means of rehearsing a narrative that in turn develops knowledge and skill that are basic to the art of nursing. The exact words that emerge during the processes of creating and recreating storylines may or may not be suitable for the actual clinical situation. Rather, the storytelling process itself enhances the nurse's ability to use narrative effectively in practice.

The *narrative* used to tell a story places the plot within a context; it conveys the feel, attitude, and mood of the story, and it integrates the storylines to form a whole, vicarious experience that is located within the story's time and space. The narrative—those verbalizations, gestures, and voice intonations that are used in practice—serve the same functions. Narratives locate the isolated experiences of the person within a larger plot, contribute to the creation of an atmosphere within which the experience can unfold, and integrates the various elements of the experience into a whole that moves toward an imagined future. For example, as you imagine various storylines that involve the scenario of Niki and her mother, you form and "bank" any number of possibilities for managing an actual situation that can be called forth when needed. You also form various "moves" (i.e., words and actions) that will constitute who you are as a nurse in similar situations. Storylines are considered fiction because, although the initial story is based on a real event, the story is embellished and enhanced as it is told. In this way, stories provide a vehicle for the rehearsal of possibilities that you might be called on to actualize in your practice at some point in the future. Storylines become etched in your memory in much the same way that actual experience remains with you and that you can call forth at a moment's notice when needed.

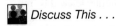 *Discuss This . . .*

Get together with a group of peers to explore developing storylines. You might begin with an anecdotal account of a real experience. The experience can be your own or one that someone observed or heard about. The first account of the experience may seem relatively simple and inadequate for representing the significance of the experience itself, and it may sound "clinical" because of the culturally acquired propensity to focus on anecdotal accounts of a sequence of events or a clinical case study.

To make a first effort less clinical and more of a story, first explore what it is about an experience that compels your attention; identify the key characters involved in the experience; and imagine each character's perspectives, motives, and intentions. Explore the context within which the experience is set and the key elements of the situation that seem important to the unfolding of the story. Imagine various endings toward which your experience could have moved or may still move. Proposing various endings provides possibilities for building tension within the story that can be significant in different ways and lead to various endings.

Next, sketch out the essential characters that you want to place within the storyline. You can shift the characters as the storyline unfolds and changes, but the characters will remain central to the storyline. Begin to write or tell the story as if you were these characters. Include those elements you explored that will create richness to the story: the story's context; the character's motives, intentions, and perspectives; the key elements of the situation; and so forth. As you begin to write and discuss the story, the elements of the storyline will begin to emerge. Imagine several different possibilities for the movement of the storyline toward an ending, and let one of your imagined possibilities become part of your story. This first narrative will become material that you can work with to recreate the storyline with other possible endings. As other possible endings are created, a richness of meaning emerges.

Creating and recreating storylines provide aesthetic narrative skills that the nurse uses as a participant in the emerging real-life stories of those for whom care is provided. The story that unfolds clinically is shaped and transformed by emerging possibilities that are situated between the past and the future. Mattingly (1994a) described this process as "therapeutic emplotment." The story that unfolds clinically is lived. The aesthetic challenge is to structure isolated episodes into a plot that moves the lived experience toward a hoped-for ending. In our example of Niki, you made a transformative move that fairly quickly brought an explosive situation to a calmer place. However, you are likely to have continuing contact with Niki, and your experience of creating transformative art/acts continues. As Niki returns to the clinic throughout her pregnancy and beyond, you will continue to participate as a player in shaping Niki's real-life story. As during that first encounter, you will use nursing as an art/act that moves the real-life story that is unfolding toward the best possible future.

In real-life stories, all participants are instrumental in the creation of the plot, the selection of the ending, and the actions that bring about changes and transformations. The plot does not happen by design; rather, it unfolds. The end that participants desire, and the uncertainty of the ending, energizes movement toward that end. A nurse's ability to participate in this aesthetic process is nurtured by skills that are developed through the rehearsal of creating and recreating storylines.

Creating conversational or written storylines that move the situation toward a desired future provides a vision of what might be and an opportunity for the rehearsal of ways in which nursing care can be enacted to energize movement in a new direction. As the actual experience unfolds, what the person and his or her family envision is shaped by everyday experiences. For example, as a nurse assists a person with taking the first steps after a traumatic injury, the possibility for mobility begins to take form, and with this possibility comes the potential for returning to a job or reengaging in a desired activity. The imagined scenarios of one's new life story gradually begin to take shape as they are formed by the mutual interactions of nurses, family members, and others involved in caring for the person.

 Consider This . . .

Consider the idea of working with someone who experienced a life-altering experience, such as a major trauma or a disabling illness. You enter the person's life story at a time when the future that the person had imagined is inalterably changed. The person and the family face a period of tension and uncertainty during which the new imagined future is a dreaded future that was never imagined before. As a nurse, you begin with small, everyday acts of nursing care. With each nursing interaction, you begin to create with the patient and family a new plot that cannot be fully anticipated in advance. On the basis of your experience and background as a nurse, you are able to help the patient and family imagine a new future. It may not be the ultimately desired future, but it may be one that they can begin to embrace. Some elements of the new future involve small, everyday things, such as learning to function with only one arm. Other elements of the new future are more complicated, such as imagining new options for making a living.

To summarize, the purpose of creating stories is twofold. First, your stories develop a deep sense of meaning and significance in human experience, and they provide a connection with human experience that only aesthetic expressions can convey. This sense of connection begins for you as you develop a story. The experiences in your stories can then become real for those who read or hear the stories that you create. Second, your stories can provide an avenue for you to explore and, in a sense, rehearse new possibilities—with new meanings and significance—for practice. If you place a dynamic in your story that explores a situation in practice that you had hoped for but never experienced, or that you imagine might be possible, your stories provide a way to experience what you have not yet come across in practice. Your stories provide a vicarious experience that helps to make potential nursing situations that have not yet been encountered seem more real.

Creating and Developing Embodied Synchronous Movement

Movement is inherent to the practice of nursing; yet little attention is given to the systematic development of movement skills other than body mechanics. Movement is generally taken for granted; people enter nursing with a lifetime of experience with moving through space and with a cultural understanding of the symbolic significance of various moves, gestures, and postures. Within the art of nursing, movement takes on a different level of significance.

As an element of the art of nursing, movement becomes the medium for the expression of meaning that parallels visual representation in the fine arts. Like the picture that conveys a thousand words, your movements as a nurse express a multitude of meanings on many levels. The communicative power of movement includes what is popularly known as *body language,* which involves movements grounded in the culture that send messages without the use of spoken language. Movement communicates who you are as a nurse, the nature of your intentions, how you regard yourself, your genuineness as a nurse and as a human, your capacity for relating to another, and your level of technical and scientific competence.

Movement, including posturing, is important for synchrony with the narrative and movement that artful nursing requires. How you move in and around a situation sets a rhythm, a style, a dynamic, a pace, and an attitude that invites or disinvites engagement. It is a fundamental symbolic marker of your abilities as a nurse artist. For example, if the way that you move into a room conveys that you are in a rush or are impatient, people's reactions to your entry will reflect their personal response to the message conveyed by your movement. Some who perceive your impatience may be apologetic for bothering you; others may feel angry that you seem to be inconvenienced by what they legitimately need and to which they feel entitled. If you do not intend to show your sense of impatience or of being rushed, your challenge is to acquire ways of moving into a situation that do not convey this message to others.

Movement makes both physical and symbolic touch possible. Without movement, touch or even symbolic touch (i.e., "touching a person's life") does not occur. The meaning of touch, which is considered vitally important in nursing practice, is conveyed through the movement toward and away from physical contact.

 Consider This . . .

> Consider a scene from the movie *Silence Like Glass.* Eva, a rising-star ballerina, faces a devastating malignancy and can no longer dance. Her dance partner, with whom she had dreamed of touring the world, comes to visit. As he is leaving, she reaches out to touch his hand in a loving gesture that also conveys the regret and sorrow of the moment. He quickly withdraws his hand from her touch, with a subtle upper body shift backward and a facial expression of repulsion. Here, if you observe just the moment of touch in a snapshot of her hand touching his, you might conclude that it was a gesture of caring and love; the fuller meaning of the episode—and his movement of withdrawal from her touch—would be lost.

Movement provides a means for a nurse to identify and define the time-space within which the care encounter will occur. For example, as the nurse enters an encounter, body moves, gestures that often include touch, and visual scanning define the space within which the nurse functions during the encounter. The nurse's moves remain primarily within a defined space until near the end of the encounter, when there is a gesture or move that is often accompanied by words that signals a retreat from the encounter.

Movement is needed for actions that protect, assist, comfort, and heal. The intentions that bring such moves into the nursing encounter are inherent within the moves and serve to define such moves. This means that moves that are intended to protect embody that intention and convey the essence of protection within the specific situation. When you consciously focus on movement, it can be deliberately shaped so that subtleties of posture and the sequence of the movement convey meanings that are intended. The intentions that energize and give meaning to movement can be perceived by others, because your intention is embedded in the style of the move and in the physical form and shape of your movement. If your movements are hurried and rushed, the form and shape of those movements suggest an intention of doing what must be done but exiting the situation as quickly as possible. Table 6.2 lists features of movement that contribute to its aesthetic quality.

Movement conveys the aesthetics of technical skill performance. Movement that just "gets the job done" is empty and mechanical. What creates an aesthetic performance is the nurse's intention to bring together the various elements of narrative and movement within the experience into a caring and healing whole in which all elements fall into the right relationship. Being able to do this requires practice (rehearsal) and well-developed skill, but without a caring and healing intention being inherent in the performance, the act of doing the technical task will be mechanical.

Intention saturates movements with meaning beyond accomplishing the skill. Intention finely tunes the style, timing, finesse, and coordination to convey artistic as well as scientific competence. Aspects of movement such as coordinated balance, finesse, style, timing, and synchrony can be rehearsed in deliberately planned exercises. Movement exercises are best rehearsed within the context of nursing, because they are guided by the situation.

Movement exercises, particularly meditative forms (e.g., tai chi, yoga), can also be used to develop the embodied movement skills of coordination, finesse, and style. The posturing and movements of such body meditations are also consistent with good body mechanics and the development of an embodied sense of balance, rhythm, and coordination.

In summary, movement is an important medium that shapes the emerging story of a lived experience. It is an avenue of communication that assists with and inspires a shift from one moment to the next. Movement is a foundational element of the art of nursing.

Rehearsal and Engaging a Connoisseur-Critic

Developing competence in transformative art/acts requires rehearsal, along with the guidance of a connoisseur-critic. Rehearsal can focus on specific aspects of narrative or movement, or it can focus on a real-life situation with all its complexity. Rehearsal of real-life situations can be performed either in a protected studio in which you role-play various situations or in a relatively safe, actual nursing situation. A *connoisseur-critic* is an experienced nurse well versed in the art of nursing and able to envision the form of artistic nursing practice. A connoisseur-critic is also committed to teaching and coaching others as they develop artistic abilities.

Engaging a connoisseur-critic to observe your rehearsal is a vital aspect of developing aesthetic ability. As the one who is performing, you cannot judge your own artistic ability. Only from an observer's critical perspective can artistic validity be perceived and

TABLE 6.2 Features of Aesthetic Movement

Defining Quality	Description
Coordinated balance	Concurrent movement of all parts of the body within a whole, smooth, integral pattern: • Includes breath patterns as a foundation for the coordination of muscle movement. Breath contributes to rhythm in movement. • Balance within a sequence of movements requires embodied knowing. You may have cognitive awareness of the sequence of movement, but the more your moves arise from embodied intelligence and not from cognitively processing, the finer and more balanced your coordination will be.
Finesse	The refinement and versatility with which moves are made: • Depends on embodied familiarity with the environment and with the objects and processes with which you work. • Requires integrating a knowing of the materials at hand with the capabilities of the body. • Comes with practice and experience and can be nurtured with rehearsal, but each individual has different aptitudes for developing finesse.
Style	The unique character that each individual brings to movement: • The particular, unique way that you use movement as you bring intention and action together. • Cannot be taught, but can be encouraged. • Can be described, but cannot be duplicated, it is an integral element of a unique self.
Timing	The rhythm, the pace of movement, and the placement of various moves within a time sequence of an unfolding experience: • Is not cognitively processed. • Is a key marker of intuitive ability; determined in the moment as an experience unfolds.
Synchrony	The ability to bring together elements of the environment with the responses of others: • Uses movement and narrative to fashion an integrated whole. • Depends on coordination, finesse, style, and timing.

judged. Through interaction with the responses of the critic, you gain insight into the integrity of your expression, deepen your knowledge of your art form, and discover avenues for moving your art into a new realm of possibility.

Connoisseur-critics have profound familiarity with and appreciation for the art form that they critique. A connoisseur has specialized knowledge of artistic expression, and his or her judgment of the practice of the art form is considered to be discriminating. Connoisseur-critics understand the technical expertise required for artistic expression.

They have studied the field that pertains to the art form and have knowledge of what the art form is directed toward as well as of the art form itself. In the case of nursing, they have studied the field of nursing and understand that nursing's art is directed toward such ends as health and healing. They also understand the processes required to bring dimensions of health and healing into being.

Connoisseur-critics also know the history of the art form and understand how it has changed over time. They are familiar with the current cultural context for the art form and the possibilities for new directions that are emerging within the art form. Given their expertise, they have developed a keenly trained "eye, ear, and feel" for the art. The intention of the connoisseur-critic is to nurture the artist's ability to obtain a new dimension of expression. This intention and its translation into action create a safe environment that nurtures the artist's skill. A skilled teacher is a skilled connoisseur-critic, and a skilled connoisseur-critic is a skilled teacher.

Skilled critics nurture critical abilities in the novice artist and shape and support the development of the reflective capacities that are necessary to refine aesthetic ability. The primary function of the connoisseur-critic in a rehearsal context is to provide guidance that moves the art form to a new level. The critic provides substantive information about well-developed aspects of the performance and elements that show promise for development, with specific guidance for taking the performance to a new level of skill. Ideally, the critic works with the artist over time so that the critic becomes familiar with the performer's unique abilities and style. Over time, the critic becomes sensitive to signals of emerging ability and engages with the artist in ways that encourage a shift toward increasing artistic competence.

The critic does not give generalized value judgments of "good" or "bad." Value judgments are empty of substantive insight about the performance. However, the critic does provide authentic indicators of the feeling response that the performance elicited as well as substantive information regarding what aspects of the performance elicited that response. For example, in response to a nurse's unexpected move that clearly turned an evolving situation in a new direction, the critic might say, "When you did that, I was worried at first because it was so unexpected and seemed so daring and out of place. But as soon as I saw what happened next, I was pleased, because you clearly made a breakthrough when you did that." Here, the value-laden responses of worry and approval are grounded in the particular perspective of the critic and explicitly linked to the nurse's actions.

When the critic observes something that could change or that needs to change, rather than render a value judgment of "bad," the critic provides specific guidance for the next step and, if possible, places the element within the context of the performer's history. For example, in response to a move that is awkward and poorly timed, the critic might say, "I sensed that you were distracted and tense today when you did what you did. One thing you might try next time is to pause and just take a deep breath before you jump into this kind of challenge. Spend a moment getting clear about your intentions as you gather your equipment, and breathe!" Alternatively, the critic might respond, "Your finesse could have been better when you performed that action. Here is a sequence of moves that you can practice during the next week that I think will help. Start out slowly, and practice breathing and establishing a rhythm and a flow."

Connoisseurship requires creativity in that the critic engages in the rehearsal with a sense of openness to insights not previously conceived. It also implies that the critic has a disciplinary focus, because the critic offers a trained perspective and expectations regarding artistic validity within a particular field. The traits that the connoisseur/critic observe are:

- *Voice intonation and expression in narrative.* The critic notices the feeling that is elicited from the narrative and notes specific elements of expression that appear to be associated with the response.
- *Substance of the narrative interactions.* The critic notices words, phrases, and narrative sequences and how they are framed within the whole.
- *Synchrony of movement.* The critic observes how movement is situated within the context and provides guidance for developing skill in areas that interfere with synchronous movement.
- *Synchrony between movement and narrative.* The critic observes the ways in which movement and words come together to form a whole within the interaction and the ways in which movement and narrative synchronize to create an artistic expression.
- *Perceived intention and emotion.* The critic senses the intention that is communicated by the nurse, which may or may not coincide with the nurse's actual felt intention. When the perceived intention (as received by the critic) and the nurse's felt intention do not coincide, the critic suggests how the nurse's movement and narrative need to shift to convey adequately the felt intention.
- *Synchrony of interaction.* The critic notices the responses of others in the situation, the rhythm and flow of the interactions, and how these reveal possibilities for the nurse to develop his or her art.

FORMAL EXPRESSIONS OF AESTHETIC KNOWING: CRITICISM AND WORKS OF ART

From the creative processes of envisioning and rehearsing, the formal expressions of aesthetic knowing emerge. These include works of art and aesthetic criticisms. Works of art as aesthetic knowledge can be made available to the broader audience within and outside the discipline. Works of art that are developed to show and symbolize artistic qualities expressed in nursing practice are an unwritten form of aesthetic knowledge. *Aesthetic criticism* is a written account that portrays the artistry of nursing. Because aesthetic criticism takes written form, it can also be shared with others.

Works of art can take a visual form, such as paintings, drawings, or photographs; a literary form, such as poetry or fiction; a more physical form that involves dance or music; or any other art form. Works of art embody and represent meaning in the experience of nursing as the artist perceives them, and they are a unique creation of the artist. Those who view, hear, or read what is expressed in a work of art also engage in the aesthetic experience of perceiving meaning in the art. The meanings perceived by the observer or reader may or may not be the same as the artist's meanings, but they can be valid meanings that inform a more complete interpretation of the art.

Aesthetic criticism, as a formalized written account of aesthetic knowledge, focuses on the transformative art/act enacted in nursing practice or on a tangible work of art representative of some nursing experience. Aesthetic criticisms highlight and bring to awareness aspects of the artistry that may not be readily perceptible to the casual observer. Aesthetic criticism provides insight into the art form, interprets the work of the nurse artist, and deepens appreciation of the nurse's art. Aesthetic criticisms are the product of a connoisseur-critic who selects the art of one or more artists as the focus for the critique. The critic reflects on the meanings as well as the technical adequacy of the art. A critique systematically explores the significance of one or more interpretations of the art and places the art in its historical and cultural context. Aesthetic criticism includes the following essential elements:

- *Historical integration.* Historical integration includes the history of the art form and the personal artistic history of the artist. The critic examines evidence of change and continuity in the artist's history and interprets its meaning. The threads that comprise the artist's history are related to the art form, and the art form is placed within the context of those threads.
- *Comparative description of the art form.* The critic examines the form that the artist takes in the artistic process and compares the artist's work with known forms of the art. By drawing comparisons, the critic substantiates the unique aspects of the artist's work and the significance of the artist's work with regard to the discipline.
- *Consideration of plausible interpretations of meaning.* The critic considers a number of plausible meanings of the art and explores what the various meanings contribute to aesthetic understanding in the discipline. The critic may develop a preferred interpretation, but the stance remains open to multiple plausible interpretations.
- *Translation of future possibility.* The critic explores the directions that the artist might take and what the work of the artist contributes to the future development of the discipline. This aspect of criticism opens the way for appreciation and inspiration, for both the artist and the other members of the discipline.

CONCLUSION

In this chapter we have explored the nature and meaning of art and aesthetics in nursing. Nursing as art has always been an important focus for nursing and various ways art has been thought of in nursing were explored. The dimensions of aesthetic knowing of critical questions, creative processes, and formal expressions were detailed and illustrated.

References

Archibald, M. M. (2012). The holism of aesthetic knowing in nursing. *Nursing Philosophy: An International Journal for Healthcare Professionals, 13*, 179–188. https://doi.org/10.1111/j.1466-769X.2012.00542.x.

Archibald, M. M., Caine, V., & Scott, S. D. (2017). Intersections of the arts and nursing knowledge. *Nursing Inquiry, 24*(2). https://doi.org/10.1111/nin.12153.

Bender, M., & Elias, D. (2016). Reorienting esthetic knowing as an appropriate "object" of scientific inquiry to advance understanding of a critical pattern of nursing knowledge in practice. *ANS. Advances in Nursing Science, 1*. https://doi.org/10.1097/ANS.0000000000000160.

Benner, P. A., Tanner, C. A., & Chesla, C. A. (1996). *Expertise in nursing practice: caring, clinical judgment, and ethics.* New York, NY: Springer Publishing Co.

Billay, D., Myrick, F., Luhanga, F., & Yonge, O. (2007). A pragmatic view of intuitive knowledge in nursing practice. *Nursing Forum, 42*, 147–155.

Chinn, P. L. (1994). Developing a method for aesthetic knowing in nursing. In P. L. Chinn, & J. Watson (Eds.), *Art and aesthetics in nursing* (pp. 19–40). New York, NY: National League for Nursing Press.

Chinn, P. L. (2001). Toward a theory of nursing art. In N. L. Chaska (Ed.), *The nursing profession: tomorrow and beyond* (pp. 287–297). Thousand Oaks, CA: Sage.

Chinn, P. L., Maeve, M. K., & Bostick, C. (1997). Aesthetic inquiry and the art of nursing. *Scholarly Inquiry for Nursing Practice, 11*, 83–96.

Chinn, P. L., & Watson, J. (1994). *Art & aesthetics in nursing.* New York, NY: National League for Nursing.

Darbyshire, P. (1994). Understanding the life of illness: learning through the art of Frida Kahlo. *ANS. Advances in Nursing Science, 17*, 51–59.

Dean, P. (2013). Nursing as art-in-action is practical as well as aesthetic. *Journal of Art and Aesthetics in Nursing and Health Sciences, 1*, 4–10.

Eisner, E. W. (1985). *Aesthetic modes of knowing: learning and teaching the ways of knowing.* Chicago, IL: University of Chicago Press.

Heidegger, M. (1962). *Being and time.* Edited by E. Robinson. New York, NY: Harper & Row.

Honan, L., Shealy, S., Fennie, K., Duffy, T. C., Friedlaender, L., & Del Vecchio, M. (2016). Looking is not seeing and listening is not hearing: a replication study with accelerated BSN students. *Journal of Professional Nursing: Official Journal of the American Association of Colleges of Nursing, 32*(5S), S30–S36. https://doi.org/10.1016/j.profnurs.2016.05.002.

Johnson, J. L. (1994). A dialectical examination of nursing art. *ANS. Advances in Nursing Science, 17*, 1–14.

Johnson, J. L. (1996). Dialectical analysis concerning the rational aspect of the art of nursing. *Image - The Journal of Nursing Scholarship, 28*, 169–175.

Kagan, P. N. (2009). Historical voices of resistance: crossing boundaries to praxis through documentary film-making for the public. *ANS. Advances in Nursing Science, 32*, 19–32.

Kramper, M., & Thawley, S. (2009). Poetry and the art of nursing. *ORL-Head and Neck Nursing: Official Journal of the Society of Otorhinolaryngology and Head-Neck Nurses, 27*, 6–11.

Lamb, J. (2009). Creating change: using the arts to help stop the stigma of mental illness and foster social integration. *Journal of Holistic Nursing: Official Journal of the American Holistic Nurses' Association, 27*, 57–65.

LeVasseur, J. J. (1999). Toward an understanding of art in nursing. *ANS. Advances in Nursing Science, 21*, 48–63.

Liehr, P., Morris, K., Leavitt, M. A., & Takahashi, R. (2013). Translating research findings to promote peace: moving from "field to forum" with verbatim theatre. *ANS. Advances in Nursing Science, 36*, 160–170.

Maeve, M. K. (1994). Coming to moral consciousness through the art of nursing narratives. In P. L. Chinn, & J. Watson (Eds.), *Art and aesthetics in nursing* (pp. 67–89). New York, NY: National League for Nursing.

Mattingly, C. (1994a). The concept of therapeutic emplotment. *Social Science & Medicine, 38*, 811–822.

Mattingly, C. (1994b). The narrative nature of clinical reasoning. In C. Mattingly, & M. H. Fleming (Eds.), *Clinical reasoning: forms of inquiry in a therapeutic practice.* Philadelphia: F.A. Davis.

Newman, M. A. (2002). The pattern that connects. *ANS. Advances in Nursing Science, 24*(3), 1–7. https://www.ncbi.nlm.nih.gov/pubmed/11890192.

Oettinger, K. B. (1939). Toward inner freedom. *The American Journal of Nursing, 39*, 1224–1229.

Pellico, L. H., & Chinn, P. L. (2007). Narrative criticism: a systematic approach to the analysis of story. *Journal of Holistic Nursing: Official Journal of the American Holistic Nurses' Association, 25*, 58–65.

Sandelowski, M. (1995). On the aesthetics of qualitative research. *Image - The Journal of Nursing Scholarship, 27*, 205–209.

Sorrell, J. M. (1994). Remembrance of things past through writing: esthetic patterns of knowing in nursing. *ANS. Advances in Nursing Science, 17*, 60–70.

Vezeau, T. M. (1994). Narrative in nursing practice and education. In P. L. Chinn, & J. Watson (Eds.), *Art and aesthetics in nursing* (pp. 163–188). New York, NY: National League for Nursing.

Wainwright, P. (2000). Towards an aesthetics of nursing. *Journal of Advanced Nursing, 32*, 750–756.

Empiric Knowledge Development

There seems to be general agreement that there is a critical need for knowledge about the empirical world, knowledge that is systematically organized into general laws and theories for the purpose of describing, explaining, and predicting phenomena of special concern to the discipline of nursing.

Barbara Carper (1978, p. 14)

The opening quote suggests that the discipline of nursing requires systematic knowledge about the empirical world—knowledge that describes, explains, and predicts events and phenomena that nurses deal with on a daily basis. Nursing, however, is often characterized as a *human science,* which means that its disciplinary knowledge focuses on phenomena and events that are very different from phenomena within the physical sciences. Understanding (and developing) shared empiric knowledge about human responses to a life-changing event is much different than understanding how solid matter responds to the application of heat or force.

 Consider This...

Early one evening, as off-duty pediatric nurse Connie prepared dinner in her suburban home, three neighbor children ran into her kitchen and asked her to come quickly because "Noah fell and is hurt." Noah is a 2-year-old neighbor boy who was born to a 15-year-old girl. He lives with his mother, Shalyn, as well as Shalyn's four siblings and parents in a recently remodeled home. As Connie reaches the living room where Noah is laying, Shalyn is near panic at the sight of her child motionless on the floor. Connie glances up, notices a loft area, and infers that Noah apparently climbed the stairs, put a stool against the loft railing, climbed over, and fell about 16 feet to the wooden floor below. At the time of Noah's fall, the only other people who were home were Shalyn and her 10-year-old brother. Shalyn heard Noah fall, but did not see how he landed. As Connie approaches Noah, she can see that his eyes are open. He has no visible injuries, and he responds with whimpers and soft crying when he was approached. Shalyn showed great relief as Noah got up and walked toward her. While Noah was being held by Shalyn, Connie was able to check his movements and pupils and palpate his head. Although he had a bump on the side of his head, Connie found nothing else unusual, despite his significant fall.

Recognizing the potential seriousness of the situation, Connie advises Shalyn to take Noah to a nearby emergency department for evaluation. Shalyn calls her mother immediately and asks her to leave work to drive them to the hospital. As Connie waits for Shalyn's mother to arrive, Shalyn says that she is worried that her father might become very angry and physically hurtful and blame her for Noah's fall. At the hospital, Noah is diagnosed with a skull fracture and kept overnight. When Noah was released, watchful waiting was recommended, and he recovered without incident. Connie called Shalyn's father that evening to verify that he understood the urgency of securing the loft so that Noah stays safe, and to determine if he was handling the situation without becoming abusive. She also checked with Shalyn to address her fears about his response.

In this case, Connie's scientific-empiric knowledge of the signs and symptoms of neurologic injury made it possible for her to assess Noah's condition immediately following the fall, knowing the effect of head trauma on motor and sensory function as well as how children might respond differently to trauma as compared with adults. Her advice to take Noah for further assessment and observation was based on scientific-empiric knowledge about how and why symptoms of head injury might not immediately be seen, and the necessity to monitor signs and symptoms of a head injury in the first 24 to 48 hours. Her empirical knowledge of patterns of domestic violence also informed her decision to check in with the family to assess whether this had become a factor. Connie's knowledge of each aspect of the situation (head injury and domestic violence) developed from her own experiences with children as well as background knowledge that had been verified and communicated to her through texts, research reports, and classroom experiences.

In this chapter we address the dimensions of empiric knowing and knowledge development—the critical questions, creative processes, and forms of expressions for the pattern of empirics. The term *empiric* has a number of nuanced, interrelated meanings. From a traditional standpoint, an empiric (noun) is an individual who relies on experience for knowledge about the world. In this way, knowledge deemed empirical was based on personal observation and experience; the person with that knowledge was an "empiric." In the clinical health care context today, an *empiric* treatment or care approach is one that has been demonstrated, through observation and experience of professionals, to be effective. There may or may not be scientific evidence to support the treatment. Empirical knowledge of this sort can be shared and transmitted. However, it does not come about through research, extrapolation from theory, nor does it originate in formal logic processes.

From a more scientific perspective on knowledge, *empiric* knowledge still refers to that which is known through sensory perception, either directly or indirectly, and what is known can be shared across observers. To be considered scientific, however, knowledge must have a degree of verifiability or authentication. Our use of the term "empiric" pertains to scientific knowledge and is knowledge that arises out of direct or indirect perceptual experience. As disciplinary knowledge, what constitutes scientific empirical knowledge is developed using a broad array of approaches. These include such things as controlled experimental studies as well as various naturalistic methods or analytic approaches. These approaches require interacting with and understanding the nature of experience as it is perceived, or represented—in language or text. This definition is broad to be sure, but the bottom line is that what constitutes empirics emanates from direct and indirect sensory perception and relies on direct and indirect perception for authentication. Not all empiric knowledge can be considered scientific. To be scientific, empirically generated knowledge must be verified using accepted professional methods. When we discuss empirics and use that term, we assume a focus on scientific-empirics rather than empirics as "knowledge from experience that seems to work."

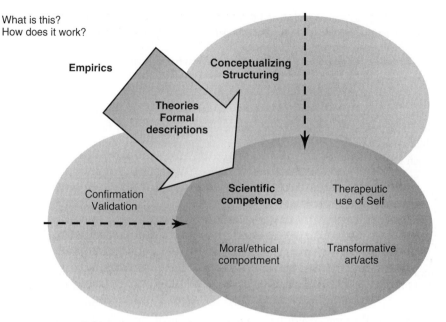

What is this?
How does it work?

Empirics

Theories
Formal
descriptions

Conceptualizing
Structuring

Confirmation
Validation

Scientific
competence

Therapeutic
use of Self

Moral/ethical
comportment

Transformative
art/acts

FIG. 7.1 Dimensions of Empiric Knowledge Development.

DIMENSIONS OF EMPIRIC KNOWLEDGE DEVELOPMENT

Fig. 7.1 shows the empiric quadrant of our model for nursing knowledge development. As the critical questions "What is this?" and "How does it work?" are asked, the creative processes of conceptualizing and structuring are initiated. As with the other patterns, these questions are also asked, not deliberatively, but more intuitively, in the moment of practice as empiric knowledge is integrated with the other patterns of knowing. The creative processes of conceptualizing and structuring provide insights and tentative "answers" to the critical questions of empirics. Out of the creative processes comes the generation or reconfiguring of formal expressions of empirics. Table 7.1 Summarizes the dimensions of empiric knowing. In this chapter we address the dimensions of critical questions, creative processes and formal expressions.

Our focus on empirical knowledge is primarily on empiric theory, however much of what follows applies to other forms of empiric knowledge as well. Formalized descriptions based on direct and indirect sensory observation, as well as empiric research reports, are other forms of empiric knowledge that arise from the critical questions and creative processes of empirics.

CRITICAL QUESTIONS: WHAT IS THIS? HOW DOES IT WORK?

The critical questions of empirics assume that some degree of objectivity exists, and that it can be understood through observation and inferences based on indirect observations.

TABLE 7.1 Dimensions of Empiric Knowledge Development

Dimension	Empirics
Critical questions	What is this? How does it work?
Creative processes	Conceptualizing Structuring
Formal expressions	Facts Models Formal descriptions Theories Thematic descriptions Empiric research reports
Authentication processes	Confirmation Validation
Integrated expression in practice	Scientific competence

In other words, the critical questions of empirics address objects, experiences, and perceptions that are assumed to be somewhat tangible. To claim something is "real" or tangible suggests that the meaning of the object, experience, or perception is similar across observers. This further implies that meaning is more located in the object, experience, or perception itself than within the person perceiving it.

 Consider This...

Suzie: "Wow, Alison, I love that aqua scarf you're wearing!"
Alison: "Thanks, Suzie; I really love aqua blue."
Suzie: "Me too! It reminds me of the Caribbean Sea and memories of Mexico."
- Is knowledge of the scarf's color empirical?
- If so, what makes it empirical?
- What determines why the scarf is said to be blue?
- Would you say knowledge about agreement on color is scientific as well as empirical?

In this example of a blue scarf, Alison and Suzi both agree that the scarf is aqua blue, and likely others would also. This suggests that aqua is a property of the scarf itself. Had Alison commented that Suzi's scarf was unattractive on her, while Suzi thought it looked attractive we would conclude that attractiveness was not an obvious inherent property of the scarf itself.

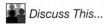 **Discuss This...**

Suppose you encounter an emotionally withdrawn child during a pediatric rotation. Recognizing this withdrawal pattern for a child in these circumstances as unusual and counterproductive, you ask: What is this? What does it mean? There could be several reasons. Discuss with your peers the possible explanations, including:

- Emotional self-protection?
- Effects of a medication?
- Pain?

Are your explanations adequate? What would you need to do to create or have an adequate explanation? What do you mean by "emotional withdrawal"?

CREATIVE PROCESSES: CONCEPTUALIZING AND STRUCTURING

The creative processes initiated by the critical questions can take various forms, each of which can lead to credible empirical knowledge. Regardless of form, creative processes will involve conceptualizing and structuring. Conceptualizing refers to thinking about and systematically considering the nature and meaning of ideas, expressing that meaning in language or symbols, and formulating empirically knowable referents for those ideas. Consider the idea of "emotional withdrawal." Conceptualizing using the processes for empirical knowledge means you will need to carefully and rigorously formulate or designate a meaning for "emotional withdrawal."

Conceptualizing can occur informally through careful thought about the meaning you discern or intend for an idea, or formally through rigorous methods of concept clarification that might be required for some types of research or theory construction. Conceptualizations can also emerge or be better understood from certain forms of inductive research inquiry. *Conceptualizing* involves creative processes of making meaning; it involves exploring a wide range of possible meanings for a concept and creating or designating a meaning that is relevant to your purpose.

Structuring refers to the organization of ideas, into various forms of empirical knowledge such as theories, descriptions, or written analyses. The *structuring* process also takes many forms but universally involves organizing concepts into a linguistic or visual structure in a way that represents them as fully as possible. Structuring can occur by using text to organize ideas into a logical or coherent form as in an interpretive study report. Or, structuring might be done by formulating hypotheses for testing as in a quasi-experimental research approach. Basically, structuring requires a language that represents the ideas the knowledge developer is working with.

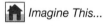 *Imagine This...*

Imagine that you have frequently observed emotional withdrawal in children undergoing chemotherapy, and are interested in finding out if therapy dogs might alleviate their emotional withdrawal. You might arrange for therapy dogs to visit with children undergoing chemotherapy, interview parents about their perceptions of their child's response, and then structure your findings in a narrative. Or, you might formulate hypotheses related to the nature and timing of exposure to therapy dogs and design an experiment to test whether certain features of timing or other variables affect response. Either way, you are structuring ideas as knowledge.

We have said that conceptualizing and structuring in the context of empiric knowledge development is a rigorous process that must be done carefully. If the meaning of the ideas you are considering is inappropriate for the context, or your approach to inquiry is inadequate, the validity of the knowledge will be questionable and authentication cannot be achieved. The next section considers the nature of concepts and techniques for conceptualizing within the context of knowledge development. While creating conceptual meaning is considered first, it should be noted that structuring may lead to clarifying conceptual meaning and both processes tend to be intermingled.

The Nature of Concepts and Conceptual Meaning

We define the term *concept* as a complex mental formulation of experience. By "experience," we mean perceptions of the world, including objects, other people, visual images, color, movement, sounds, behavior, and interactions; in other words, we refer to the totality of what is perceived. Experience is considered empiric when it can be symbolically shared and verified by others with sensory evidence.

Fig. 7.2 shows the three sources of experience interacting to form the meaning of the concept: (1) the word or other symbolic label; (2) the thing itself (object, property, or event); and (3) the feelings, values, and attitudes associated with the word and with the perception of the thing. As any one of these elements changes over time, the concept itself changes.

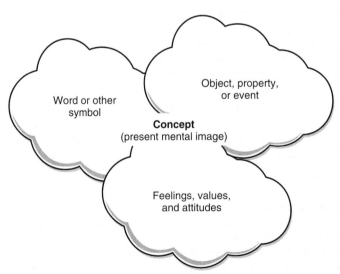

FIG. 7.2 Sources of Experience Forming Conceptual Meaning.

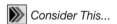 *Consider This...*

> Consider the concept of *mouse*. Until the 1980s, this word symbol was almost exclusively connected to a little critter that wreaks havoc in people's basements and prompts screams of terror in movies. In a very short time frame, this word symbol came to signify not only that little critter but also a very different object: a device that is used to navigate a cursor on a computer. At first, this device was thought to be optional and mainly useful for the playing of games. However, it quickly became not optional but necessary (which is an attitude or feeling), and certainly not an object that elicits screams and screeches. Almost any word could have been chosen for this little object, but its originators selected the word *mouse,* which derives from the resemblance of early models that had a cord attached to the rear part of the device (suggesting a tail) to the common rodent "mouse." More recently the concept of a mouse as it relates to computer navigation has changed from something that was once necessary to something that is no longer required once track pads for navigation were introduced.

The same word may be used to represent more than one concept or mental image. For example, the word *cup* may be used to represent several different kinds of objects or ideas. Each use of the word carries with it different perceptions and meanings. If the object is a fancy teacup, a very different mental image forms than if the object is the cup into which a golf ball falls on a putting green. When creating, designating, or deciding conceptual meaning, you examine the range of meanings signified by a word symbol, and make a reasoned decision about what elements of meaning are important for your purpose.

All concepts can be located on a continuum from the more *empiric* (i.e., more directly experienced) to the *abstract* (i.e., more mentally constructed) (Jacox, 1974; Kaplan, 1964). In one sense, all concepts are both empiric and abstract. They are empiric because they are formed from perceptual encounters with the world as it is experienced, but they are abstract because they are mental images of that experience.

Some concepts are formed from very direct experiences that can be more readily verified by others. Others are formed from experiences that are commonly recognized but inferred indirectly. Fig 7.3 illustrates this continuum. Relatively empiric concepts are ideas that are formed from the direct observation of objects, properties, or events. As concepts become more abstract, they are inferred from indirect evidence. The most abstract concepts are mental constructions that encompass a complex network of subconcepts.

The most concrete empiric concepts have direct forms of measurement. Concepts formed around objects such as a cup or properties such as temperature are examples of highly empiric concepts, because the object or property that represents the idea (i.e., the empiric indicator) can be directly experienced through the senses and confirmed by many different people. Properties such as height and weight can be measured with standardized instruments.

As concepts become more abstract, their observational signifiers (i.e., their empiric indicators) become less concrete and less directly measurable. The assessment of an abstract concept depends increasingly on indirect means. Although an indirect assessment or observation is different from direct measurement, it is still

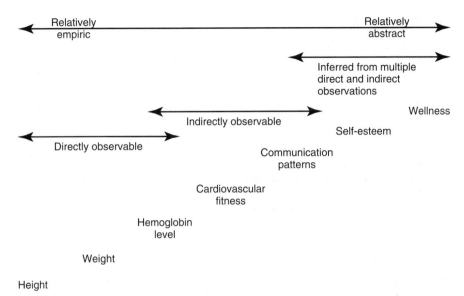

FIG. 7.3 Empiric–Abstract Continuum.

considered a reasonable indicator of the concept. An individual's hemoglobin level is representative of a concept that cannot be directly observed but that can be indirectly measured with the aid of laboratory instruments, which is a less direct form of measurement.

Cardiovascular fitness is an example of a concept in the middle range on the empiric–abstract continuum. Concepts increase in complexity in this range, and several empiric indicators must be assessed. Because no actual object that can be called "cardiovascular fitness" exists, a definition is required if we are to know what it is. Although definitions for less empirically based concepts are thoughtfully formulated, these are arbitrary because many different definitions could be chosen. As concepts become increasingly abstract, definitions become more dependent on a meaning for the concept that is created in relation to the purpose for defining it.

Self-esteem is an example of a highly abstract concept for which there is no direct measure. The instruments or tools that are developed to assess self-esteem depend on definitions that serve a specific purpose and are built on many behaviors and personality characteristics that experts agree are associated with the concept. Ideas about these characteristics may be derived from a theory, scholarly writings, or from creating conceptual meaning. Each behavioral trait that is contained in a self-esteem measurement tool can be considered a partial indicator of self-esteem. When the composite behaviors and personal characteristics are built into an assessment tool, it is usually a more adequate indicator of the abstract concept than any one behavior alone. The composite score obtained from the tool is then considered to be a measurement that has been constructed as an empiric indicator.

Highly abstract concepts are sometimes called *constructs*. Constructs are the most complex type of concept on the empiric–abstract continuum. These concepts include ideas with a reality base so abstract that meaning is constructed from multiple sources of direct and indirect evidence. An example of a construct is *wellness*. Although the idea of wellness exists, it cannot be directly observed. Fig. 7.3 illustrates the idea that highly abstract concepts are constructed from other concepts. All concepts shown on the continuum (as well as others) can be included in the concept of wellness.

Some abstract concepts have little meaning outside of the context of a theory. For example, Levine (1967) coined the word *trophicogenic* to mean "nurse-induced illness." Abstract concepts may also acquire additional meanings through gradual transfer into common language usage. Freud's concept of *ego* is an example. The word *ego* once had no common meaning outside of Freud's theory, but now almost everyone who speaks American English knows the meaning of the phrase "a big ego."

A single object, property, or event can also be represented by several different words. Each word conveys a slightly different meaning and often reflects nuances that relate to socially derived value meanings. For example, the words *jalopy, puddle-jumper, Beemer,* and *Hot Wheels* all refer to one basic thing: an automobile. The use of any of these words to describe an automobile conveys the perspective of the person who is using the word, as well as the features of the object itself.

Feelings, values, and attitudes are inner processes that are associated with concepts. For example, the word *mother* carries feelings, values, and attitudes that form from human experience with an actual person. Varying experiences with a certain mother (the person) account for the range of feelings that people associate with the word *mother*. At the same time, the meaning of the concept *mother* is formed from shared cultural and societal heritages. A concept such as *mother,* which can carry simple and specific or highly complex meanings, changes in its level of abstraction, depending on the context of usage. For example, a specific and simple meaning might be in the context of a questionnaire when a yes or no box is provided for responders to check indicating if they are a biological mother (i.e., have given birth). This simple and specific meaning contrasts with the meaning of mother if one is trying to discern the characteristics of early childhood mothering that is protective, nurturing, and enduring.

! Why Is This Important?

Nurses often claim that they tend to be very "concrete"—that they do not relate to theoretic abstractions. At the same time, nurses regularly address experiences such as *grief, anxiety,* and *hopelessness,* all concepts that are highly abstract. These concepts come to be seen as more "concrete" because the behavioral manifestations that we associate with them have been commonly accepted.

Although it usually is not possible or necessary to identify precisely where concepts fit on the empiric–abstract continuum, it is important to understand that concepts vary in the degree they are connected to what is perceived as experience and the extent to which their meaning is mentally constructed. Many nursing concepts are highly abstract. When you begin to work with an abstract concept, it is natural to wonder why it is difficult to grasp the meaning of the term and understand all that is conveyed by the concept.

Methods for Creating Conceptual Meaning

We talk about *creating* conceptual meaning because, in the context of knowledge development in nursing, concepts are often highly abstract and a meaning needs to be created from among a set of competing and nuanced meanings. Even when the concept is quite empirically grounded, designating a meaning is still an act of creation because even more empirically based concepts can have multiple meanings.

Creating conceptual meaning produces a tentative definition of the concept. We emphasize *tentative* because the definition can and may need to be revised. This does not mean, however, that "anything goes" or that any definition that suits the author will do. The use of *tentative* here means that the definition is open and can be changed as new insights and understandings come to light, or as circumstances change.

There are various methods for creating conceptual meaning, each of which has advantages and drawbacks (Beckwith, Dickinson, & Kendall, 2008). These techniques are designated as concept clarification, concept development, or concept analysis. Most of the methods have been used for several decades and can be usefully employed systematic, reliable methods. Norris (1982) described several methods for concept clarification. Walker and Avant (2010) detailed a method of concept analysis based on the work of Wilson (1963). Morse (1995) proposed methods of concept development and analysis that draw on qualitative and quantitative research approaches to validate meanings projected by analytic processes. Moscou (2008) described a method of concept analysis based on research evidence. An "evolutionary" method of concept analysis proposed by Rodgers and Knafl (2000) recognizes that conceptual meaning is dependent on context. Morrow (2009) described a creative process for selecting and conceptualizing meaning on the basis of the contemplation of a painting, then placing the meaning within a nursing framework. Bonis (2013) described an approach to concept analysis that focuses on detecting differences in the conceptual understandings embedded in different disciplines, so that nurses can better judge the value of borrowing research instruments from other disciplines.

Our approaches to creating conceptual meaning are similar to some of the processes described by other authors, but our approach assumes that meanings are created for a particular purpose and do not remain static but rather change over time and in different contexts. Therefore, it is not possible to make a claim that a concept is "mature" or sufficiently developed. Meanings are not inherent in objects or in a reality that exists independently; rather, they are shaped and formed in relation to a particular purpose and a particular context. For example, consider again the example of the word *mouse* and the two very different conceptual meanings that it carries. The conceptual meanings you would bring with you to a pet store and those you would bring to a computer store intending to purchase a mouse are shaped by the purpose of your shopping trip and the type of store that you enter to achieve this purpose.

When creating meaning, a wide variety of sources and methods can be used. Some are more formal and rigorous; others less so. Whether you go through a formal process of concept clarification, use a standard definition, or rely on professional literature to establish meaning depends on your purpose. There is no recipe or specific method to follow, and the approach to creating meaning can shift according to the purpose for which your concept is intended or used. The following sections provide guidelines that you can select, adapt, and blend as guided by your purpose. Not all concepts require formal methods for establishing meaning. When necessary for one's purposes, however, these approaches are extremely important and valuable. In these next sections, we consider more formal methods for creating conceptual meaning.

Regardless of your approach to creating conceptual meaning, you start with the designated concept. Concept selection is guided by your purpose and expresses values related to your purpose. For example, your purpose might be to work with the concept *dependence* for a research project. Eventually, you will need a clear conceptualization of dependence as well as ideas about how to measure or assess it. Another purpose might be to differentiate between two closely related concepts, such as *sympathy* and *empathy*. In this case, your concern is to create definitions that differentiate on the basis of a thorough familiarity with the meanings that are possible.

Another reason for creating conceptual meaning is to examine the ways in which concepts are used in existing writings. For example, the concept of *intuition* frequently appears in nursing literature, with many different but related meanings. The meanings that are conveyed reflect different assumptions about the phenomenon. As you become aware of these meanings, you become familiar with meanings that are consistent with your own purpose.

Other purposes behind creating conceptual meaning include generating research hypotheses, formulating nursing diagnoses, and developing computerized databases for clinical decision making. Creating conceptual meaning is also a valuable process for learning critical-thinking skills (Kramer, 1993). When you keep your purpose as clear as possible, you have an anchor that provides a sense of direction when you seem to be lost.

! Why Is This Important?

Because nursing has many broad, wholistic, and inclusive interests, it is easy to lose sight of the fact that a nursing perspective brings important insights to conceptual meaning. When choosing concepts, in addition to your purpose, the role and context of nursing is important to the choice. As you create conceptual meaning, it is important to make choices that help ensure meanings are useful to nurses as they manage human responses and help persons to move toward health. The important question is not, "Is this a nursing concept?" but rather, "Is this concept of interest to nursing, and is the meaning created useful for nursing's purposes?"

Sociopolitical considerations will also influence your choice of a concept and your approach to understanding it, often in ways that are subtle and difficult to perceive. For example, if you choose to examine the concept of *transition* for daughters who must place their mothers in nursing homes, you may eventually be lead to consider the consequences of women's caretaking within a society that devalues its elders and women's caregiving work.

Some concepts are not appropriate as a focus for the process of creating conceptual meaning. Some are too empirically grounded, and others are too expansive to yield a useful outcome. Concepts that represent empirically knowable objects (e.g., antiembolic stockings) are usually not good choices, because they are highly empirically grounded and can be demonstrated by a display of the thing itself. You do not need to examine the concepts to understand their meanings, and having criteria for recognizing them will not help you clinically in any significant way. Broad concepts such as *caring* and *stress* pose another set of problems. Because these types of concepts are so vast, creating meaning can result only in a broad understanding that omits necessary detail and that may be misleading. This is not to say that creating conceptual meaning for very narrow or broad concepts is never useful, and for some purposes, it may be justifiable. In our experience, the concepts that are most often amenable to the creation of conceptual meaning are those in the middle range. It often is helpful when choosing a concept to place it within the context of use, stress as associated with first-time mothers, to narrow its scope in relation to your purpose. In this case, stress still remains the concept of interest but you situate it within a context that will limit your exploration of meanings.

Once you have selected or encountered a concept that you believe needs to be subjected to formal processes of creating conceptual meaning, processes for creating conceptual meaning can be initiated.

Sources of Evidence

The sources that you choose and the extent to which you use various sources depend on your purposes. Early in the process of gathering evidence for the concept you have chosen, tentative criteria are proposed, and those criteria are refined in the light of additional information provided by continued gathering of evidence. We recommend beginning the process of criteria formulation early so that useful information is not lost. *Criteria* are succinct statements that describe essential characteristics and features that distinguish the concept as a recognizable entity and that differentiate this entity from other related ideas. Establishing tentative criteria using an exemplar case is a useful beginning strategy.

Exemplar Case. An exemplar case is a description or depiction of a situation, experience, or event that satisfies the following statement: "If this is not *x (insert your concept),* then nothing is." The case can be drawn from nursing practice, literature, art, film, or any other source in which the concept is represented or symbolized. The case is selected because it represents the concept to the best of your present understanding. When you deal with more abstract nursing concepts, exemplar cases of abstract concepts involve experiences and circumstances that are described in words. Exemplar cases may be created from your own experience, or you may find cases in the literature that have been constructed or described by others. However, you should always trust your own judgment about whether cases found in the literature are useful. You may find a case that is said to represent your concept, but you may decide it is not an adequate representation for your purposes.

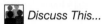 *Discuss This...*

Discuss developing an exemplar case for the concept of *mothering* with a group of your peers.
- Start with this scenario as an exemplar case: An infant cries, and an adult picks up the infant.
- Is this an adequate case to represent mothering? If not, why not?
- What circumstances, behaviors, motives, attitudes, and feelings would need to be included in your case so that everyone can agree that it is an exemplar case of mothering?

When you create your own exemplar case, it is important to work with your ideas and revise your description until you are satisfied that the case fully represents your concept. In the exemplar case of mothering, the adult initially might be portrayed as female. Later, you might portray a male in the same case. In the absence of any evidence one way or the other, you might tentatively decide that the idea of mothering that you are creating will be deliberately limited to instances that involve women. Because your decision is tentative, you can change your construction for another purpose or circumstance.

While you are working with exemplar cases, pose the following question: What makes this an instance of this concept? The responses to this question form the basis for a tentative list of features that must be present for mothering to occur. These features will become criteria that are designed to allow you to recognize the concept and to differentiate it from related concepts. In the case of mothering, the features serve to distinguish your concept (for example, mothering) from similar concepts (such as caring, nurturing, or helping).

Definitions. Two additional sources that provide information about conceptual meaning are dictionary definitions and usages of the concept you are exploring. Dictionary definitions are often circular and do not give a complete sense of meaning for the concept, but they do help to clarify common usages and ideas associated with the concept. They are also useful for tracing the origins of words, which provides clues about core meaning.

Existing theories and professional literature can provide definitions that extend beyond the limits of common usage. The way that concepts are used in the context of professional literature convey meanings within the domain of the discipline. For example, the term *mother* as defined in the dictionary reflects the social and biologic role of parenting and includes a few characteristics of the role, such as authority and affection. In the context of psychologic theories, however, the meanings that are conveyed include values, roles, functions, and characteristics of people such as parenting, physical care, responsibility, and power.

Visual Images. Visual images such as photographs, cartoons, calendars, paintings, and drawings are useful sources for creating conceptual meaning (Morrow, 2009). Images may be explicitly labeled or named as the concept of interest, or you may judge them to reasonably represent it. Suppose you find a painting that the artist has labeled "Sorrow." The artist's linking of the visual image to the concept through language provides further information about the meaning of the concept, enriches the range of meaning, and helps to minimize any bias inherent in your own views of the meaning of the concept. In some instances, you or others might deliberately create images that represent the concept that is being clarified rather than use existing sources.

Whether you personally create and examine an image or ask others to create images, the idea is to compare them for similarities and differences and reflect that information against your tentative criteria. Often, visual imagery will highlight some aspect of the concept that is significant. Visual imagery of depression, for example in drug ads, often depicts women; this suggests the condition is female specific. Visual images that represent concepts well also highlight difficulties with expressing meaning using words. A photograph may express rich dimensions of the concept of *dignity,* yet the essence of dignity expressed by the photo is impossible to describe—an example of how aesthetic expressions of concepts contribute to empiric knowledge.

Popular and Classical Literature. A variety of literature resources can provide information about conceptual meaning. Literature reflects meanings that arise from the culture and provides rich sources of exemplar cases for concepts. Classical prose and poetry are often good sources of meaning for concepts used in nursing. For example, images of love and longing may be found in the poetic works of Emily Dickinson. Louisa May Alcott's classic *Little Women* provides information about the nature of intimacy and caring. The popular current literature is also a source of valuable data about conceptual meaning. Popular self-help books on topics such as overcoming negative thinking and codependency often can clarify commonly understood (or misunderstood) conceptual meanings. Fairy tales, myths, fables, and stories can provide relevant insights whereas usages expressed in popular jargon and cartoons may highlight borderline meanings.

Music and Poetry. The imagery of music or poetry may be useful for the creation of conceptual meaning. You can find music or poetry by seeking out lyrics or titles that name the concept under consideration. The music itself or the title or lyrics may reasonably suggest the concept. Music and poetry can effectively convey meanings through rhythm, tones, lyrical or linguistic forms and metaphors, or musical moods that reflect experiences in life events with which nurses deal. For example, the Shaker folk tune "Simple Gifts" suggests criteria for concepts of authenticity, genuineness, centeredness, and community. The tune itself conveys a sense of inner happiness and peace; the lyrics reflect relationships between inner peace and the ability to build strong relationships. The popular Cole Porter song "Don't Fence Me In" conveys through its musical mood, rhythm, and lyrics what it feels like to be confined emotionally and projects a yearning to be free.

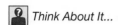 *Think About It...*

> Jot down some criteria for the concept of mothering, then search the Internet for "songs about mother." How do they refine your ideas about the concept of mothering? How has the imagery in those songs changed over the years?

Professional Literature. Professional literature often provides meanings that are pertinent to the practice of nursing. For example, philosophers as well as nurses have written about the concept of *presence* as a way of being with another. When the work of a scholar in another discipline coincides with your experience as a nurse, the scholar's work can augment your conceptual meaning. When you find contradictions with your experience as a nurse, this prompts you to clarify your own insights about the phenomenon.

Anecdotal Accounts and Opinions. Peers, coworkers, hospitalized individuals, other professional workers, and people who are not connected to nursing can provide valuable information about the meaning of a concept. It may be useful to seek others' opinions if your direct experience with the concept is limited. Nurses who work with the concept daily may be able to shed light on nuances of meaning. For example, a nurse who works with people whose lung function is severely compromised might observe that anxiety, although usually characterized by increased activity, evokes a different reaction in these patients. Rather than random activity, anxiety may be accompanied by a deliberate quieting of behavior to conserve energy. Asking knowledgeable others to share their opinions and understandings grounds your meaning in everyday perception and tests professional meanings in relation to everyday assumptions about a phenomenon.

Testing Your Criteria. As you examine your sources of evidence, you begin the process of testing the soundness of your conceptualization of whatever conceptual meaning you are creating in relation to your purpose. Some meanings may seem reasonable or plausible but not well suited to your purpose. For example, someone who is interested in *mothering* as it pertains to a foster mother may not find useful information contained in the 1915 song that spells out M-O-T-H-E-R (see http://parlorsongs.com/issues/2000-5/2000-5.php for lyrics and information about this song).

Contrary Cases. Contrary cases are those cases that are certainly not instances of the concept—they are the antithesis of the exemplar case that the process begins with. For more concrete concepts, contrary cases are relatively easy. A saucer or a spoon can be presented as things that are not cups, and green is certainly not the color red. For the concept of *hopelessness, hope* could be presented as a contrary case.

As you consider contrary cases, ask the following: What makes this instance different from the concept that I have selected? By comparing the differences between exemplar and contrary cases, you will begin to revise, add to, or delete from the tentative criteria that are emerging. In constructing a narrative that describes hope, you might notice that a certain type of body position with walking movement seems to be associated with hopelessness. If you are having difficulty with constructing a contrary case, ask someone to suggest a scenario that is definitely not what you are trying to describe. Sometimes you can locate a contrary case in the literature. Contrary cases that contribute to meaning often reveal important aspects of the exemplar case that are hidden in assumptions you may be making about the concept.

Related Cases. Related cases represent a different but similar concept. Related cases may share several criteria with the concept of interest, but one or more criteria will be particularly associated with the exemplar case and will distinguish the exemplar case from the related cases.

For the concept of *mothering,* you could create a related case of child tending, such as care provided by a nanny, that would be similar to the exemplar case. You might make a child care worker the adult or substitute an elderly person for the infant. Again, you consider differences and similarities between the exemplar case and the related cases and revise the tentative criteria to reflect your new insights. For example, you might conclude that mothering requires an investment in the ongoing welfare of the infant, whereas nannying or tending does not, rather in instances of tending investment in the child's welfare is time limited.

Borderline Cases. A borderline case is found when the same word is used in a different context. For example, if you are examining the concept of *fatigue* in chronic illness, a useful borderline case of the use of the term *fatigue* would be "military fatigue clothing." To offer a "cup of cheer" is an exemplary borderline usage of the term *cup.* This highlights the feature of cups as being capable of holding something. For the concept of anxiety, when a 5-year-old child jumps up and down and exclaims, "I'm so anxious for my birthday to be here!" the meaning of *anxious* is not the same meaning that concerns nurses. What the child's usage does convey is the physical agitation that accompanies the experience of anxiety within the context of nursing practice.

Slang terms and terms used to describe technologic operations or features are rich sources of borderline cases when they are first entering the language. After they become well accepted, they are no longer borderline; they move to more central conceptual meanings, and they may even become exemplary cases. During the early 1990s, the word *web* probably would have prompted a mental image of something that a spider creates, and a reference to the Internet would have been considered a borderline case. By the end of the 1990s, the word *web* (i.e., World Wide Web) was so fully associated with the Internet that it might have become a model case of *web.*

For the concept of *mothering,* a borderline case might be a computer motherboard, and you might choose this borderline usage to help clarify features of the concept of *mother* that can be seen as foundational to the concept of mothering. These features could also include the central importance of the mother in some cultures for defining the scope of relationships or structuring the energy of all relationships within the system.

Paradoxic cases are variants of borderline cases that are useful to highlight the central meanings of concepts. Paradoxically, these cases embody elements of both exemplar and contrary cases. For example, when exploring the meaning of *dignity*, you might create a case in which actions that violate dignity occur to preserve a central feature of dignity. Your case might be the emergency cardiopulmonary resuscitation of a person in a public space to preserve the life of that person. Such a case is paradoxic in that it violates some criteria for dignity but highlights the importance, indeed precedence, of worthiness as a feature of dignity by highlighting actions that aim to maintain the individual's worth (e.g., life and health) regardless of circumstances. You may invent other varieties of cases during the process of creating conceptual meaning. How the cases are classified or the number and variety of sources, including cases, is not critical. Rather, their important function is to assist you with discerning the range of possible meanings important for creating a meaning that is useful for your purpose. Although creating conceptual meaning is a rigorous and thoughtful process, it is centrally important to remember that sources of evidence are somewhat arbitrary, and are historically and culturally situated. What you call them is not essential to the process; what is important is the meaning that you derive from the conceptual exploration and the investigation.

Exploring Contexts and Values. The values and meanings for concepts that grow out of personal experience do not occur in a vacuum; rather they occur in social contexts that have embedded cultural meanings that influence the mental representations of experience. For example, consider the values and meanings surrounding the concept of *judgment* if you are a student taking an examination, or a magistrate preparing to impose a sentence. When you explore conceptual meaning across a variety of contexts, you likely will be made aware of meanings and values that shape meanings that you previously had not considered.

One way to explore conceptual meaning across various contexts is to place your exemplar cases in different contexts and ask: What would happen in a different situation? For example, if you place an exemplar case of the color red in the context of a magazine advertisement, what symbolic meaning is conveyed? In the context of traffic signs and symbols, what meaning does the color now convey? What about a woman wearing a red suit in a boardroom where everyone else is dressed in dark suits? What might you learn about mothering in the context of a same-sex household? In a single-father or -mother household? As you consider various possible combinations of context, you will illuminate how meanings are influenced by context.

Placing the concept in a subtly differing context also reveals values. The concept of *mothering* has a relatively positive connotation for many people. Most people agree that humans require "good" mothering to grow and develop adequately. However, people differ widely with regard to what they consider to be good mothering; these differences are often associated with the cultural context. For example, people probably would disagree about whether encouraging a child's obedience to rules or encouraging independent decision making is good mothering. What is considered mothering, and good and bad mothering, reflects deeply embedded cultural values. When you consider your exemplar case across different social contexts, you create an avenue for perceiving important meanings that are grounded in differing values and cultural contexts and you can make deliberate choices about the importance those meanings.

Formulating Criteria for Concepts

For cases where concepts require formal processes of creating conceptual meaning, we suggest using criteria as an expression of conceptual meaning. Criteria provide a sensitive and succinct form for conveying essential conceptual meaning. Criteria are particularly useful as tools to initiate other processes of empiric theory development, including designating ways to assess or measure the concept. As we have said, criteria for the concept emerge gradually and continuously as you consider definitions, various cases, other sources, and varying contexts and values. As you develop the criteria, you will naturally refine them so that they reflect the meaning that you intend. Criteria often express both qualitative and quantitative aspects of meaning and should suggest a definition of the concept. Because criteria are more complex than a limited word definition, they amplify the meaning and suggest direction for the processes of developing empiric knowledge, including theory.

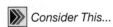 *Consider This...*

For concrete objects, the criteria may be relatively simple but they have the same challenges as more complicated abstract concepts. For the concept of a cup, examples of criteria might include the following:
- The object is cylindric or conic in shape.
- The object is capable of containing physical matter.
- The height normally is between 3 and 7 inches, and the widest diameter is 3 to 4 inches.
- When the object contains liquid, it can safely hold hot liquids.

Notice that this set of criteria is phrased so that a disposable foam cup or a golfing green cup can be included. This choice is guided by the purpose. If you needed to make sure that the golfing green cup was not included as a cup, you might revise the criteria to include "the object is capable of being held in the hand, regardless of what it contains." This criterion places a limit on the volume and weight of the cup and implies that it must be a portable object.

Developing criteria for more abstract concepts is a more complex process, and the criteria are thus often more abstract. Criteria for the concept of *mothering* might include the following:
- The mothering person must have visual contact with the person who receives the mothering in a manner that can be observed.
- The person who receives the mothering must be physically touched by the mothering person.
- Some positive feeling must be experienced by the mothering person and by the person who receives the mothering.
- There must be a reciprocal interaction between the mothering person and the person who receives mothering.
- Vocalization by the mothering person must occur.

These criteria do not limit the mothering person by gender, age, or species. If the purpose of applying the criteria is to distinguish between instances of mothering and fathering, these criteria would need to be revised to specify at least gender role. If the purpose is to differentiate between mothering and neglect, they might be adequate.

The following question arises during the course of creating conceptual meaning: How do I know that the meaning that I have created is adequate? You can examine your conceptual meaning for adequacy in relation to the processes that are used to create meaning as well as the conceptual meaning that you have created. Fuller (1991) suggested examining the process and the product of conceptualization in terms of both validity and reliability. A conceptualization is *valid* if it is based on multiple examples that are fully representative of the range of meanings for the concept, if you used multiple interpretive stages during the clarification process, and if the essential structure (or pattern) of the concept can be understood from the criteria. The conceptualization is *reliable* if the concept can be consistently recognized on the basis of the criteria that you have created. You may never know for sure that the meaning is adequate; however, the meaning can be considered adequate if it reflects a reasonable and communicable understanding that is useful for your purposes. If your aims reflect valued nursing goals, if you have been careful when choosing and using resources, and if you understand why you have made the choices that you have, you will have created an adequate and useful meaning. Additional processes for knowledge development will provide a check on conceptual meaning and will contribute to further refinements.

CREATIVE PROCESSES: STRUCTURING EMPIRIC KNOWLEDGE

In addition to conceptualizing, structuring is a basic creative process within the empiric pattern. Structuring empiric knowledge requires systematic and rigorous approaches. Research is a central means of structuring empirical knowledge and developing empiric theory. As hypotheses link empirical referents for testing, knowledge is generated about how the concepts as represented are related (e.g., conceptualized and defined). Structuring can also occur through inductive methods, such as grounded theory, as information emerges from interviews. More interpretive and naturalistic methods also involve structuring. Structuring can also occur apart from research by carefully considering and making judgments about how concepts are related. There is no shortage of professional literature devoted to research methods for generating empiric knowledge. However, methods for generating empiric theory as a form of empiric knowledge are less well understood and approaches vary. Because of this, we focus on empiric theory development in this text.

Structuring Empiric Theory

Structuring empiric theory involves forming systematic linkages between and among concepts. Many approaches can be used (Alligood & Tomey, 2013; Dubin, 1978; George, 2011; Grace & Perry, 2013; Masters, 2014; Newman, 1979; Reynolds, 2007).

The choice of a particular approach depends on your purposes, what you already know or assume to be true, and your underlying philosophic ideas about the nature of nursing knowledge. If you begin with an entirely new idea about something, with very little reported about it in the existing literature, the form of the theoretical relationships that you construct may be a categorization of the concepts into a relational taxonomy that essentially describes your ideas. If you begin with an idea that builds on other theorists' descriptions or a body of research, you might develop a theoretic structure that provides explanations of the complex interrelationships among concepts. If you are structuring theory as an outcome of grounded research, the interrelationships between data clusters guide the theoretic structure that you create. It should be noted that approaches to empiric theory generation, indeed the nature of theory itself, varies across disciplines as well as within the discipline of nursing. There is no accepted template for generating or characterizing "theory" in nursing. Our approach to structuring and contextualizing empiric theory are described in detail in the next sections and include the following:

- *Identifying and defining the concepts.* Concepts are important elements that convey the focus and meaning of the theory. Definitions of concepts can evolve from the processes of creating conceptual meaning, they can be thoughtfully borrowed from other theories, or they can be formulated from other sources. Definitions should indicate as clearly and concisely as possible the theoretic meaning of important concepts within the theory.
- *Identifying assumptions.* Assumptions are the basic underlying premises from which and within which theoretic reasoning proceeds.
- *Clarifying the context within which the theory is placed.* Contextual placement describes the circumstances within which the theoretic relationships are expected to be relevant. Clear statements about context are particularly important if the theory is to be used in practice.
- *Designing relationship statements.* Projected relationships between and among the concepts of the theory, taken as a whole, provide the substance and form of the theory.

Identifying and Defining Concepts. Structuring theory requires that you identify the concepts that will form the basic fabric of the theory. The concepts can come from life experiences, clinical practice, basic or applied research, knowledge of the literature, and the formal processes of creating conceptual meaning that were just described. Often, theory emerges because of a conviction that existing knowledge and theories are not adequate to represent an experience.

Some concepts are better suited for theory development than others. Concepts that are extremely abstract carry broad meanings and refer to a wide range of experience. They usually are not suitable as a beginning point for theory development. For example, concepts such as *social structure, stress,* and *caring* refer to such a broad range of experiences that relating them meaningfully is extremely difficult.

If concepts are extremely narrow and concrete, they refer to only a narrow range of experience, and the level of abstraction may not be sufficient for theoretic purposes. For example, concepts such as *toothache* or *post appendectomy surgical pain* apply to relatively few instances of pain. *Chronic pain* and *acute pain* may be more suitable concepts from which to develop theory. What is considered a suitable level of abstraction for theory varies in the field of nursing. The recent trends toward middle-range, situation-specific theory and evidence-based practice provide useful guidelines for decisions about the level of abstraction required for theoretic concepts.

As the concepts are specified or begin to form, early ideas about the structure of their relationships begin to emerge. There are usually one or two primary or central concepts around which the theoretic relationships build. Thinking about possible relationships helps to clarify what concepts the theory needs to include. Previous research, existing theories, philosophies, and personal experience provide a background for forming theoretic relationships. Initially, you might simply note concepts that you think are related on the basis of your experience, what you find in the literature, or ongoing research.

Assumptions also influence conceptual structure. For example, an assumption that is inherent in most empiric theory is the concept of linear time, which in turn determines the relationship linkages that various concepts have with one another. Often value assumptions underlie theory—for example, a theory accounting for how music influences discomfort during diagnostic procedures may assume that alleviating discomfort is good.

As initial ideas are formed about the relationships among concepts, the concepts themselves become clearer, and processes of creating conceptual meaning might be useful to make the meanings explicit. Some concepts might be grouped together and assigned more abstract terms to compose a different, perhaps new, concept. This occurs especially when theory is structured and conceptualized with inductive theory development processes such as grounded theory. For example, you might begin to see that self-identifiers of female caregivers such as *weak, fearful, inadequate, dependent,* and *unworthy* could be grouped to become components of the more abstract concept of *caregiver powerlessness.*

As the concepts of the theory are identified and conceptualized, theoretic definitions emerge. Theoretic definitions form the basis for and reflect empiric indicators and operational definitions for concepts needed for research, and they convey the general meaning of the concept. Empiric indicators are different from theoretic definitions in that they specify as clearly as possible how the concept is to be assessed in a specific study.

! Why Is This Important?

Theoretic definitions provide a basis for understanding concepts and relationships in any number of situations, whereas empiric or operational definitions limit meaning to the specific observable tools used in research. For example, a theoretic definition for the concept of *mothering* might read as follows:

Mothering: An interaction between a human adult and a child that conveys reciprocal feelings of attachment. The interaction is behaviorally expressed by reciprocal visual contact, touching, and vocalization.

This theoretic definition gives a general idea of the concept's empiric indicators, which are sometimes referred to as *operational definitions.* The first part of the mothering definition provides a general meaning for the term, and the second part suggests behaviors associated with the concept that can be assessed. Empiric indicators would specify observational tools or measurements that would be used in a research study. Visual contact and touching could be measured by making video recordings and counting the numbers of times the mother and child have direct eye contact, and numbers of times unnecessary touch occurs. Vocalizations could be empirically observed using voice recordings that measure intensity and pitch of the sound.

Notice that the theoretic definition serves the purpose of providing the essential meaning of the concept, whereas the empiric indicators refer to how this meaning is observed and assessed in a particular research study.

Identifying Assumptions. Assumptions are underlying givens that are presumed to be true. Philosophic assumptions form the grounding for a theory. If they are challenged, the substance of the entire theory is also challenged on philosophic grounds. Assumptions that could be empirically assessed but that are not within the context of the theory also affect the value of the entire theory. For example, a theory intended to promote self-care in people who are providing care for the elderly may assume that the caregivers desire to be self-caring. Although this assumption could be empirically assessed, for purposes of the theory, it is reasonable to assume that this is true. If not true and the caregivers have little or no desire to be self-caring, the theory will not be helpful, and another approach will be required.

Stated assumptions may be easy to recognize, but many assumptions are implied or not stated and thus may be difficult to recognize. Commonly accepted truths can be viewed differently within a theoretic context, and they may need to be made recognizable even if they seem self-evident. For example, if a theory includes the concept of grief, certain underlying assumptions about the nature of life and death would influence the essential ideas of the theory, and these assumptions need to be stated. A theory of grief that is based on a view of death as a transition to another form of life will likely be different from a theory of grief when death is assumed to be the end of life.

Rogers (1970) explicitly stated her assumption that humans are unified wholes who possess their own integrity and who manifest characteristics that are more than and different from the sum of their parts. On the surface, this statement seems perfectly reasonable and sensible, but it is significant because it is an assumption of wholism that is not common to all nursing theory and conceptual models. As an assumption, it does not require empiric evidence, but it is fundamental to the relationship statements that Rogers proposed.

Assumptions influence all aspects of structuring theory as well as other forms of empirical knowledge. If the assumption of wholism is used as a basis for a theory of mothering, interrelated concepts must be consistent with a wholistic view of human experience. Patterns of behavior that reflect the whole would be subsumed in the theoretic concepts; these might include patterns of movement and communication. By contrast, if humans are assumed to be biologic and social organisms that are a "sum of parts," then the assumption is that mothering can be understood by assessing a number of indicators such as physical responses to touch and vocalizations, stated cultural beliefs about mothering, and response of mother to distress in the child.

Clarifying the Context. Empiric theory should be placed within a context if the theory is to be useful for practice. If a theory of mothering is meant to apply only to the interactions of women and children in Western cultures, these limits on the applicability of the theory must be considered and stated. As the theory is extended, it might be useful for other cultures and for other types of intimate relationships such as adult–child, adult–adult, and adult–companion–animal interactions.

Contexts that are very broad or very narrow reflect the range of applicability of a theory. An attempt to structure a theory for many cultures may not be useful for any culture. Conversely, a theory that is structured within the context of a single institution (e.g., one specific hospital) may not be useful for other settings. Historically, as nursing incorporated an emphasis on middle-range theory, the context for which theories were developed narrowed. Broad frameworks or conceptual models that addressed phenomena such as adaptation (Roy, 1999) or conservation (Levine, 1967) were considered theory and are still useful in many nursing situations. Middle-range theories tended to focus on phenomena that were limited to some nursing situations but that were commonly recognized in nursing, such as uncertainty and hopelessness. Situation-specific theory narrowed context even further to particular situations of uncertainty or hopelessness (Im & Meleis, 1999). To be situation specific, a middle-range theory of hopelessness or uncertainty would need to be modified for use across different contexts, for example differing cultural contexts or for different age groups.

Designing Relationship Statements.   Relationship statements structurally interrelate the concepts of the theory. The statements range from those that simply relate two concepts, to relatively complex statements that account for interactions among multiple concepts. Theories usually contain several levels of relationship statements, which comprise a reasonably complete explanation of how the concepts of the theory interact. The relationships begin to take form as the concepts are identified and emerge, but the process of designing the relationship statements requires specific attention to the substance, direction, strength, and quality of the interactions that occur among concepts.

Consider a relationship statement that might be formulated about the concept of mothering. A theorist might propose that, as an adult's visual contact with an infant increases, the infant's visual contact with the adult will also increase. This relationship statement speculates that one event (increased adult visual contact) precedes a second event (increased infant visual contact). This relationship also describes a substantive interaction (visual contact) as a component of mothering. It implies direction (an increase) as part of the interaction.

A more complex relational statement addresses further dimensions of quality, contexts, and circumstances that are proposed. Such a statement might take the following form:

Under the conditions of *C1* through *Cn,* if *x* occurs, then *y* will occur.

A way to illustrate the concept of mothering might take the following form:

When an adult mothering figure and an infant are in close proximity (C1),
and
when the adult has a negative feeling toward the infant (C2),

and

when the frequency of physical contact is limited (C3),

then,

if the adult's frequency of visual contact decreases,

the infant's frequency of visual contact will also decrease.

A relationship may also be designed to introduce new concepts to the potential theory. Initially, such a relationship might read as follows:

> If the infant's frequency of visual contact is not sufficient to satisfy the mother, the adult's frequency of visual contact will increase in a conscious effort to engage the infant in interaction.

This relationship introduces the subjective value of "sufficient to satisfy." The idea of sufficiency is not objectively identifiable or empirically observable. As the theory is developed further, possible empiric indicators for "sufficient to satisfy" might be created, or this dimension of the theory might be viewed as something to be subjectively assessed. In this way, the theory stimulates the creation of new empiric knowledge.

In general, structuring processes for empirical theory as well as other theory-like empirical knowledge forms such as conceptual models or frameworks involves identifying concepts of importance to nursing and understanding the meaning of those concepts. Formal processes for creating meaning may be required for some purposes or adequate meanings may already be available in the professional literature. Concepts are linked in relation to one another, the context for which the theory is intended is identified and underlying assumptions are made explicit. We have presented general guidelines useful in structuring empiric theory. It is important to understand the process is messy and involves twists and turns that change and alter what is being created.

EMPIRIC KNOWLEDGE FORMS OTHER THAN THEORY

Our emphasis is on empiric theory as a valuable and primary empiric knowledge structure. However, our approaches for conceptualizing and structuring theory can also be used to generate other forms of empiric knowledge. Other forms include empiric research reports; findings from naturalistic, interpretive inquiry; and rigorously structured descriptions within the realm of empiric knowledge. Traditionally empiric knowledge has referred to knowledge generated through experimental and observational research methods associated with traditional science. This characterization of empirics continues to this day, but we view empirics as broader.

Although it is difficult to know where to draw the line on what constitutes "empiric" knowledge, we have drawn it in relation to knowledge generated either directly or indirectly through rigorous and controlled observation, whether those observations tend to be more factual or more interpretive. In our view, empirics requires the possibility of confirmation and validation, which involves agreement across observers that the interpretation or observation is a "correct" or reasonable one. Again, we acknowledge that not everyone would interpret empiric knowledge so broadly.

There are numerous approaches to structuring empiric knowledge. We have not detailed methods for conceptualizing and structuring that accrue from various research or analytic approaches as there is a vast literature detailing proper procedures for generating these various types of empiric knowledge (Polit & Beck, 2016). The accuracy and rigor of these methods for structuring and conceptualizing empiric knowledge is well accepted.

As we have said, there are techniques for generating theory in the disciplinary literature, but there is not agreement about these techniques or even what empiric theory is. It is for these reasons that we have focused on structuring and conceptualizing knowledge that is expressed as empiric theory as we have conceptualized it.

CONCEPTUALIZATIONS OF THEORY

Because theory is defined in many different ways within and outside of the discipline of nursing, understanding what it is can be confusing. Each definition can be functional, depending on how you are using the term. Theory has common, everyday connotations that is apparent in phrases such as, "I have a theory about that," or "My theory about *x* is...." These uses imply that theory is an idea or feeling or that it explains something. In this text, we use a definition that is consistent with the more everyday meanings of theory: as a collection of ideas or explanatory hunches. However, our definition goes beyond this to a characterization of theory as something that is deliberately designed for a specific purpose.

Beliefs about the nature of empiric theory in nursing differ because they arise in part from the various fields of inquiry from which nursing knowledge is developed. Some nursing theorists come from traditions in which the ideal of theory is logically linked sets of confirmed hypotheses. Others view theory as loosely connected ideas that are conjectured but not confirmed. Still others think of theory as beliefs and values about human nature and action. As a result, the nursing literature contains varying definitions of theory, but this diversity serves to stimulate the further understanding and development of theory. The following four definitions in the nursing literature emphasize different perspectives and different underlying values that involve theory. These definitions each highlight important aspects of theory that we draw on in our own definition:

- *A logically interconnected set of confirmed hypotheses* (McKay, 1969). This definition implies a specific form of expression that is based on rules of logic. It also requires that hypotheses be tested and confirmed with the use of methods of scientific-empiric research to generate theory.
- *A conceptual system or framework that is invented to serve some purpose* (Dickoff & James, 1968). This definition emphasizes the purpose for which a theory is created. The term *invented* implies a creative process that bypasses the type of testing and confirmation that McKay suggests. This definition emphasizes the importance of the theory having a purpose.
- *An imaginative grouping of knowledge, ideas, and experiences that are represented symbolically and that seek to illuminate a given phenomenon* (Watson, 1985). This definition also emphasizes creativity. For Watson, the purpose of creating theory is to enhance understanding of a given phenomenon—that is, a theory has the

purpose of understanding what a phenomenon is, and such theory may or may not have direct application in practice.

- *Conceptual and pragmatic principles that form a general frame of reference for a field of inquiry* (Ellis, 1968). This definition does not address a specific type of purpose for theory, and it does not suggest any particular method for developing theory. For Ellis, theory provides a philosophic view that guides inquiry in a discipline.

From our perspective, theory is a creative and rigorous structuring of ideas. The ideas, as concepts, are expressed by word symbols that form a conceptual structure. The structure is created using methods that draw on the creativity of the theorist. The concepts contained within the theory must be defined, and they must have a logical relationship with one another to form a coherent structure or pattern. Empiric theory is purposeful; that is, theorists create the theory for some reason. Theoretic purposes may take many different forms, but the purpose needs to be clearly evident.

Theory is not a finalized prescription or a formula for practice; it cannot describe exactly what can be objectively observed. Instead, theory projects tentative ideas that open new perceptions and possibilities with regard to what might be beyond the common surface understandings of the world. Theory is grounded in assumptions, value choices, and the creative and imaginative judgment of the theorist. You may or may not share the values and views of the theorist, but your exposure to the theory and the views that it reveals can expand your own thinking about your experience, your profession, and the direction of your own work. The conceptualization and structuring processes we describe creates theory consistent with our definition which follows:

> *Empiric theory:* **A creative and rigorous structuring of ideas that projects a tentative, purposeful, and systematic view of phenomena.**

The word *creative* underscores the role of human imagination and vision in the development and expression of theory; it does not mean that "anything goes" or that theory is improvised. As we have shown, the creative processes required to develop theory are rigorous, systematic, and disciplined, thereby yielding a well-developed conception that bears the mark of the creator. In our view, theoretic statements are always tentative and open to revision as new evidence and insights emerge. The statements are developed toward some purpose or within a specific context. Our definition does not require that a hypothesis be tested before the statements can be considered as theory. Ideas that the creator systematically develops on the basis of experience and observation can be considered as theory before formal testing occurs.

We have defined *theory* for the purpose of explaining to you, the reader, our view of what theory is, how to develop it, and how to evaluate it. Definitions of related terms help to make clearer the meaning of the central term (in this case, *theory*). Our definitions of several related terms for the context of this book are provided in Table 7.2. The definitions of related terms may not be universally accepted, but we believe that these are reasonable and reflect common meanings. In addition, no matter how rigorous the attempt to differentiate like terms by providing definitions, there will be elements of shared meaning among them.

TABLE 7.2 Conceptual Definitions of Terms Related to the Concept of Theory

Term	Definition
Science	An approach to the generation of empiric knowledge that relies on accessible sensory experience to create knowledge and to form understanding. The term also refers to the results or products generated when the systematic methods of empirics are used.
Philosophy	A discipline that discerns the nature of the world and of knowledge and knowing and that involves ways of discerning reality and principles of value. Philosophy relies on logic and reasoning rather than empiric evidence to create knowledge.
Fact	That which generally is held to be an empirically verifiable object, property, or event, which means that the phenomenon is experienced and named consistently and similarly by others in a given similar context.
Model	A symbolic representation of an empiric experience in the form of words, pictorial or graphic diagrams, mathematical notations, or physical material (e.g., a model airplane).
Theoretic or conceptual framework	A logical grouping of related concepts or theories that usually is created to draw together several different aspects that are relevant to a complex situation, such as a practice setting or an educational program.
Paradigm	A worldview or ideology. A paradigm implies standards or criteria for assigning value or worth to both the processes and the products of a discipline as well as for the methods of knowledge development within a discipline.

CONCLUSION

For empirics, the critical questions "What is this?" and "How does it work?" initiate the creative processes of conceptualizing and structuring. The creative processes occur in relation to the purposes of inquiry, the underlying assumptions being made, and the context in which the critical questions are asked. Empiric theory has specific characteristics that form the basis for our definition of theory. These characteristics provide a taxonomy for describing and critically reflecting theory which is detailed in Chapter 8.

References

Alligood, M. R., & Tomey, A. M. (2013). *Nursing theorists and their work* (8th ed.). St. Louis, MO: Elsevier-Mosby.

Beckwith, S., Dickinson, A., & Kendall, S. (2008). The "con" of concept analysis. A discussion paper which explores and critiques the ontological focus, reliability and antecedents of concept analysis frameworks. *International Journal of Nursing Studies, 45*, 1831–1841.

Bonis, S. A. (2013). Concept analysis: method to enhance interdisciplinary conceptual understanding. *ANS. Advances in Nursing Science, 36*, 80–93. https://doi.org/10.1097/ANS.0b013e318290d86e.

Carper, B. A. (1978). Fundamental patterns of knowing in nursing. *ANS. Advances in Nursing Science, 1*, 13–23.

Dickoff, J., & James, P. (1968). A theory of theories: a position paper. *Nursing Research, 17*, 197–203.

Dubin, R. (1978). *Theory building* (rev. ed.). New York, NY: The Free Press.

Ellis, R. (1968). Characteristics of significant theories. *Nursing Research, 17*, 217–222.

Fuller, J. (1991). *A conceptualization of presence as a nursing phenomenon.* Salt Lake City, UT: University of Utah.

George, J. B. (2013). *Nursing theories: the basis for professional nursing practice* (6th ed.). Pearson Education London.

Grace, P. J., & Perry, D. J. (2013). Philosophic inquiry and the goals of nursing: a critical approach for disciplinary knowledge development and action. *ANS. Advances in Nursing Science, 36*, 64–79.

Im, E.-O., & Meleis, A. I. (1999). Situation-specific theories: philosophical roots, properties, and approach. *ANS. Advances in Nursing Science, 22*, 11–24.

Jacox, A. (1974). Theory construction in nursing: an overview. *Nursing Research, 23*, 4–13.

Kaplan, A. (1964). *The conduct of inquiry.* New York, NY: Thomas Y. Crowell Co., Inc.

Kramer, M. (1993). Concept clarification and critical thinking: integrated processes. *The Journal of Nursing Education, 32*, 1–10.

Levine, M. E. (1967). The four conservation principles of nursing. *Nursing Forum, 6*, 93–98.

Masters, K. (2014). *Nursing theories: a framework for professional practice.* Burlington, MA: Jones & Bartlett Publishers.

McKay, R. P. (1969). Theories, models and systems for nursing. *Nursing Research, 18*, 393–399.

Morrow, M. R. (2009). Being judicious: a creative conceptualization. *Nursing Science Quarterly, 22*, 103–107.

Morse, J. M. (1995). Exploring the theoretical basis of nursing using advanced techniques of concept analysis. *ANS. Advances in Nursing Science, 17*, 31–46.

Moscou, S. (2008). The conceptualization and operationalization of race and ethnicity by health services researchers. *Nursing Inquiry, 15*, 94–105.

Newman, M. A. (1979). *Theory development in nursing.* Philadelphia, PA: F.A. Davis Co.

Norris, C. M. (1982). *Concept clarification in nursing.* Rockville, MD: Aspen Systems Corp.

Polit, D., & Beck, C. T. (2016). *Nursing research: generating and assessing evidence for nursing practice* (10th ed.). Philadelphia, PA: Lippincott, Williams and Wilkins.

Reynolds, P. D. (2007). *A primer in theory construction.* Needham, MA: Allyn & Bacon.

Rodgers, B. L., & Knafl, K. (2000). *Concept development in nursing: foundations, techniques and applications.* St Louis, MO: Saunders-Elsevier.

Rogers, M. E. (1970). *An introduction to the theoretical basis of nursing.* Philadelphia, PA: F.A. Davis Co.

Roy, S. C., & Andrews, H. A. (1999). *The Roy Adaptation Model.* Prentice Hall.

Walker, L. O., & Avant, K. C. (2010). *Strategies for theory construction in nursing* (5th ed.). Norwalk, CT: Appleton & Lange.

Watson, J. (1985). *Nursing: human science and human care: a theory of nursing.* Norwalk, CT: Appleton-Century-Crofts.

Wilson, J. (1963). *Thinking with concepts.* London: Cambridge University Press.

Description and Critical Reflection of Empiric Theory

We converse with one another of knowledge, research, assumptions and so forth, overconfident that we understand.

Norma Koltoff (1967, p. 122)

The processes for developing empiric theory—a common formal expression of empiric knowledge—include deliberative processes of critical reflection that assures members of the discipline that we understand what the theory is expressing. We have identified specific reflective tools to guide the process of clarifying meanings that are conveyed in an empiric theory. No matter the stage of development for empirical knowledge, including theory, anyone who is curious about a theory's meanings continue to ask: "What is this?" and "How does it work?" These questions not only stimulate the development of empiric knowledge but serve as an organizing framework for deliberately examining it.

In this chapter we retain an emphasis on theory as an empiric knowledge form because of its generalizability across multiple similar nursing situations. Its value, however, depends upon soundness of development and meaning in relation to the purposes for which it is used. The processes of describing and critically reflecting theory address questions of soundness in relation to purpose and lead to a clearer understanding of the nature of a theory as well as implications for further development. This is important if you are going to use a theory in research or in practice.

The opening quote from Koltoff supports the imperative to examine carefully the meaning of a theory when it is used to guide nursing practice and knowledge development. When you read a particular theory that has the potential to guide your research or practice, it is reasonable to believe that you understand what it means. To a certain extent, you likely do grasp much of its meaning, but the possibility exists that you are inserting meanings, making assumptions, or creating purposes for its use that might not be consistent with the theory.

 Think About It...

Suppose you are working in oncology and have an interest in comfort theory as a way to help people who are going through chemotherapy. As you read a theory that addresses the nature of comfort, what enhances comfort, and the projected outcomes of comfort for the persons you care for, it is important to understand clearly what the theorist means by the term *comfort*. For example, knowing what the theorist means and understanding the theorist's underlying assumptions about comfort are important for judging whether the theory will be useful in your practice. If comfort as described by the theorist is not even possible for persons receiving chemotherapy, the theory may not be useful to you. If the theorist assumes that comfort can be achieved but, in your situation, individuals are destined to remain uncomfortable, the theory again may not be useful.

The processes of description and critical reflection can be used to scrutinize theory to determine not only if it is useful for your purposes but also if it can be modified to be useful. Just because a theory might not totally fit your situation does not mean that it cannot be used to guide care. The critical issue is knowing how the theory does and does not reflect your situation so that decisions about its use can be deliberatively made. In our "think about it" example of the meaning of comfort, if the definition of *comfort* proposed in a theory is not exactly appropriate for your situation but the assumptions and the other features of the theory are, you may rightfully decide that the theory could be used to guide actions that promote comfort in a way that is appropriate for persons receiving chemotherapy.

Description and critical reflection are also basic to understanding the degree to which theory might be used as a component of evidence-informed practice. Indeed, the use of *evidence-informed practice* as an alternate term for *evidence-based practice* invites the use of well-developed theory. We believe that theory can and should serve to inform clinical practice decisions and activities. Theory that has been developed in conjunction with empiric generalizable research, carefully formulated through analytic thought, and subsequently critiqued in relation to a clinical purpose may be most valuable in guiding clinical outcomes in a desired direction. Well-constructed theory has the advantage of being generalizable across similar situations within the domain to which it applies. Theory, as a more general guide than isolated research findings, underscores the importance of considering context of care and allows for individualization of care practices to the unique situation of the patient or client (Thorne & Sawatzky, 2014).

! Why Is This Important?

When you are serious about using a theory as a basis for clinical practice or for guiding research, it is critically important to examine the theory carefully and not assume that you understand the nature of the theory. Without careful examination, care decisions guided by the theory will be less than effective, and research outcomes that are grounded in or that extend the theory will likely be flawed. In addition, if not carefully examined and understood in relation to the purpose of its use, a theory remains underdeveloped with regard to its usefulness for the discipline of nursing. It is through the processes of description and critical reflection that disciplinary theory is both evaluated and refined (Im, 2015; Liehr & Smith, 2017).

The definition of empiric theory that we use in this text points to the elements of a theory that can form the basis for describing what the theory is all about. Our definition is as follows:

Theory: A creative and rigorous structuring of ideas that projects a tentative, purposeful, and systematic view of phenomena.

The descriptive components that this definition suggests include the following:
- *Purpose:* If a theory is purposeful, a purpose can be found. The purpose of a theory may not be stated explicitly, but it should be identifiable.
- *Concepts:* If a theory represents a structuring of ideas, the ideas will be in the form of concepts that are expressed through language.
- *Definitions:* If the concepts of a theory are integrated systematically, their meanings will be conveyed by definitions. Definitions vary with regard to precision and completeness, but conceptual meaning should be identifiable and consistent in a theory.
- *Relationships and structure:* If the concepts are related and structured into a systematic whole, the overall whole of the theory is identifiable by examining the network of interrelationships among concepts.
- *Assumptions:* If a theory is tentative, assumptions form the underlying taken-for-granted truths on which the theory was developed, thus leaving open possible theoretic interpretations that can come from different sets of assumptions.

WHAT IS THIS AND HOW DOES THIS WORK? THE DESCRIPTION OF THEORY

Describing a theory is a process of posing questions about the components of the theory as suggested by our definition, then responding to the questions with your own reading or interpretation of the theory. Some elements will seem clear, some will depend on tentative interpretations, and some will remain unclear. Despite ambiguities, the process of describing theory creates a description that can then form the basis for critical reflection. This chapter focuses on theory as a form of empiric knowledge to be described and reflected on critically. You should note, however, that many of the questions we propose to describe and reflect theory could be used in relation to other forms of empiric knowledge as well.

What Is the Purpose of This Theory?

The general purpose of a theory is important because it specifies the context and situations in which the theory is useful. Purpose can be approached initially by asking, "Why was this theory formulated?" The responses to this question provide information that pertains to theoretic purposes.

Some purposes are specific to the clinical practice of nursing. In these theories, the concepts of the theory include nursing actions and behaviors that contribute to the purpose. Pain alleviation and restored self-care ability are examples of purpose that require clinical practice and suggest that nursing actions are part of the theory. Note that these purpose statements have a value orientation of alleviation and restoration. These ideas imply change toward a certain goal rather than just change for the sake of change. Such value connotations are important to notice when describing the purpose of a theory.

Some purposes may not require the direct clinical practice of nursing but are useful for understanding phenomena that occur in the context of nursing practice. These purposes can contribute to the achievement of practice purposes, or they may not be directly relevant to practice goals. For example, consider a theory with the central purpose of explaining the variables that affect blood flow velocity in the skin. Clinical practice is not necessary to explain blood flow velocity, but a theory with this purpose might be linked to a theoretic explanation of how blood flow velocity influences the incidence of decubitus ulcers or the extent of peripheral neuropathy in people with diabetes. A theory that explains skin blood flow velocity and the factors that affect it might have the potential to help practitioners prevent skin breakdown and peripheral neuropathy.

Theoretic purposes that do not require direct clinical nursing actions but that are of concern to nursing also may involve professional issues in nursing. For example, the purpose of an empiric theory might be to describe the features of organizations that empower nurses. This valued and necessary purpose is not directly related to the specific nursing actions of giving care, but it is certainly useful for changing practice.

It is important to clarify whether purposes are embedded in the theoretic structure or they are reasonable extensions of the theory. For example, consider a theory of mother–infant attachment that links together the following concepts: (1) the birth or adoption experience, (2) maternal support systems, (3) the degree of bonding, and (4) healthy infant development. The linkages are formed in a way that suggests that maternal attachment is influenced by the nature of the birth or adoption experience, which determines the extent of maternal support and bonding; it goes on to suggest that these features, if positive, encourage healthy infant development. In this example, healthy infant development is an example of a clinical outcome or purpose that is structured within the theory.

Suppose the theorist stated that the purpose of the theory was quality of life of the family unit, but the theorist did not explain how the concepts within the theory interrelate to create a certain quality of life. Quality of life as a purpose would constitute an extension of the theory because the concept is not located within the structure of the theory. Purposes that are embedded within the structure of the theory are usually explicit. Purposes that are reasonable extensions of the theory are important for understanding the clinical usefulness of the theory, although they are not clearly linked to the central concepts within the theory. Often, purposes that are extensions of theory are linked to the concepts and structures of the theory by implicit assumptions. Purposes outside the context of the theory also suggest directions for the further development of the theory. In the example just cited, research or logical reasoning would be indicated that links healthy infant development with quality-of-life indicators.

Purposes within a theory may be found for different individuals or groups of individuals who might use or benefit from the use of the theory. For example, if a theory is developed to address the clinical goal of alleviating pain, the theory can be examined for purposes that are appropriate for the individual nurse, the physician, the person receiving care, and the person's family. Consider a theory that is developed with a clinical purpose of alleviating fatigue associated with cancer therapy. The theoretic purpose for the nurse might be distinctly different from that implied for the person receiving nursing care. The nurse's purpose might be to design a plan of care that minimizes stressors associated with care provision. The purpose for the person receiving care might be to rest and to provide responses that indicate the effectiveness of the system for minimizing fatigue. Taken together, these two purposes might be viewed as an overall purpose of creating a nurse–patient interactive process that minimizes patient fatigue.

In addition to whether or not purposes can be found for various individuals who use or who are affected by the theory, you can ask questions related to the scope of the theory's purpose. For example, does the overall purpose focus on an individual, a family, a group, or society in general? An organized society or an expanded collective consciousness is an example of a broad purpose that can be applied to relatively unbounded groups of people. Purposes such as environmental health or political activism may apply to whole communities or may be linked to definable groups within those communities. When there are multiple purposes within a theory, the scope of those purposes may vary. You may find narrower-scope purposes for individuals and families and broader-scope purposes for a community. When multiple purposes within a theory are found, if clarity is not compromised, you should be able to order purposes in a hierarchy that flows toward one central purpose.

The following question often arises: "How are purposes to be separated from the concepts of the theory?" Purposes that are part of the matrix of the theory are also concepts of the theory. One approach to identifying which concept is also the central purpose is to describe or designate the concept toward which theoretic reasoning flows. This is related to the structure of the theory. Ask the following: "What is the end point of this theory?" and "When is this theory no longer useful?" Responses to these questions provide clues about purpose and help to clarify the context in which the theory can be used. In the theoretic framework of Hall (1966), for example, the theory would cease to be valuable when the client has achieved self-actualization, which may be deemed the overall purpose. This purpose of self-actualization within the structure of Hall's theoretic framework represents the end point of theoretic reasoning. Within the context of Hall's theory, self-actualization is a purpose that requires nursing practice. Outside the context of Hall's theory, self-actualization is a purpose shared with other professions.

Think About It...

Reflect on a purpose that guides your practice of nursing. Do you frequently seek to alleviate pain, or calm someone's anxiety, or help families deal with the uncertainty of living with a chronic illness, or reduce risk factors in a community? What theoretic ideas inform your practice around this purpose? Can you identify a theory that has been developed in the literature that addresses your purpose? Think about the challenges you face in your practice, and whether or not the theoretic ideas you identify might give you some guidance.

What Are the *Concepts* of This Theory?

Concepts are identified by searching out words or groups of words that represent objects, properties, or events within the theory. You can begin to describe concepts by listing key ideas and tentatively identifying how they seem to interrelate. As you begin to discern relationships, your perception of the key concepts of the theory will become clearer. One initial difficulty that is faced when identifying concepts is determining which concepts are integral to the theory and which are part of some supporting narrative. There is no easy way to deal with this challenge. By beginning to identify concepts and then deriving interrelationships, decisions can be made about which concepts are central to the theory.

As you identify important theoretic concepts, ask questions about the nature of the concepts and their organization. Is there a major concept with subconcepts organized under it? Are there several major concepts with subconcepts organized under them? Are the concepts singular entities? Are some concepts singular entities and others organized with subconcepts? What are the relationships and interrelationships between and among concepts? Are some concepts mentioned that do not seem to fit the emerging structure? What is the relative scope of the various concepts? After the concepts are identified and such questions addressed, the relationships and structure will begin to emerge.

Other questions deal with the number of concepts. How many concepts are there? How many might be considered major concepts? How many are minor concepts? Do not become stuck trying to distinguish between major and minor. Rather, notice whether one or a few concepts really stand out as important while others seem less important, and consider why this is the case. As you consider the organization and number of concepts, address qualitative features of the concepts as well. Do the concepts represent abstractions of objects, properties, or events? Is it possible to identify what they represent? Are the concepts more empirically grounded, or are they more abstract? Which type of concept—more empiric or more abstract—seems to prevail? Are the concepts fairly discrete in meaning, or do several have similar meanings? When similar meanings for concepts exist, do they all seem to express a single idea, or do they differ? How are they different? Concepts that are alike may represent either one central idea that is fairly clear or several different images. For example, the concepts of *rehabilitation, restoration,* and *recovery,* which share common meanings, may appear in the same theory with similar meanings or with different meanings.

Ask questions about how concrete or abstract the concepts of the theory are. The nature of the concepts in a theory helps you to identify how general the theory is or to determine the range of situations in which the theory can be applied. Theories that focus on very broad, abstract concepts (e.g., caring) can be applicable to a very wide range of situations; these theories are sometimes labeled as "grand" theories. When the concepts tend to be descriptive of more specific situations, they can be labeled as "middle-range" theories. The labels or categories are not important in themselves; what is important to note is the potential for the concepts to be useful in practice, under what circumstances, and for what purposes.

The nature of the concepts also provides an indication of the potential for the further development of the theory. If the concepts are so abstract that they cannot be defined sufficiently for empiric investigation, then the potential for development as an empiric theory is limited.

When you are addressing the question of a theory's concepts, the concepts within it must be examined carefully for quantity, character, emerging relationships, and structure. The description of concepts is crucial because the quantity and character of those concepts form an understanding of the purpose of the theory, the structure and nature of theoretic relationships, the definitions, and the assumptions.

What Are the *Definitions* in This Theory?

A definition is an explicit meaning that is conveyed for a concept. Definitions exist to clarify the nature of the abstraction constructed by the theorist in a way that others can comprehend. Definitions suggest how word representations of an idea (concept) are expressed in experience.

It is often difficult to determine from a listing of key words the concepts that are basic to the theoretic structure and that comprise definitions and assumptions. Carefully reading the theory and relying on your own judgment should provide this information.

Concepts may be defined in a list of definitions or in narrative form in the text, but not labeled as definitions. It is not always easy to recognize narratives as definitions, because narratives are not labeled and may contain information that is not directly pertinent to the definition of the concept.

Concept definitions can also be implied by how the theorist uses the conceptual terms in the context. For example, if a theorist uses the concept of *wholism* but this term is not explicitly defined, you can examine the use of the term and infer the meaning or definition. If the theorist identifies and describes various dimensions of wholistic health, the definition of *wholism* might be akin to "the sum of the parts." If the theorist does not use parts or dimensions when speaking of wholistic health, the theorist may be using a definition that is more closely associated with wholism as being more than the sum of the parts.

Because concepts may have both *explicit* and *implicit* definitions, ask the following: How are concepts defined: explicitly, implicitly, or both? Are implied definitions consistent with explicit definitions? Can common language meanings be taken as the meaning intended? Would a common language approach lead to differing interpretations of the meanings of the concepts?

Another way to describe definitions is to characterize the extent to which the definitions are *general* or *specific*. Both explicit and implicit meanings may be general or specific. Assess how general or specific the definitions are. How clearly does the definition suggest an associated empiric experience? Is the definition specific about what a phenomenon is, or does it suggest what its use is? Does it provide possibilities for empiric indicators that represent the phenomenon?

For the abstract concepts that are found in many nursing theories, specific definitions are difficult to formulate. Attempting prematurely to create specific meanings for abstract concepts may interfere with exploring a wide range of possibilities that lead to the discovery of richer or alternative meanings. Definitions that specify general features can conjure specific mental images of the actual experience. An early definition that is broad and nonspecific encourages the exploration of many possible meanings. General meanings are preferred in broad-scope theories or theories that are not likely to be empirically tested. Most definitions have both specific and general features. It is important to attend to how definitions are both specific and general.

After the definitions are identified, ask the following: Are similar definitions used for different concepts? Are differing definitions used for the same concept? Are some concepts defined differently than common convention would define them? Are definitions expanded as the narrative proceeds? Is it difficult to judge whether definitions are provided at all? Can definitions fit other terms within or outside of the structure of the theory?

What Are the *Relationships* in This Theory?

Relationships are the linkages among and between concepts. The nature of relationships in theory may take several forms. Often the relationship statements that are uncovered may be peripheral to the core of the theory.

As concepts are identified, ideas about relationships between and among them begin to form. Suppose you uncover the following relationship statement: "The individual is composed of three dimensions and is an integral part of the environment." This statement suggests that the individual is related to an environment and that there are three interrelated subcomponents of the individual.

When a tentative identification of the relationships is made, ask the following: Are there concepts that stand alone and that are unrelated to others? Are there concepts that are interrelated with other concepts in several ways and others that are related in only one or two ways? Are there concepts to which several other concepts relate but that, in turn, are not related to other concepts?

The ways in which the relationships emerge provide clues regarding the theoretic purposes and the assumptions on which the theory is based. Some concepts may be linked to the theory by assumptions, which may explain why the concept seems to fit within the matrix of the theory but why a theoretic relationship that contains the concept is not explicitly stated.

The theoretic purpose may be represented by the linear relationships of several concepts that converge on one specific concept that, in turn, is not linked to any other concepts; in other words, the linkages end with a specific concept. As linkages between concepts are identified, you can address the nature and character of the relationships. If a relationship is unclear, ask yourself what relationships might be possible, and ask about their associated characters; your ideas can provide clues for the further development of the theory.

Examine the *nature* of the relationships. Are the relationships basically descriptive, or do they explain something about the phenomenon of interest? Do they create meaning without explaining it? Do they impart understanding? Is there evidence that some relationships are predictive? Relationships within theory that create meaning and impart understanding often link multiple concepts in a loose structure. In other forms of description, concepts are interrelated without elaboration on how and why conceptual relationships are arranged. Concepts that are interrelated often explain how empiric events occur and may provide some detail about how and why concepts interrelate. Prediction implies "if-then" statements about the occurrence of empiric phenomena. When empirically based predictions of human behavior are shown to be valid, they are usually based on explanation.

The statement, "Individuals are composed of three dimensions," is mainly descriptive. It implies that one concept—the individual—is composed of three parts called *dimensions*. If this sentence was expanded to, "The individual is composed of three dimensions that overlap and share common core areas," the statement becomes more explanatory. It proposes that each dimension has a shared area with another dimension, and that an area is shared by all three. If the phrase "an interrelated whole" were to be added, the "how" of the relationship becomes even clearer because the dimensions must overlap to integrate the "parts" of the individual.

Predictions are fairly easy to detect. Sentences that translate into "if-then" statements are predictive. It is not possible to make such a statement from the sentence, "The individual is composed of three dimensions," unless it would be the following, which is implied: "If there are not three dimensions, then it is not an individual." The statement, "The individual is an interrelated whole composed of three dimensions that overlap and share common areas," implies that disturbances in one sphere would be reflected in other spheres. However, this prediction is implied and not explicit.

Suppose the statement read as follows: "Because the individual is an interrelated whole that is composed of three dimensions that overlap and share common areas, a disturbance in one dimension is reflected by disturbances in other dimensions." This statement is clearly predictive.

▶▶ Consider This...

The distinctions among *description, explanation,* and *prediction* are not always clear, but these distinctions add to your understanding of the theory. Generally, the term *description* means that the statement projects what something is or the features of its character. *Explanation* suggests how or why it is. *Prediction* is used to project circumstances that create or alter a phenomenon. Our use of the terms *descriptive, explanatory,* and *predictive* when describing the nature of theoretic relationships refers only to the form of the theory from a purely analytic standpoint. For the purposes of describing a theory, research findings are not required to confirm the nature of relationship statements as descriptive, explanatory, or predictive. The clarity you gain in understanding these theoretic distinctions provides guidance for developing research.

What Is the *Structure* of This Theory?

The structure of a theory gives overall form to the conceptual relationships within it. The structure emerges from the relationships of the theory. Consider these two concepts within a theory: the *individual* and the *environment*. In one theory, the individual is part of the environment; in another theory, the individual is separate from the environment. In both theories, there is an identifiable relationship between the individual and the environment, but the structure of the relationship differs.

Although your responses to questions about the relationships of the concepts of a theory usually suggest the theory's form, in some cases they do not. Many theories do not contain a single discernible structure in which all concepts will fit into a coherent, unified network. There may be several, perhaps competing structures that cannot be reconciled. Determining the structure of the theory will be difficult if the network of relationships is unclear or extremely complex. Fig. 8.1 illustrates a sample of four

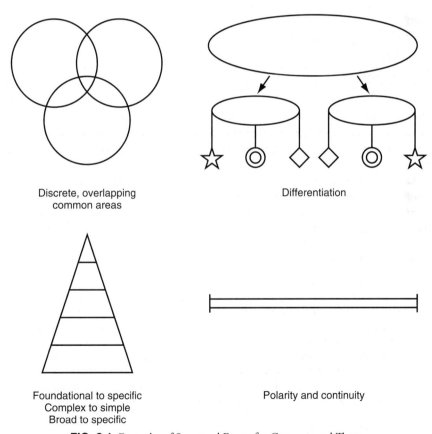

Discrete, overlapping
common areas

Differentiation

Foundational to specific
Complex to simple
Broad to specific

Polarity and continuity

FIG. 8.1 Examples of Structural Forms for Concepts and Theory.

structural forms and the ideas that these suggest. Some theories may reflect one or more of these structures, whereas others will not. Individual concepts within theories may be structured in these forms. Structural forms are powerful devices for shaping our perceptions. As you describe a theory, do not expect that it will fit into one of these four structures. The theory may fit, but many more structures are possible. Conversely, during the process of theory development, these are only examples of various structures that might evolve during the process of relationship structuring.

 Discuss This...

> Discuss with your peers how you might structure the following relationship statement: "Individuals are composed of component parts." This statement only suggests a structure in which parts are perceptible, and any image on Fig. 8.1 could easily represent it, except the image that suggests polarity. Suppose each of these structures represents the broad theory of health. The triangular drawing suggests that health is composed of a series of related subconcepts that vary in breadth or simplicity. It also suggests foundational concepts on which other subconcepts are built. The base level might be genetic integrity, which could be followed by organ or system health, and finally by the health of communities or societies. A theory that deals with how genetic health forms the basis for individual, collective, and societal health might be structured in this way.
>
> Discuss some of the ideas that you are interested in, or that you encounter in your nursing practice. Discuss what factors might go into each of these structures to describe, explain, or predict your phenomena.

The overlapping circles in Fig. 8.1 depict discrete components that have common areas between and among them. Health might be viewed as having biophysiologic, psychoemotional, and sociocultural aspects. If a person is biologically well but psychoemotionally unwell, the diagram suggests that the psychoemotional illness will affect biophysiologic wellness. Psychoemotional ill health could result in biophysiologic consequences. Basically, the overlapping circles illustrate that health is composed of separate components, but that sharing occurs between any two components as well as among all three. The structure, as illustrated, suggests equality with regard to importance, overlap, and sharing among the three subunits.

Applying this idea to the horizontal line drawing on the figure shows health being represented as a continuum in a linear relationship with illness. When health is placed on a continuum with illness at the opposite end, health and illness are conceptualized as a continuous variable, and degrees of health and illness are possible. The extremes of a continuum also suggest that health is the absence of illness and that illness is the absence of health. If health is viewed as a concept that can coexist with illness, health and illness can be represented by a continuum. However, if health and illness are not considered as continuous concepts, they do not fit this structural form.

The fourth structural form conveys the idea of differentiation by dividing major concepts into subconcepts. For this structural form, health might be differentiated into its mental and physical components. Physical health could be further divided into bodily or anatomic health and functional or physiologic health, with some comparable divisions such as emotional and spiritual for mental health. Differentiation can proceed indefinitely. Some concepts lend themselves to differentiation more easily than others. *Needs* is a concept that can be easily differentiated, whereas the concept of *wholism* cannot.

Conceptually unrelated or distinctly different concepts cannot be structured as a continuum. A relationship between gender and social practices could not be represented on a continuum. Gender and social practices could be structured as overlapping circles, as two conceptual entities that influence one another, or in a structure in which social practices shape gender. As you study the examples of structure, note how different concepts fit some structures more easily than others, and how some concepts such as *wholistic health* cannot be represented well by any structure. In fact, none of these structures for representing health may make sense to you, because the structures may be inconsistent with your personal ideas about the nature of health.

As relationships are explored, the overall theoretic structure and the structures of individual components begin to emerge. To address questions of structure, begin by asking the following questions: What are the most central relationships? What are the direction, strength, and quality of those relationships? Can I draw a model that shows the structure of the theory? What is the order of appearance of relationships within the narrative? Do relationships appear to move toward or away from the theoretic purpose? Do relationships coalesce the concepts or differentiate them? Does the theorist diagram the structure?

After the structures of the major or central relationships are identified, other aspects of structure can be described: How are other structures united with the central or core relationships? Can all the relationships be structured? Do the structures take multiple forms? Are competing or partial structures suggested? Does the theorist provide diagrams that illustrate aspects of structure?

After you have linked together concepts and purposes in relationships, it becomes possible to describe the entire structural form of the theory. Notice how the relationships move as the theory unfolds. A theory that defies structuring can sometimes be approached by simply outlining the order in which the concepts are presented. Outlining can provide insight about how ideas are organized. Some recognizable structure is essential to theory because structure flows from relationships.

What Are the *Assumptions* in This Theory?

Assumptions are those basic givens or accepted truths that are fundamental to theoretic reasoning. To uncover assumptions, a central question can be asked: "What is the author taking as an accepted truth?" This question can be asked after the purposes are determined, the concepts are structured by relational statements, and the definitions are described.

Sometimes the theorist states assumptions explicitly. If so, ask the following: "What are the explicit givens?" and "What do they assume?" Statements that are explicitly labeled as *assumptions* may not be the same as the assumptions that are basic to the theory. The extent to which explicitly labeled assumptions are assumptions and not something else must be examined. It is often difficult to separate assumptions that are implicit or integrated into the narrative of the theory from relationship statements, but they can be identified. As with explicit assumptions, ask the following: "What are the implicit givens?" and "What do they assume?"

Explore your ideas about the assumptions of the theory further. What individual, environmental, nursing, and health-related assumptions are made? Are the assumptions competing or compatible? Are there several assumptions about one phenomenon and few about another? Are the assumptions made at the outset, between and within relationships, or in relation to the purposes of the theory?

Assumptions may take the form of factual assertions, or they may reflect value positions. *Factual assumptions* are those that are knowable or potentially knowable through perceptual experience. *Value assumptions* assert or imply what is right, good, or ought to be. Often, an empirically knowable assumption (e.g., "It is assumed for the purposes of this theory that people want information") contains important underlying value assumptions. The assumption that people want information (which could be empirically verified) may further imply that information is good, which cannot be verified empirically. The value assumption that "it is good to have information" leads to further questions about what sort of information is good. It is important to examine factual assumptions by asking, "What value does this factual assumption reflect?" It is also important to examine all the other components of theory. What does this concept, definition, relationship, structure, or purpose assume?

After you discern the assumptions, the values that are held by the theorist can be explored. What does the theorist assume to be valuable, good, right, wrong, or worthwhile? Are there value-laden terms and phrases in the definitions of the concepts and in the supporting narrative of the theory? Who is assumed to be responsible for the experiences or circumstances depicted in the theory? Who benefits from the circumstances or experiences of this theory? These questions often give clues to values that form fundamental assumptions. For example, the Freudian theoretic notion of *penis envy* implies that penises are body parts that are so valued as to be enviable, and that a person who does not have a penis will experience this value-laden emotion. A useful approach to uncovering hidden values is to imagine possibilities other than those presented in the theory. If these alternative possibilities are plausible but unconventional, you have uncovered important value assumptions. Imagining the idea of *womb envy*, which is not a part of Freudian thinking but is a plausible alternative possibility, indicates that you have uncovered an important androcentric assumption from which the theory builds.

Describing or discerning assumptions are often grounded in beliefs so taken for granted that they are difficult to recognize. Sometimes it is not possible to agree personally with and accept a theory because it is so unusual or strange. Uneasiness or discomfort with a theory may be a clue to assumptions that are unlike your own beliefs or values. After assumptions are recognized, the theory that contains them can be understood on its own terms.

FORMING A COMPLETE DESCRIPTION

In summary, we propose the following six questions for describing a theory:

1. *What is the purpose of this theory?* This question addresses why the theory was formulated and reflects the contexts and situations to which the theory can be applied.
2. *What are the concepts of this theory?* This question identifies the ideas that are structured and related within the theory.
3. *How are the concepts defined within this theory?* This question clarifies the meanings of concepts within the theory. It questions what empiric experience is represented by the ideas within the theory.
4. *What is the nature of the relationships within this theory?* This question addresses how concepts are linked together. It focuses on the various forms that relationship statements can take and how they give structure to the theory.
5. *What is the structure of the theory?* This question addresses the overall form of the conceptual interrelationships. It discerns whether the theory contains partial structures or has one basic form.
6. *On what assumptions does the theory build?* This question addresses the basic truths that are believed to underlie theoretic reasoning. It questions whether those assumptions reflect philosophic values or factual assertions.

A general approach to describing theory is to read the work and then begin to consider the descriptive questions. All the questions are not necessarily answerable for a single theory. However, as you answer the questions that apply to the theory under consideration, concepts will be tentatively identified, and the purpose of the theory will emerge. As definitions become evident, you will begin to see relationships. From the nature of the relationships, you will be able to address questions regarding the structure of the theory. Responses to the questions about assumptions provide a level of awareness of meanings that will help you form an understanding of the theory. After an initial description of the components, each component can be reexamined and revised.

For any theory, it is often not easy to describe theoretic purposes and assumptions. Concepts and their definitions may be more readily identifiable, especially if they are fairly explicit. Discerning relationships and structure is often problematic when describing theory, but these traits, too, will be present.

Forming a complete description of a theory requires the systematic and critical examination of the work. When approached seriously, every word, phrase, and sentence must be examined and reexamined for meaning. Ideas that emerge in response to the descriptive questions often lead to uncertainty and the revision of earlier ideas. After a time, the description does begin to take shape, and fewer changes occur. There will always be some tentativeness in your descriptions, because your description requires your own interpretive insights with respect to the theorist's ideas, and these insights change. If you are not able to reach a tentative resolution with respect to the fundamental nature of a theory after reasonable study and thought, the best course of action is to propose your ideas for the revision and further development of the theory. Your continuing uncertainty indicates that further theoretic development must occur.

Despite uncertainty and tentativeness, it is important to rely on your own judgment about the nature of a theory and not to assume that published descriptions and analyses are more accurate or authoritative than yours. When you complete a description and critical reflection with care and precision, your conclusions should be trusted to be an accurate understanding of the theory.

HOW DOES IT WORK? THE CRITICAL REFLECTION OF THEORY

After a theory is described, critical questions can be addressed to develop information about how well developed a theory is or how adequate it is in relation to its purposes. Note that describing and critically reflecting theory are fundamentally different processes. Description can be compared with a more objective process of setting forth facts about the theory by asking, "What is this?" By contrast, critical reflection involves ascertaining how adequate a theory is in relation to some purpose. In this section, we identify questions that can be used as part of critical reflection. As you question the worth of a theory, you will form insights that will help you to know how that theory might be used and further developed.

As you study and read different nursing theories, you may think, "This does not seem right," "Maybe I could change my practice along this line," or "This is really exciting." When these types of thoughts occur, you are comparing the theory with some personal and perhaps unrecognized ideas about what is important for theory. Each person's ideas of the adequacy of a theory are influenced by a personal perspective of what is valuable or good. For research, you might agree, "This could be helpful." For practice, you might think, "Maybe I could use this." For idea stimulation, you might think, "This really gives me some exciting new ideas." In these instances, you have formed an impression of the value of the theory from your personal values about practice, research, and critical thinking. Your values are important components that are integrated into a more formal critical reflection process.

Critical reflection contributes to understanding how well the theory relates to practice, research, or educational activities. Members of a discipline form ideas about what questions to ask and what responses are generally accepted if a theory is to be seen as valuable for the discipline. Just as there are many ways to describe theory, there are many critical questions that can be asked about the functional value of theory, and there are many responses to these questions. When these questions are asked, members of a discipline can consider what responses they tend to value and why. The questions that we pose are consistent with generally accepted methods for evaluating theories that have been described in the nursing literature (Alligood & Tomey, 2013; Barnum, 1998; Ellis, 1968; Fawcett, 2005; Hardy, 1974). However, our approach differs from other accepted methods in that we focus on asking questions to consider in relation to your own purposes, rather than a standard that a theory is expected to meet. Each of these questions revolve around standard characteristics of adequate theories. However, the answers to these questions can vary widely depending on your circumstances and the purposes for which you intend to use the theory. In our view, the judgment of the worth of a theory is relative to your purpose and how the theory can contribute to what you envision for nursing practice.

The questions for critical reflection are as follows:

- How clear is this theory?
- How simple is this theory?
- How general is this theory?
- How accessible is this theory?
- How important is this theory?

There are no correct answers to these questions, and the questions do not imply the responses. For example, "How clear is this?" does not necessarily mean that a theory should be perfectly clear or that clearer is necessarily better. Rather, when you address this question, you are using it as a tool to examine whether the level of clarity of the theory is adequate for the theory's purpose. As you engage in discussions about the questions, you can form a consensus with your colleagues regarding where to go next with the theory. These insights can best be formed in discussions among people with diverse perspectives. For example, although a theory that challenges assumptions about practice is somewhat unclear, it may be an important theory for changing nursing practice and providing new concepts. The lack of clarity allows for imagining new possibilities, which may be part of the theory's strength.

Although each of the five critical reflection questions is fundamentally different, the questions are interrelated. For example, one question addresses accessibility, and another addresses generality. If seen as general or broad in scope, a theory may be less accessible (i.e., less related to perceptual experience) than a narrower (i.e., less general) theory.

Responses to the questions used to create a description affect your responses to the critical reflection questions. For example, to decide how clear, accessible, or general a theory is, you need to describe the purpose of the theory, what concepts are included, and how those concepts are structured. As your description of the theory is formed, you can begin the process of critical reflection. The ideas that you develop from this process contribute to your own critical insights and to substantive discussion that gives direction for further theory development. The issues to consider as you address each of the questions for critically reflecting theory are described in the following sections.

How *Clear* Is This Theory?

When determining how clear a theory is, you will be considering semantic clarity, semantic consistency, structural clarity, and structural consistency. *Clarity*, in general, refers to how well the theory can be understood and how consistently the ideas are conceptualized. *Semantic clarity* and *semantic consistency* primarily refer to understanding the intended theoretic meaning of the concepts. *Structural clarity* and *structural consistency* reflect an understanding of the intended connections between concepts within the theory as well as the whole of the theory.

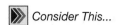 *Consider This...*

> To help understand the subset criteria of semantic clarity, consider a diagram or figure representing a theory in a professional journal article. Examine the boxes or spheres and the concepts named in the figure, and the lines or arrows that connect the ideas within the figure. *Semantics* concerns meaning. *Semantic clarity* refers to how clearly the concepts within the figure are implicitly or explicitly defined, usually in the narrative explanation of the theory. *Semantic consistency,* on the other hand, examines if the meaning proposed for those concepts is used the same way throughout the explanation or description provided with the figure. As you begin to read the article describing the theory, a concept's meaning when first encountered may be quite clear, but when you reach the conclusion the writer seems to be using the concept in a way that refers to something a bit different although both meanings, when considered individually, may seem pretty clear. This divergence of meanings sets up semantic inconsistency. On the other hand, the meaning of concepts may be unclear, although the reason for this unclarity and the unclarity itself is consistent. This is an example of *semantic unclarity* with semantic consistency. This distinction may seem trivial but is important. When you detect *unclarity* in a theory with regard to conceptual meaning, making this distinction means you will have a sense of whether the unclarity occurred because the concept was poorly defined or because the concept took on different meanings throughout the theory, or both. If the source of unclarity is understood, it can be corrected or recognized as problematic in relation to intended uses.

Structural clarity addresses the conceptual linkages within the theory, whereas *structural consistency* refers to the extent to which linkages remain stable throughout the description of the theory and without contradictions. In the example of the figure or diagram of the theory, structural clarity would address whether or not the connecting lines or arrows between the boxes (relationships among and between concepts) support a coherent understanding of the entire theory. Structural clarity also means that individual relationships between concepts are clear, particularly within the narrative portion of the theory. Structural consistency addresses whether the linkages between concepts are similarly presented throughout the theory, and it can be assessed by examining the narrative of the theory in relation to the figure. If the theory narrative proposes that two important concepts are interrelated, but this is not obvious in the figure, structural clarity is lacking. If it appears from the figure that two concepts are linked, but you find the narrative seems to link those concepts differently, you have found structural inconsistency.

In summary and most importantly, *semantics* involves conceptual meaning, *structure* involves conceptual linkages, and both are subcriteria within *clarity.* Understanding the conceptual meaning or linkages is a tool for deciding if and how you might use the theory, and what would be needed to use it appropriately for your purposes.

Semantic Clarity. The definitions of concepts in the theory are important aspects of semantic clarity. Definitions help to establish empiric meaning for concepts within the theory. If concepts are not defined or are not completely defined, the empiric indicators for the idea become less clear. When concepts are clearly defined, empiric indicators can be more easily identified. Clarity implies in part that when different nurses read the theory, a similar empiric image comes to mind when the word for the concept is used. If there are no definitions or if only a few of the concepts are defined, clarity is limited.

The types of definitions that are used within theory affect semantic clarity. Definitions that reflect both specific and general traits enhance clarity, whereas a general or a specific definition alone often limits clarity. Specific definitions usually lend clarity, because they provide clear and accurate guidance for the intended empiric indicators for a concept. General definitions contribute a contextual sense of meaning for concepts and lend a richness of meaning that is not possible with specific definitions. Considering the extent to which each type of definition contributes to clarity of meaning can help you to form your own ideas about the adequacy of the theory for your purpose.

Clarity may be obscured by the borrowing of terms from other disciplines or the use of common language terms that carry broad general meanings. Words such as *stress* and *coping* have general common language meanings, and they also have specific theoretic meanings in other disciplines. If words with multiple meanings are used in a theory and not defined, a person's everyday meaning of the term is often assumed rather than the meaning within the theory; therefore, clarity is lost. Clarity is enhanced when the concept's definition is consistent with common meanings of the term in the profession.

Clarity is affected when words that have no common meaning are used, or when the theorist invents or coins words to represent some idea. Coined words can help to convey a meaning for which there is no word, but they also can detract from clarity, especially when a more familiar word or phrase would suffice. It would be possible to generate an entire theory about quizzendroids, plankerods, and ziots. The theory could be logical and consistent, but it would be unclear because the words are invented and do not signify recognizable objects, properties, or events. Although exaggerated, this example demonstrates the effects on clarity when vague or strange words are used, when words are not defined, or when words with many possible meanings are used and not defined.

Semantic clarity can also be affected by excessive verbiage. Normally, the use of varying words to represent similar meanings is a writing skill that can be used to avoid the overuse of a single term. In a theory, however, if several similar concepts are used interchangeably when one would suffice, there is excessive verbiage, and the clarity of the theory's presentation is reduced rather than improved. In a theory, varying the word for an important concept interjects subtly different meanings. For example, interchanging the words *restoration, rehabilitation,* and *recovery* for the same concept affects clarity, because each word has a slightly different meaning and suggests different contexts of use.

Clarity is also affected when excessive narrative is included. Semantic clarity may be decreased by excessive examples; however, the judicious use of examples usually aids clarity. Diagrams can enhance or obscure clarity. To enhance clarity, diagrams should be self-explanatory and simple in expression, because overly complex illustrations discourage comprehension. In general, the alternative mode of providing information in the form of diagrams helps to clarify the ideas in the theory.

An economy of words, the provision of key definitions, and the wise use of examples and diagrams lend clarity. Absolute semantic clarity can never be achieved, nor is it necessarily desirable. Because of the limitations of language, no matter how clearly the theorist represents theoretic meaning, it will not be perceived uniformly by all readers.

Semantic Consistency. Semantic consistency is a second feature to consider with respect to the question of clarity. A theory that implicitly or explicitly defines concepts inconsistently gives competing messages with regard to meaning. Semantic consistency means that the concepts of the theory are used in ways that are consistent with their definition. Sometimes a definition is explicitly stated, but somewhere within the theory, another meaning is implied. When key words are not explicitly defined, their implied meanings may be inconsistent from one instance of use to the next. Occasionally, words are explicitly defined but in different ways. Inconsistencies that occur when terms are defined explicitly are fairly easy to uncover, but other types of inconsistencies may be more covert.

The consistent use of basic assumptions is also important to the achievement of consistency. The theory's purpose, the definitions of concepts, and the relationships need to be consistent with the stated and unstated assumptions of the theory. Examples and diagrams can also be considered in the light of the assumptions of the theory. For example, suppose a basic theoretic assumption is the unity of the individual and the environment and that both change simultaneously and irreversibly through time and space. This assumption is consistent with a definition of health as expanding consciousness, but it is inconsistent with a theoretic conceptualization of health as a state of adaptation. Adaptation typically implies conforming or adjusting to environmental stimuli to fit within the environment. The concept of *adaptation* tends to suggest the assumption that events external to the person are primary determinants of health, and that the person and the environment are separate entities. The unity of the individual and the environment is a concept that can be used to convey an assumption that humans and the environment are interconnected and that they change simultaneously. Simultaneous change negates the idea of conforming or adjusting to stimuli as health; rather, it implies incorporating change, becoming a different person, and increasing options and awareness of choice.

For clarity, the purposes of the theory must be consistent with all other components. A purpose of health that is achieved by deliberate nursing actions may be at odds with the basic assumption that health is deterministic. As you become aware of inconsistencies, you will uncover other meanings that are conveyed in the definitions and the other components of the theory.

When reflecting on consistency, examine your descriptions for each component of the theory, and consider where there are consistencies and inconsistencies within and among the descriptive elements of the theory. Definitions must be examined for consistency with one another and in relation to assumptions. Structure is sometimes inconsistent with relationships. If a theory is extremely inconsistent, it is difficult to continue the process of critical reflection regarding the theory. Some semantic inconsistencies within theory are more common early during the theory's development and leave room for new possibilities for further development. However, inconsistencies at the basic roots of a theory (e.g., between assumptions and goals) have implications that will affect the entire theory and that must be addressed.

Structural Clarity. Structural clarity is closely linked to semantic clarity. Structural clarity refers to how identifiable and apparent the connections and reasoning are within theory. The descriptive elements of structure and relationships provide important information for addressing this dimension of clarity.

In a theory with structural clarity, you can readily identify and recognize the underlying conceptual network. With structural clarity, concepts are interconnected and organized into a coherent whole. If you cannot discern the structure of the theory, you begin to search for those structural elements that are related and for gaps that occur in the flow of the theory. If all major relationships are included within a single structure, clarity is enhanced. Clarity is lost when significant relationships are not contained within a coherent structure. Pieces of relationships, rudiments of structure, or concepts that stand alone are evidence that parts have not yet been integrated into the whole during development of the theory.

Structural Consistency. Structural consistency refers to the consistent use of structural form within a theory. Often a theory, especially a more middle-range theory, is built around one predominant structural form, such as a form that differentiates concepts, structures concepts linearly, or structures concepts in a hierarchy. Sometimes, one structural form provides an overall general profile for major relationships within theory, and more minor components of the theory take a different structural form. Whatever structure or structures are used to link together concepts and relationships, their consistent use throughout the theory serves as a structural map that enhances clarity. A theorist may begin with a structural movement that is linear. If this structure is reflected in the linkages among elements of the theory, you will observe a high level of structural consistency. A shift in reasoning to a structure that integrates concepts (e.g., Venn diagram of overlapping circles) may be confusing, or the structure might function well within a structural scheme that is linear.

In summary, "How clear is this theory?" can be asked as a means of exploring the ways in which a theory is or is not clear and comprehensible and what its level of clarity means for the development and use of the theory. The ideas of semantic and structural consistency and clarity can be used to guide the discussion of issues of clarity, because inconsistencies provide double messages that confound clarity. A very general (broad-scope) theory may be quite ambiguous but still useful for the stimulation of new ideas. For example, a middle-range theory of hopelessness may have aspects that are vague but that may still be important to help nurses understand the experience. However, the ambiguity of that same theory may affect its usefulness for guiding research. Becoming aware of the ways in which clarity is obscured in the light of your purpose makes it possible to design ways to develop further the theory's clarity. The degree to which a theory must be clear depends on how the nurse intends to use it.

How *Simple* Is This Theory?

Simplicity means that the number of elements within each descriptive category—particularly concepts and their interrelationships—are minimal. *Complexity* implies many theoretic relationships between and among numerous concepts. A theory with nine concepts has significantly greater theoretic complexity than a theory with only three concepts. Adding even one or two concepts to a theory greatly increases the potential for theoretic interrelationships and, subsequently, complexity. The desirability of simplicity or complexity can vary with the stage of theory development. In grounded theory or phenomenologic descriptions, there may be considerable complexity as the theory begins to emerge. As the theory develops, however, relationships and concepts coalesce, and the theory becomes simpler. Regardless of the approach to theory development, some concepts created early during the process eventually may be deleted or changed. Theories reflect varying degrees of simplicity. In nursing, some situations suggest the need for relatively simple and broad theories that can be used as general guides for practice. Other situations suggest simple but more empirically accessible theories to guide research. Still other situations suggest the need for theories that are relatively complex because of the value that such theories have for enhancing the understanding of extremely complex practice situations.

How *General* Is This Theory?

The *generality* of a theory refers to its breadth of scope and purpose; a general theory can be applied to a broad array of situations. The term *parsimony* is sometimes used as a synonym to describe the trait of theoretic simplicity, but the concept of parsimony also includes the idea of generality. A *parsimonious theory* is conceptually simple (i.e., it contains few structural elements), but it accounts for a broad range of empiric experiences.

The scope of concepts and purposes within the theory provides clues with regard to its generality. A theory that contains broad concepts will encompass more empiric indicators than a theory that contains very narrow concepts. The concepts of *humans* and *universe* could be interpreted as organizing almost every empiric indicator possible. A comprehensive theory that involves these two concepts would be highly general. A theory that interrelates the individual and the physical environment is less general, but still fairly broad in scope. The concept of the *individual* implies that the theory is concerned with a single person. The use of *physical* as a modifier for *environment* conveys the notion of part of the environment only. Information about individuals in communities could not be understood within this theory. A theory that addresses the characteristics of acutely ill people in the intensive care unit environment is even less general, and the scope of concepts subsequently narrows.

Questions that address the generality of a theory include the following: To whom or what does this theory apply, and when does it apply? Does the purpose pertain to all health care professionals? Does it apply to people in general? Does the purpose apply to specific specialties of nursing and only at given times? The more limited the scope of application of the theory, the less general is the theory.

Whether generality is viewed as desirable depends on your purpose for the theory. General theory is quite useful for generating ideas or hypotheses. Nursing theories that address broad concepts (e.g., individuals, society, health, environment) have a high degree of generality and are useful for organizing ideas about universal health behaviors. Theories that address a specific human experience (e.g., pain) are less general and, because of their relative specificity, are useful for guiding practice in a clinical setting.

How *Accessible* Is This Theory?

Accessibility addresses the extent to which empiric indicators for the concepts can be identified and to what extent the purposes of the theory can be attained. If a theory is to be used for explaining some aspect of practice, its theoretic concepts must be linked to the empiric indicators that are available in practice. *Empiric indicators* are perceptually accessible experiences that can be used in practice to assess the phenomena described by the theory and can help determine whether the purposes of the theory are realized in a way that the theory suggests.

Only selected dimensions of highly abstract concepts may be empirically accessible. If the concepts of a theory do not reflect empiric dimensions, or if the empiric dimensions are obscure, the concepts may be ideas that cannot be explored or understood empirically.

 Consider This…

> Consider the example of a theory about rehabilitation and interaction. The theoretic definitions of the concepts are clues to the accessibility of the theory. Without definition, the words *rehabilitation* and *interaction* can assume many dimensions of meaning. If the concepts are defined, the ways in which they are to be empirically accessed is clearer. If the definitions point to the measurements or observable behaviors that can be associated with rehabilitation and the specific types of interactions that promote rehabilitation, then the theory can be judged to be relatively accessible in a clinical context.

Increasing the complexity of a theory often increases its empiric accessibility. As subconceptual categories are clarified, empiric indicators become more precise. Suppose that the concepts of *rehabilitation* and *interaction* are related within the same theory. The theory is judged to have a high degree of generality and simplicity because the concepts are broad and few in number. Designating five subconcepts for each concept would increase the theory's complexity. Those five subconcepts are likely to have more precise empiric bases than are the broader concepts. With empirically accessible subconcepts, the empiric accessibility of the theory increases. If a concept does not have an empiric basis at the outset, specifying subconcepts for larger wholes does not increase empiric accessibility.

Research testing requires the empiric accessibility of concepts. It also confirms those concepts that are clinically relevant and accessible. For example, if *rehabilitation* is defined in a research project as "able to complete activities of daily living independently," you have established a clear link between the idea of rehabilitation and a reasonable clinical observation. If the research supports the hypothesis derived from the theory, it also provides evidence of empiric accessibility for the concept of rehabilitation.

The empiric accessibility of the concepts contained within a theory is basic to validating theoretic relationships and making use of the theory in practice. Although grounded approaches to generating theory assume empiric accessibility, the extent to which empiric accessibility is important can vary. Considering the theory's purpose will help you to make judgments about how empirically accessible a theory should be. Theory that provides a conceptual perspective for clinical practice may not require much empiric accessibility. If a theory is to be used to guide research, empiric accessibility is important. If a theory will be used to shape nursing practice, concepts need to be empirically accessible in the clinical area. If concepts are not empirically grounded, creating conceptual meaning may provide direction for the empiric indicators that are needed for research.

How *Important* Is This Theory?

In nursing, the importance of a theory is closely tied to the idea of its clinical significance or its practical value. An important theory is forward looking; is usable in practice, education, and research; and is valuable for creating a desired future. The central question to be answered is, "Does this theory create understanding that is important to nursing?" Some nursing theories guide research and practice; some generate radically new ideas about health and caring; and some differentiate the focus of nursing from other service professions.

If a theory contains concepts, definitions, purposes, and assumptions that are grounded in practice, it will have practical value for enhancing theory-based research that can become research evidence that is integrated into evidence-informed clinical decisions. A theory that has limited empiric accessibility may not have practical value for research, but it can stimulate ideas and spark political action that improves practice.

One approach to addressing the question of importance is to reflect on the theory's basic theoretic assumptions. If the underlying assumptions are unsound, the importance of the theory is minimal. For example, if a theory is based on a view of the individual as *parts,* its importance for wholistic nursing is minimal. If a theory is based on an assumption of *wholism* and it moves the understanding of wholism to a new dimension, it likely is to be highly important to nursing.

Theories that have extremely broad purposes may be essentially unattainable and therefore have limited value for the creation of clinical outcomes. This same theory may be important for generating ideas and challenging practice.

The importance of theory depends on the professional and personal values of the person who is addressing the question. Asking, "Do I like this theory?" and "Why do I like it or not like it?" will help you to identify the values that you hold for yourself, your practice, the profession, and the theory. Contributing your ideas about what is important for nursing through careful deliberation and discussion with nurse colleagues will help clarify the direction that a theory should take to achieve important professional purposes.

FORMING A COMPLETE CRITICAL REFLECTION

In summary, the five questions to consider when critically reflecting on the description of a theory are as follows:

1. *Is this theory clear?* This question addresses the clarity and consistency of the presentation. Clarity and consistency may be both semantic and structural.
2. *Is this theory simple?* This question addresses the number of structural components and relationships within the theory. Complexity implies numerous relational components within the theory; simplicity implies fewer relational components.
3. *Is this theory general?* This question addresses the scope of experiences covered by the theory. Generality infers a wide scope of phenomena; specificity narrows the range of events included in the theory. Generality in combination with simplicity yields parsimony.
4. *Is this theory accessible?* This question addresses the extent to which concepts within the theory are grounded in empirically identifiable phenomena.
5. *Is this theory important?* This question addresses the extent to which a theory leads to valued nursing goals in practice, research, and education.

WHEN ARE THOROUGH DESCRIPTION AND CRITICAL REFLECTION IMPORTANT?

As you might expect, there is no easy answer to the previous question, except to say, "You will know." When you are serious about appropriately using theory and begin the work of understanding any given theory, you will soon understand why considering it carefully is important. The use of any theory for any purpose should not be done unknowingly. Deciding to what extent theory ought to be examined in relation to its intended use comes with an understanding of and practice with the processes of description and critical reflection.

We believe that completing at least one guided and thorough description and critical reflection, even as an exercise, is important for appreciating the complexity of developing and using theory for shaping practice outcomes. It also underscores the problems of attempting to use theory without a good general understanding of it. Misuse of theory for shaping practice outcomes can range from harmful to worthless. The analytic skills developed in this process also transfer to other areas and may mitigate tendencies to think understanding is present when it is not.

CONCLUSION

For knowledge developers the process of description and critical reflection is important for general understanding of the theory. Description and critical reflections are centrally important for establishing that the whole of the theory fits the context of use.

References

Alligood, M. R., & Tomey, A. M. (2013). *Nursing theorists and their work* (8th ed.). St. Louis, MO: Elsevier-Mosby.

Barnum, B. J. S. (1998). *Nursing theory* (5th ed.). Boston, MA: Lippincott-Raven.

Ellis, R. (1968). Characteristics of significant theories. *Nursing Research, 17*, 217–222.

Fawcett, J. (2005). Criteria for evaluation of theory. *Nursing Science Quarterly, 18*, 131–135.

Hall, L. E. (1966). Another view of nursing care and quality. In K. M. Straub, & K. S. Parker (Eds.), *Continuity in patient care: the role of nursing* (pp. 47–60). Washington, DC: Catholic University Press.

Hardy, M. E. (1974). Theories: Components, development, evaluation. *Nursing Research, 23*, 100–107.

Im, E.-O. (2015). The current status of theory evaluation in nursing. *Journal of Advanced Nursing, 71*(10), 2268–2278. https://doi.org/10.1111/jan.12698.

Koltoff, N. J. (1967). The use of the laboratory. *Nursing Research, 16*, 122.

Liehr, P., & Smith, M. J. (2017). Middle range theory: a perspective on development and use. ANS. *Advances in Nursing Science, 40*(1), 51–63. https://doi.org/10.1097/ANS.0000000000000162.

Thorne, S. E., & Sawatzky, R. (2014). Particularizing the general: sustaining theoretical integrity in the context of an evidence-based practice agenda. *ANS. Advances in Nursing Science, 37*, 1–10.

Knowledge Authentication Processes

The experience of looking at human behavior is much like running head on into a cloud—a cloud whose origin and subsequent direction is unknown. Before the impact, you can see the cloud—dynamic and three dimensional; but when you reach out to grab a handful to test, you come away with nothing visible but your clenched fist. You may have been buffeted a bit by the dynamic forces within the cloud but aside from this, it moves on still visible, still dynamic, and still three dimensional. Then your thoughts run something like this: "I can see the cloud; I can feel the forces it contains, but how do I really study it when it refuses to lend itself to anything more than a fleeting encounter?

Marjorie R. Wright (1966, p. 244)

This opening quote underscores the challenges of authenticating knowledge in nursing. Nursing is often described as a human science where what is studied is changing and affected by a myriad of factors that cannot be known. This alone makes authenticating knowledge challenging. Adding the complexities of authenticating knowledge associated with the nonempiric patterns of knowing creates additional challenges and complexities. In this chapter we address authentication processes that draw on the established methods of authentication arising from each unique pattern of knowing, but we return over and over to bring into focus the whole of knowing. To paraphrase Wright's quote: "We can see the whole, we can feel the forces it contains, but how do we really study it when it refuses to lend itself to anything more than a fleeting encounter?" We do not claim to have an adequate response, but we do believe that by drawing on the authentication of each pattern of knowing, we may at least build a path to what we are seeking.

The formal expressions of knowledge within each of the knowing patterns needs to be authenticated in order to be accepted as significant and useful for the discipline. Authentication is important for determining how well the knowledge functions in relation to the purpose for which it was created. In this way, authentication serves as a "green light" for implementation and also provides direction for ongoing development that improves the knowledge structure.

Table 9.1 shows the authentication processes for each of the patterns of knowing. Authentication processes focus on the formal expressions of knowledge within each pattern, and draw on established methods of scholarship.

While each pattern has different methods for authenticating formal knowledge expressions within the pattern, authentication processes within any of the other

TABLE 9.1 Dimensions Associated With Each of the Patterns of Knowing

Dimension	Emancipatory	Ethics	Personal	Aesthetics	Empirics
Critical questions	Who benefits? What is wrong with this picture? What are the barriers to freedom? What changes are needed?	Is this right? Is this responsible?	Do I know what I do? Do I do what I know?	What does this mean? How is this significant?	What is this? How does it work?
Creative processes	Critiquing Imagining	Clarifying Exploring	Opening Centering	Envisioning Rehearsing	Conceptualizing Structuring
Formal expressions	Action plans Manifestoes Critical analyses Visions for the future	Principles and codes	Personal stories Genuine Self	Aesthetic criticism Works of art	Models Formal descriptions Theories
Authentication processes	Social equity Sustainability Empowerment Demystification	Dialogue Justification	Response Reflection	Appreciation Inspiration	Confirmation Validation
Integrated expression in practice	Praxis	Moral and ethical comportment	Therapeutic use of Self	Transformative art/acts	Scientific competence

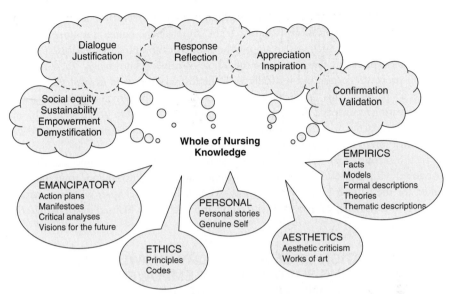

FIG. 9.1 Interrelationship Between Authentication Processes and Formal Expressions of Nursing Knowledge.

patterns can become important when knowledge expressions are authenticated. For example, if you are using the processes of dialogue and justification to examine ethical knowledge it may be important to consider whether a set of principles being examined is sustainable or empowering, which is a consideration for authentication within emancipatory knowing. If confirming and validating an empiric theory of hopelessness, one might engage the processes of appreciation and inspiration within the aesthetic pattern to understand if the theory does inspire appreciation of the nature of hopelessness. Basically, formal expressions of knowledge within any pattern may be strengthened when authentication processes within other patterns are used in relation to the expression. In this manner, authentication processes ultimately contribute to the whole of knowing by helping ensure that when knowledge is integrated in practice (e.g., becomes the whole of knowing), the desired outcomes can be better achieved. We do not claim that authentication processes across all patterns will always be useful in relation to a formal expression of knowledge. We do believe that authentication processes within all patterns should be at least considered for appropriateness when formal knowledge expressions are authenticated.

Fig. 9.1 provides a conceptual image of the ways in which the authentication processes associated with each pattern can be brought to bear on any formal expression of nursing knowledge.

As illustrated in the figure, the formal expressions of nursing knowledge that we have associated with each pattern of knowing (shown along the figure's lower level) point to a collective of formal expressions that constitute the whole of nursing knowledge. This collective of formal expressions is shown at the center of the figure. The upper level of cloudlike structures depict overlap among the authentication processes and also point to the formal expressions that constitute the whole of nursing knowledge. These authentication processes correspond vertically with the formal expression examples associated with each pattern. This figure illustrates that while each pattern has unique ways of authenticating knowledge that are appropriate within that pattern of knowing, authentication approaches within any other pattern may be useful, and may be adapted for authentication of knowledge within other patterns.

In the sections that follow, we focus first on the authentication processes that are associated with each of the patterns of knowing, examining the authentication methods suited for the pattern from which it arises. We conclude the chapter with explanation of ways in which each pattern's authentication approaches can be used to strengthen the whole of knowing.

AUTHENTICATION OF EMANCIPATORY KNOWLEDGE: DEMONSTRATING SUSTAINABILITY, EMPOWERMENT, SOCIAL EQUITY, AND DEMYSTIFICATION

Within the pattern of emancipatory knowing, critical questions related to freedoms and benefits initiate the creative processes of critiquing and imagining. These in turn generate formal knowledge expressions such as action plans, manifestos, critical analyses, and vision statements. Authentication of emancipatory knowledge examines social equity, demystification, empowerment, and sustainability. The outcome of authentication, in turn, is critically questioned, the process reinitiates, formal expressions alter, and authentication continues.

The disciplinary processes for authenticating emancipatory knowledge include challenging and affirming the *sustainability* of real change, and determining the extent to which *empowerment* and *social equity* occur, as well as the extent to which previously hidden circumstances that have created injustices have been *demystified*.

The fundamental method that we propose for authenticating emancipatory knowledge is drawn from the work of Paulo Freire's (1970) concept of "testing untested feasibilities." Since emancipatory knowing, by definition, is at the center of knowing and expressed as praxis (refer back to Fig. 1.1) the processes of testing untested feasibilities can be relevant for any of the fundamental patterns of knowing.

The process of testing untested feasibilities is accomplished in a group—usually a small group of people who share a recognition of a particular problem related to justice, powerlessness, or unfair barriers (any of those situations that emancipatory knowing is concerned with). The testing process begins with a close examination of the formal expression of emancipatory knowledge—the manifesto, action plan, vision for the future or critical analysis of an existing political/social reality. This examination focuses on the question: What needs to change, and how can it change? The group then turns attention to imagining possible actions that could begin to create the desired change:

They identify feasible actions that have not been put into action before, or that might have been attempted, but might be adopted again.

Determining untested feasibilities engages authentication processes that arise from other patterns of knowing, since all patterns of knowing contribute to the critical examination and selection of any untested feasibility. The group addresses each of these feasibility dimensions:

- Is this action ethically sound? Any potential action is only feasible if it is responsible and right given the situation. The processes of dialogue and justification are used to ensure that any potential feasible action is ethically sound as a means of changing the unjust situation (see "Authenticating Ethical Knowledge" section for more detail).
- Is this action consistent with each person's self-authenticity? When personal knowing and emancipatory knowing come together, each person is called upon to examine his or her personal motives and to develop confidence to fully support the emancipatory intent of potential action. This means setting aside paternalistic motives that privilege the needs and desires of any individual or group over the needs and desires of those who are disadvantaged.
- Can this action lead to a cohesive "whole" in which each part of the situation is in harmony with all others? The group examines the potential action for its transformative potential, opening the way for possibilities that have not been previously imagined.
- Do we have a clear understanding of the facts that are relevant to the situation? Is the existing data reliable? Does existing data support our potential action? Myriads of facts need to be examined in the process of testing untested feasibilities, such as the economic realities of the situation, epidemiologic or demographic data related to the injustice you are addressing. It is important to clearly separate fact from impressions or assumptions about a situation. In doing so, you can identify areas around which you need to first obtain factual data before proceeding.

Having arrived at one or more potential actions, the next step is to actually test the actions—to implement the action or actions to determine their feasibility in terms of the authenticating dimensions of sustainability, social equity, empowerment, and demystification. Often these benchmarks cannot be confirmed in short periods of time, but it is possible to determine progress in relation to these ideals.

- Sustainability: Does the action lead toward the social change that was envisioned, and does it last?
- Social equity: Is there movement toward demonstrable elimination or reduction of conditions that create disadvantage for some and advantage for others?
- Empowerment: Is there growing ability of individuals and groups to exercise their will, to have their voices heard, and to claim their full human potential?
- Demystification: To what extent are formerly hidden dimensions of the situation made visible?

At any time there are indications that an action is not moving toward the ideals of authentication, the group returns to the process of examining the projected untested feasibilities, and refining, adjusting, or replacing the action that was initially selected to test. The group proceeds to test the feasibilities now seen as having potential for change, informed by the insight and experience gained in the previous action or actions.

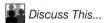 *Discuss This...*

A graduate nursing student named Carson is completing his master's thesis by addressing what motivates elders to purchase nutritional supplements. Carson has noticed that the advertising of nutritional supplements is being intentionally directed at older individuals. Carson knows that much of this advertising promotes expensive supplements that have limited if any benefit, and in many cases makes false claims about alleviating several life quality problems associated with aging. One day while shopping for groceries Carson overhears two of his elderly neighbors, Helen and Trudy, discussing the benefits of the latest advertised supplement which is not only expensive, but also (he knows) ineffective and perhaps harmful. While Carson hesitates for a moment, he decides to approach them, initiate a discussion about their need for product, and share his thoughts about the product being unnecessary and potentially harmful. As he turns around to see what Helen and Trudy do, he notices them returning the product to the store shelf. He smiles to himself, satisfied he has done the right thing.

Discuss the following questions with your peers:

- Were Carson's actions motivated by a concern for social justice?
- What, in addition, might Carson do to strengthen a focus on social justice for vulnerable elders?
- What actions might be most important for nursing in the long run? Explain each.
- What knowledge and knowing within other patterns were (or might be) operating in this situation?

The case example of Carson is limited and initially involves only a conversation between him and two neighbors, but the possibility for authentication is still present. Sustainability might be assessed by talking with Helen and Trudy in a few weeks and determining if they were still convinced of the product's ineffectiveness and not using it. Also, Carson can determine if they have alerted others to the nature of the product, based on what Carson had told them. Suppose Trudy and Helen had indeed stopped using the products and also had began to question other heavily advertised supplements as being useful. This suggests they have moved to a place where their knowledge meant they were not being disadvantaged by spending limited income on useless products. Empowerment and demystification would come, with the insight of knowing that certain products have limited value; and that purchasing them simply "lines the pockets" of some large corporation at their own expense. As "movers and shakers," if Helen and Trudy had conducted a seminar at the local senior center alerting other seniors to what they had learned, this further suggests the criteria of sustainability, social equity, demystification, and empowerment that was not only happening for Helen and Trudy, but was expanding into other groups and populations.

AUTHENTICATING ETHICAL KNOWLEDGE: DIALOGUE AND JUSTIFICATION

Within the pattern of ethical knowing, the critical questions related to what is right and responsible initiate the creative processes of exploring and clarifying. These in turn generate formal knowledge expressions such as principles and codes that are subjected to authentication using processes of dialogue and justification. The outcome of authentication, in turn, is critically questioned, the process reinitiates, formal expressions alter, and authentication continues.

It is within the processes of dialogue and justification that knowledge is more deliberatively examined with reference to the perspectives of justice and care. Through these processes, ethical knowledge is examined and refined, and becomes part of the disciplinary heritage that individual nurses subsequently carry into practice. This knowledge is revisited and challenged as the need arises by asking the critical questions: "Is this knowledge right?" and "Is it responsible?" With these questions, nurses consider whether disciplinary forms of ethical knowledge guide right and responsible ethical decisions. These questions engage the clarifying and exploring processes that we have described with the use of dialogue and justification.

Dialogue requires a community of those who are challenged by an ethical problem. They come together as a community—face to face, online, or through exchanges in the professional literature—to examine established ethical perspectives, principles, and codes (Btoush & Campbell, 2009; Freysteinson, 2009; Quaghebeur & Gastmans, 2009). As a group, they strive to understand alternative points of view more fully. On some issues, they come to a point where they can accept, reject, or modify the knowledge form. On others, the dialogues continue over long periods of time.

Traditionally, ethical knowledge forms have been examined for internal logic as a standard of validity. Although internal logic is important for coherence, it is an insufficient standard for establishing the value of ethical knowledge in nursing. With dialogue, ideally multiple voices over time will be integrated into justification processes. The choice of the word *justification* suggests no particular framework for establishing the value of an ethical knowledge form.

Justification processes for ethical knowledge forms in nursing can appeal to the authority of historical values associated with nursing, existing moral/ethical knowledge, currently held values, and values and moral knowing consistent with an envisioned future. For example, the value of caring might be cited as an important historical factor that can be used to justify caring in nursing; in other words, caring as a historically embedded duty justifies caring as a contemporary value. Principles of nonmaleficence or autonomy, as baccalaureate students generally learn, might be called on to justify ethical knowledge. In addition, an envisioned future may form a critical template against which to reflect ethical knowledge. This occurs when we question whether caring is an ethic that will help us to achieve professional autonomy and identity. It is assumed that the collective voice of nursing will be the best hope for the emergence of appropriate and productive justification frameworks as the basis for re-envisioning the form of ethical knowledge.

We have chosen an eclectic approach to forming and justifying ethical principles because we believe no single perspective is entirely useful for all situations. Rather, the more likely scenario is that multiple justification perspectives will be used. Care must be balanced with a concern for justice; rules must be used in the context of doing the least harm or benefiting people in some way.

>> *Consider This...*

As an example of how care and justice might emerge with the use of the processes of dialogue and justification, suppose that you and your peers are examining a situation beginning with a deontologic perspective that provides a rule for ethical action. The situation involves a mother who is suspected of inflicting physical harm on her young child.

The 2-year-old girl, who is currently being hospitalized for an emergency appendectomy, has bruises and marks that you believe are the result of being struck. However, the mother attributes them to the caregiver, who, you subsequently learn, is the child's grandmother. Although old and new bruises are seen, the child has no broken bones and appears to be quite healthy otherwise.

Assume that the rule being discussed is that of *nonmaleficence:* doing no harm. This is a principle that is generally followed by you and the professional group with whom you work. You and others initially suggest that doing no harm in this case means establishing the source of the child's bruises and subsequently protecting the child from further injury. As the dialogue proceeds about how to report concerns to child protective services or to ask the mother more pointedly about the bruises and their source, the dialogue and justification processes take an unexpected turn, and you begin to realize that doing no harm in this situation is becoming fairly complex.

The social worker on your team reveals that the mother is unmarried, must work outside the home to support herself and her child, and out of necessity is leaving the child in the care of the grandmother to minimize child care expenses. The mother cannot afford paid child care because she needs her income to meet expenses, including renting an apartment that keeps her whereabouts hidden from a former partner who abused both her and the child in the past.

A staff nurse states that he has talked with the grandmother during a recent visit. He offers the information that, although the child's grandmother is well meaning and loving, she was recently confined to a wheelchair because of a progressive, long-term debilitating muscular disease. The staff nurse believes that the grandmother may bruise the child inadvertently by bumping her against the wheelchair or other household items as she provides care. An intern on the team shares that the grandmother had voluntarily offered in a conversation with her that, on occasion, the child had slipped from her arms to the floor, and the grandmother was worried that this may have caused the child's appendicitis. The intern, from talking with the grandmother, believes that generally she manages to care for the child properly, and certainly she intends to be a good caregiver to help her daughter.

Given the ongoing dialogue, it is becoming apparent that it might actually be harmful to the young child not to allow the grandmother to provide care during the day, if it means the child's return to the mother's care, the loss of the mother's income, the discovery of the mother and child by the abusive partner, and the risk of harm to both.

Although this example is somewhat contrived, the message is that dialogue and justification led the team to question the initial thinking about what was right, in that unconsidered approaches to protecting the young child from harm could likely result in unintended consequences of harm.

Justification and dialogue raise the question of what values and actions should prevail. What about the rule of doing no harm? Should the rule be violated to produce a greater good? The answers are never totally clear, but open, reasoned, and knowledgeable dialogue seems to be an effective approach to making the best decision that is possible. For the situation of the mother and her 2-year-old child, perhaps the best decision might be—assuming that the bruises are unintended, not seriously life threatening, and occurring because of the grandmother's physical condition—to let the grandmother continue to care for the child and to teach her care techniques that minimize the risk of physical harm to the child. As the situation changes (e.g., if the child is or may be seriously injured while in the grandmother's care), a different decision will emerge from the justification and dialogue processes. In the example, it is knowledge within the pattern of emancipatory knowing that would suggest a core solution. Such knowing would require critical analysis and action involving, for example, the sociopolitical context that contributed to the situation of a single parent with no options for financial support or safe child care.

Many different groups with a variety of justification perspectives carry out the justification and dialogue processes to develop ethical knowledge over time. Ethical knowledge is often communicated in a vacuum, and we know little about how it is actually used or applied. Arguments for one type of approach versus another are academically interesting, but positions become blurred, and the conditions within the work environment of nurses are often ignored.

As analyses and understandings subsequent to the process of dialogue and justification find their way into the disciplinary literature and other venues where dialogue can occur, ethical knowledge forms will achieve legitimacy in relation to practice. It is unlikely that anything that could be considered "final" will ever evolve, because ethical knowledge is never used in the same context. However, the ideal of generating ethical knowledge from practice and refining that knowledge, with the intent that it will be returned to practice, needs to be the goal.

Through dialogue and justification, many perspectives can be brought to bear on ethical knowledge. The open questioning and dialogue that considers the context of working nurses is nursing's best hope for usable and effective ethical knowledge and moral behavior. It is through justification processes that an understanding of ethics and morality in nursing will be approached and will allow the knowledgeable and committed action required for praxis to emerge.

AUTHENTICATING PERSONAL KNOWLEDGE: RESPONSE AND REFLECTION

Within the pattern of personal knowing, the critical questions related to doing what is known and knowing what is done initiate the creative processes of opening and centering. These in turn generate formal knowledge expressions of a genuine Self and personal stories that are subjected to authentication through response and reflection processes. The outcome of authentication, in turn, is critically questioned, the process reinitiates, formal expressions alter, and authentication continues.

It is through the processes of response and reflection that the Self and personal stories that reflect the Self can be examined. Response and reflection in relation to the self come from being in the world with others. The Self is perceived as unique by others and brings to each interaction a dynamic that is recognized and known. As people respond to one another, they give messages that affirm, disappoint, celebrate, or negate aspects of the expressed Self. Responses are taken in, felt, and internalized. When responses are internalized, reflection on their meaning can follow. The person may return to critical questioning and to the creative processes of opening and centering with the use of journaling and meditation. The person also may reflect on the responses in other ways and take in meanings that arise anew from the interactive experiences.

In addition to responses that are received from interactions that occur during the course of daily experience, insights from meditation, journaling, and other self-knowing practices can be shared with trusted friends and colleagues who are willing to listen and to respond to what is offered. Drew (1997), when exploring nurses' meaningful experiences and expanding self-awareness, found that sharing the story of an experience with another person enlarged, solidified, and deepened the meaning of the experience in a way that improved therapeutic interactions.

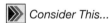 *Consider This...*

One morning Cindy's alarm did not awaken her, causing her to rush about to get ready for her clinical experience. Making it "on time" left a wake of debris in the apartment she shared with two other nursing students. After a particularly difficult day, Cindy returns to a cool and grumpy Annie, who is about to leave for an evening class, and Emily, who is studying. As Cindy prepares a cup of coffee, Annie gets up to leave for her evening class and promptly trips on a pile of clothes and pair of shoes Cindy has left by the front door. At this, Annie explodes, telling Cindy how selfish and unconscientious she is to leave such a mess and not address it immediately when she returned home. Annie screams that this is not the first time this has happened, it is a pattern and it reflects pure inconsideration of her roommates. Not only is her room a mess, but also her stuff is left lying around and the organization of the refrigerator and shelves which they have agreed on is disregarded as Cindy just stuffs whatever into any place without paying attention to where it is. In short, Annie unloads on Cindy citing incidences of inconsiderate, selfish, and unconscientious behavior, with Emily nodding in agreement. Cindy retreats to her room, devastated and sobbing. Annie leaves for her class and Emily returns to her reading.

Fortunately, Cindy, Annie, and Emily have all been introduced to the personal pattern of knowing in their nursing program. Once Cindy calms down, she reviews what they have learned about opening and centering, and the importance of meditation and journaling. She journals about her feelings in response to Annie's anger, and faces the reality of Annie's accusations leveled in the height of anger, even though she hardly thinks of herself as selfish or inconsiderate. As Cindy thinks back on her behavior she begins to write about her typical day and how she moves through it; she notes her interaction patterns with her roommates; and recognizes her impatience and intolerance for the detail of housekeeping. She recognizes that clutter does not bother her like it does other people, but on the other hand she dislikes dust and grime and cleans the apartment once a week, a job that neither Annie nor Emily do. The next morning, Cindy asks Annie and Emily to have dinner together to talk about what happened the evening before. They agree, and together have a candid and frank discussion about the situation.

Their discussion is difficult, but as they reflect on their experiences and respond to one another, they all gain a deeper understanding of themselves, and of one another. They each agree to shift how they manage housekeeping tasks and their personal responsibilities in doing so.

This example illustrates how response and reflection can contribute to personal growth. In this example, Cindy takes the time to be open to the meaning of her experience with her roommates, centers on her own deep inner values and intentions, and then invites Annie and Emily to engage in discussion to gain deeper understanding. As a result, their interactions and actions shift in a way that creates a more healthy situation. It is this kind of dedication to one's own personal knowing, in all areas of one's experience, that makes it possible for nurses to tap into this vital source of knowing. The authentication process for personal knowing is ongoing, just as the example of Cindy's experience with her roommates illustrates. This is the key to addressing the questions "Do I know what I do?" and "Do I do what I know?".

 Think About It...

Bring to mind an experience in your professional or personal life when someone you respect has given you feedback that heightened your awareness of who you are and how you are perceived to others around you. Perhaps this person affirmed a characteristic that you value and that made you feel good about yourself (you are generally kind and understanding). Or he or she might have reflected a characteristic that you would rather not be known for (you are overly judgmental or critical). Reflect on this experience to explore, with all the honesty and candor you can muster, how his or her impression fits with who you know yourself to be, and the nature of your character that you wish to convey to the world. Write a brief story that tells an imaginary or real situation in which you express yourself as you want to be known in the world. Over a couple of days, return your focus to your story to reflect on what it means as you develop your actions (what you do) to be consistent with who you know yourself to be (what you know).

AUTHENTICATING AESTHETIC KNOWLEDGE: APPRECIATION AND INSPIRATION

Within the pattern of aesthetic knowing, the critical questions related to what is meaningful and significant initiate the creative processes of envisioning and rehearsing. These in turn generate formal knowledge expressions including written criticisms and works of art that are subjected to authentication by questioning whether expressions are appreciated for what they are and whether they inspire a deeper understanding of what is represented. The outcome of authentication, in turn, is critically questioned, the process reinitiates, formal expressions alter, and authentication continues.

As nurses share and communicate insights that are derived from the creative processes of envisioning, rehearsing, and then formally expressing the artistry of nursing, others in the discipline respond to the formal expression of art and the meaning that it provides in relation to the discipline of nursing. In the sphere of aesthetics, the authentication of aesthetic knowledge involves appreciation and inspiration.

In the pattern of aesthetics, the authentication of aesthetic knowledge requires responses of appreciation and inspiration. Appreciation means that others affirm that they see meaning in the art/act or in the artistic representation, and that the meaning conveyed is appropriate and important for the discipline of nursing. Inspiration means that the work brings forth new meanings and possibilities for understanding the experience that it represents, and that it moves the viewer or observer toward the experience that is represented. In other words, observers are moved to bring something represented in the art/act into their own practices, or to draw on insights represented by the art/act to inform their own practices.

Formal expressions of aesthetic knowing are unique in temporal time and space and that are grounded in the wholeness of human experience. Thus, the authentication processes of appreciation and inspiration reflect back on the artistic experience that is represented and on the symbolized meanings inherent in its representation.

There are three guiding principles for the authentication processes of the appreciation and inspiration of aesthetic knowledge. These principles ask the following:

- Is the artistic expression a unique, creative expression that is grounded in the immediacy and enduring wholeness of human experience?
- Does the artistic expression expand and enrich the plausible meanings of the experience?
- Does the artistic expression illuminate possibilities for the future?

Unique features serve to distinguish artistic expressions from any other type of expression and serve to reveal possibilities in human experience and expression that have not existed before and that will not be replicated. An expression of aesthetic knowing in nursing is authenticated when you and others in the discipline come to appreciate something about nursing not previously appreciated, and are inspired to consider new possibilities for your own practice and for the nursing discipline. The expression is also authenticated if it inspires you and others to change the Self and learn in some way or to integrate new creative possibilities into your practice.

Works of art, as aesthetic expressions, are perceived immediately—in the moment—and call forth human responses that inspire in some way. To say they are forms of knowledge that are responded to "immediately" means that you perceive them all at once; they are not mediated by language or other symbols. In perceiving, you have a distinct response, which is your "appreciation"—whether it is positive or not. For example, when you see a painting that connects with you about some aspect of nursing, the feeling response of "it just speaks to me" is immediate and in the moment. You do not read the painting line by line like you would a book. Rather, you notice a painting all at once. Your eye movements scan and interpret the painting, and it touches something within you—an experience forms your appreciation or inspires you. You are drawn to dwell on the painting and begin to notice nuances of expression in the art. The capacity to call forth human responses in the moment and to draw the observer into a deeper experience of the art reflects a work of art's power to reflect something that is significant but common in the human experience.

 Think About It...

Zane returns to his senior seminar following a 2-week absence because of the sudden death of his parents in an automobile accident. During this time of grief he was responsible for legal arrangements related to his parent's estate as well as arranging for the care of his 14-year-old brother. Upon his return, the instructor senses the importance of the moment and after talking with Zane privately, invites him to share any thoughts and feelings with the class. Zane talks about the shock of the event, as well as the grief and exhaustion he felt as he moved through the needed tasks associated with managing his parent's death and making arrangements for his brother. At one point Zane reaches into his pocket and produces a piece of paper. His voice quivers as he tells his peers that this poem really spoke to him and helped him deal with the loss of his parents and then begins to read from the paper. His voice breaks as he reads and tears come, but he finishes, and returns the paper to his pocket.

> Nature's first green is gold,
> Her hardest hue to hold.
> Her early leaf's a flower;
> But only so an hour.
> Then leaf subsides to leaf.
> So Eden sank to grief,
> So dawn goes down to day.
> Nothing gold can stay.

Nothing Gold Can Stay by Robert Frost (n.d.)

Although this short poem can be interpreted in multiple ways, think about the experience of grief that Zane has shared and ponder whether this poem might be appreciated and inspirational in relation to understanding the experience of death and grief.

Remaining in tune with and appreciating works of art that represent human experience enhances nurses' capacity for connoisseurship—the ability to recognize and affirm significant transformative arts/acts. Connoisseurship is required to engage in aesthetic criticism that reveals meanings and insights that arise from the art/act, meanings that extend beyond the impressions of any one person's perceptions.

 Discuss This...

Take a look at Richard Prince's campy *Nurse Paintings* and read the review of the paintings by Sandy and Henry Summers on the "Truth About Nursing" website (http://www.truthaboutnursing.org/media/va/nurse_paintings.html). With a group of colleagues who have also viewed this work, discuss your own responses to the paintings. What do the paintings convey aesthetically about nursing? What human responses do they call forth? What do they reflect that is significant? What do they inspire you to think and do? Consider your own thoughts and feelings in comparison to the Summerses' review.

Unlike works of art, aesthetic criticism usually takes a written form. These criticisms are authenticated in a way similar to that of works of art, but the whole of the criticism is not appreciated all at once in the moment as a painting or sculpture might be. However, authentic aesthetic criticisms can be both appreciated and inspirational. When you reflect on a well-written criticism, new possibilities for your nursing art and its possibilities for nursing come into awareness, just as they do when works of art are authenticated. Although aesthetic criticisms are formalized expressions of aesthetic knowing that are written, it should be noted that appreciation and inspiration could also come about when you and a connoisseur-critic engage in a nursing encounter. To summarize, a response that is elicited by an aesthetic art form—whether a work of art or an aesthetic criticism—deepens the observer-participant's appreciation of the experience that is represented and creates new meanings and possibilities for the expression of nursing art to an extent that would not otherwise be possible.

AUTHENTICATING EMPIRICAL KNOWLEDGE: CONFIRMATION AND VALIDATION

Within the pattern of empirical knowing, the critical questions "What is this?" and "How does it work?" initiate the creative processes of conceptualizing and structuring. These in turn generate formal knowledge expressions such as empiric theory and formal descriptions that are subjected to authentication by questioning whether such expressions can be confirmed or validated to represent what they claim to represent. The outcome of authentication, in turn, is critically questioned, the process reinitiates, formal expressions alter, and authentication continues.

Authentication processes for empirics vary in degree of rigor as well as with the knowledge form. Confirming and validating the nature of directly observed objects, such as agreeing on the color of a scarf with a friend, may involve minimal rigor, while carefully examining the elements of a theory can be a time-consuming and tedious process. In empiric knowledge development, research is a common way to confirm and validate knowledge, but reasoned, critical review of descriptions of empirical knowledge as well as looking at outcomes for clients or patients when knowledge is used is also a means of validation. These methods, taken together, provide a strong foundation that strengthens nursing practice in relation to the general principles provided by empiric knowledge.

We use both confirmation and validation to characterize authentication processes within the empiric pattern. Their meanings are similar, yet there are important differences. *Confirmation* is the term reserved for the authentication of more qualitative and naturalistic forms of empiric research findings, whereas the term *validation* is used to refer to authentication processes for more quantitative, measurable forms of empiric research findings. Qualitative and naturalistic inquiry processes may result in knowledge that can already be considered confirmed because they are direct reports of human experience, depending on the inquiry method used as well as the nature of the findings. However, these forms can still be subjected to critical review or research validation. Alternatively, additional clinical confirmation may be needed for some qualitative and naturalistic research findings.

In this section, we describe research and critical review approaches for confirming and validating empiric knowledge. There are excellent sources that provide extensive explanation of rigorous approaches to research, so in this text our focus is primarily on the use of research methods to confirm and validate conceptual underpinnings required to refine concepts and theoretic relationships. We also describe the approaches that help ensure any given research project fulfills sound standards. We use the term *theory* in a way that is consistent with our broad definition but also intend these processes to include a wide range of empirically grounded knowledge structures.

Refining Concepts and Relationships

Research can be useful to examine conceptual meaning and theoretic relationships among and between concepts. This type of research focuses on the correspondence of the ideas of the empiric knowledge form with perceptible sensory experience (Dubin, 1978; Glaser & Strauss, 1967; Newman, 1979; Polit & Beck, 2016; Reynolds, 2007). Because empiric concepts are abstractions of what can be observed or perceived during experience, a translation must be made from the theoretic to the empiric (i.e., deductive approach) and from the empiric to the theoretic (i.e., inductive approach).

To function as viable structural elements of empiric knowledge, including theory, concepts must adequately represent the perceptual experience intended. Both quantitative and qualitative descriptive approaches can be used to obtain evidence that is useful for refining empiric indicators. Such research may suggest the need to revisit creating conceptual meaning in an attempt to better represent the experience. Investigations designed to develop and refine empiric indicators and operational definitions of concepts are crucial for confirming and validating conceptual relationships.

Validation of relationships that connect two or more concepts is directly influenced by the nature of the empiric indicators for the concepts that are being related. Validation and confirmation involve qualitative and quantitative approaches. Replication requires repeating the confirmation or validation activities in other contexts. Relationships, including those in theory, cannot be proven to be true, but it is possible to show empiric support for proposed relationships. If the evidence does not support proposed relationships, the ideas they represent cannot be sustained. Alternative explanations are then considered on the basis of the empiric evidence.

Refining concepts and conceptual relationships draws on one or more of the following subcomponents:
- Identifying empiric indicators for the concepts
- Empirically grounding emerging relationships
- Validating relationships with the use of empiric methods

Identifying Empiric Indicators. Empiric indicators and operational definitions are used to represent concepts as variables in empiric research, and can also be derived for concepts as an outcome of some inductive research approaches. Formally structured theory can propose empiric indicators, but until those indicators are put into operation in research, they remain speculative. Challenging empirical indicators for concepts in actual research makes it possible to refine the knowledge structure.

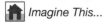 *Imagine This...*

Consider the following abstract relationship statement:

As the adult's eye contact increases, the infant's eye contact will increase.

Imagine that a research project is designed to obtain empiric evidence about the designation of eye contact as an empiric indicator of mothering. Details such as length of gaze and frequency of eye contact could be specified for the relatively abstract concept of *eye contact.* To use these indicators, the researcher would create a method for observing and timing the length of gaze and the frequency of eye contact. Imagine how you might go about doing this.

Part of the process for identifying empiric indicators, especially when primarily deductive processes are used, is to state operational definitions. *Operational definitions* specify the standards or criteria to be used when making the observations. For example, an operational definition of the term *gaze* might be "a steady, direct, visual focusing on an object that lasts at least 3 seconds." This definition indicates what gaze is (the empiric indicator for visual contact), the characteristics that must be present to call a behavior a *gaze* (direct visual focusing on an object), and a standard time parameter that distinguishes a gaze from other related behaviors, such as a glance or a look.

It is difficult to identify empiric indicators for concepts that are more abstract than the concept of *eye contact.* Many concepts related to nursing, such as *anxiety, body image,* and *self-esteem,* are highly abstract and cannot be directly measured. Tests and tools have been constructed to provide an indirect estimate of traits such as these. The inability to measure them directly does not mean they are nonexistent or cannot be assessed. The empiric challenge is to refine ideas about, and evidence for, empiric indicators so that the strength of the relationships can be explored.

Many of the concepts that are important for nursing are highly abstract, and even the actual experiences are not clearly perceived. Subsequently, the problem of finding adequate empiric indicators becomes complex and difficult. For example, *anxiety* is an abstract concept that can be theoretically defined. However, when we explore the experience of anxiety, we find that although people recognize what we mean by the term *anxiety,* the actual experiences of anxiety are elusive to describe. Nevertheless, if the concept is important for nursing, empiric knowledge development depends on diligent efforts to make clear, as accurately as possible, the link between the abstract concepts and the human experience the concepts represent. These examples underscore the value of creating conceptual meaning for adequate theory in nursing.

One approach that can be used to derive empiric measures for abstract nursing concepts is to use multiple empiric indicators to form useful research definitions. For example, anxiety might be measured with a self-report tool. The tool can be constructed to include many sensations that are generally indicative of anxiety. An operational definition of the concept of *anxiety* then becomes "what is assessed with the use of the tool."

Anxiety may also be assessed empirically by observing a person's behavior and appropriate physiologic indicators of neuroendocrine function. In this case, operational definitions would include specific ways to measure the behaviors observed and the specific range of laboratory test results associated with anxiety. All these empiric indicators are possible.

❗ Why Is This Important?

It is important to recognize that not just any approach to measurement will do. Dictionary definitions or other forms of description of concepts might suggest empiric indicators, but for scientific confirmation and validation, you need to turn to the knowledge source from which your concept is derived. When concepts are operationalized, they must be defined and measured or assessed consistent with the meaning of the theory or empirical knowledge in which they are embedded. For example, if you are working with the concept of *caring* in the context of Jean Watson's "human care theory," it would be counterproductive to use a tool to assess caring behavior that was developed based on Kristin Swansons's "theory of caring" (Sitzman & Watson, 2013; Swanson, 1990).

Empirically Grounding Emerging Relationships. The process of empirically grounding emerging relationships involves connecting experiences with representations of those experiences. When an abstract conceptual relationship is taken as the starting point, the investigator designs a study to explore or test the hypothetic relationship framed in terms of the empiric indicators for the concepts. Several investigations may be required to confirm that the relationship proposed is accurate. When the investigations provide sufficient empiric evidence that conclusions can be drawn about the relationship, the investigator can return to the concepts within the knowledge structure and refine the theoretic statements or other relationships to reflect what has been supported empirically.

An investigator can also begin by exploring a selected empiric situation as a starting point, with the goal of finding the concepts and relationships that accurately represent a situation that is not yet clearly understood but that is recognized as important to the discipline of nursing. The investigator selects a social context in which the phenomenon under consideration is likely to occur and observes the interactions and circumstances of that context. From the observations, the investigator derives relationship statements that are grounded in the available empiric evidence. A variety of inductive approaches can be used to ground emerging relationships (Creswell, 2013; Denzin & Lincoln, 2012; Glaser & Strauss, 1967; Lincoln & Guba, 1985).

Validating Relationships Using Traditional Empiric Methods. Validating theoretic and other conceptual relationships requires creating a design that tests the descriptive and explanatory powers of a designated relationship. If validating relationships within theory, relationships are proposed after a theory is structured (i.e., deduction). When the purpose of the research design is to generate conceptual and eventually theoretic relationships, the relationships may be considered to be confirmed and ready for replication and additional confirmation in other settings.

A key to the *deductive* validation of conceptual relationships is to use a design that ensures that the proposed relationship is actually the one that occurs and thus accounts for the study findings. For example, if a study concludes that a mother's gaze prompts an infant's gaze in return, the researcher needs to consider ways to be sure that it is actually the mother's gaze that accounts for the infant's behavior. Typically, the researcher designs the study so that other factors that could influence the behavior of the infants in the study (e.g., sensory experiences such as noise, touch, or visual distractions that might affect the process of visual interaction) are accounted for or held constant.

The purpose of deductively validating any relationship statement is to provide empiric evidence that the relationships proposed in the theory are adequate within a specific situation. With each approach to design that is used, the research question or hypothesis is revised to suit the type of design that has been selected. Empiric evidence based on many different research design approaches provides a strong basis for judging the adequacy of the theory. If theoretic statements are deductively tested and are not supported by empiric evidence, one or more of the following four possibilities can account for the disparity between the theory and the empiric findings:

- *The meaning of the concepts is not adequately created.* The process of creating conceptual meaning can be used to determine whether the definitions and meanings of the concepts under study are clear and whether they are well differentiated from related concepts. If they are not, theoretic revisions can be made, which may result in new approaches to empiric study.

- *The relationship statement is not adequately structured.* The processes of theory structuring and contextualizing can be used to examine the logic or form of the statements. Given the benefit of the empiric evidence, new insights into the form and structure of the theory may emerge. The theorist can revise the theoretic relationship statements on the basis of these insights.

- *The empiric indicators for the concept are not adequate.* The empiric evidence might point to new possibilities for empiric indicators or suggest revisions of the existing indicators. This process is particularly important when the empiric indicators represent highly abstract concepts and are constructed out of speculative ideas about how the concepts can be observed empirically.

- *The definitions are inadequate or inconsistent.* Typically, conflicting research results are attributed to faulty definitions and the related measurement problems of empiric research. This is a possibility, but accurate assessment depends on adequately conceived concepts, sound theoretic statements, and adequate empiric indicators. If these are all in place, it is then reasonable to consider problems with measurement or with assessment of the concept.

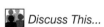 Discuss This...

Within your study group of three or four classmates, select a concept you think is important for nursing. Without conferring, define the concept and develop a set of empirical criteria you will use to assess or measure the concept. Share your criteria with one another, note differences, and discuss their adequacy for representing the concept.

Where and how do they differ? Would they be useful across contexts? If you were a research assistant would they be easy or difficult to assess or measure?

When *inductive* methods are used to refine concepts and theoretic relationships, the relationships may be considered valid and confirmed if sound research procedures and processes are used to generate them. When relationships are deduced from inductively generated theory, they can be explored in similar settings or extended into new contexts. When this occurs, problems with faulty concepts, relational statements, empiric indicators, and operational definitions will become evident.

Developing Sound Validation Research

Research processes for confirmation and validation can be assessed for soundness at each stage. The following serves as a guide for evaluating the approach to research based on confirmation and validation of knowledge.

- Research elements such as problem statements, purposes, and hypotheses are clearly related and reflect those elements of the knowledge structure being validated.
- The literature review used to survey research findings and justify the need for validation research is pertinent and complete.
- The means of obtaining data, the selection of the sample for study, the research design, and the analysis of the data are appropriate in relation to the purpose.
- The analysis of data must be consistent with the purposes of the research and be appropriate to the research design.
- Results reported do not exceed the limits of design or findings; appropriate recommendations for ongoing research are suggested.

Confirmation and Validation Using Critical Analysis and Reasoned Thought

Not all theory or empirical knowledge needs confirmation and validation before use in the practice situation. If, after carefully looking at and understanding what is proposed, it seems reasonable and useful the knowledge may be used in the clinical setting. In fact, this happens frequently as knowledge becomes available. There is always a judgment made in relation to using empirical knowledge in clinical settings and much of what goes into that judgment has been considered in this chapter.

AUTHENTICATION AND THE WHOLE OF NURSING KNOWLEDGE

As we said at the beginning of this chapter, while each pattern of knowing has unique and specific approaches for authentication of knowledge, formal expressions of nursing knowledge may benefit from the use of authentication processes associated with other pattern of knowing.

When emancipatory authentication demonstrates the ideals of sustainability, social equity and empowerment are brought to bear on other forms of knowledge expression, that knowledge is being examined in relation to its potential for praxis. For example, if an empiric theory or an ethical principle sustains conditions of privilege for some and disadvantage for others, that empiric theory or ethical principle is of questionable practice value and should not be further developed without addressing its deficiencies. If one's personal Self harbors inherent social or ethnic biases, examining Self in relation to its contribution to social inequities or empowerment of others may lead to changes that remove those impediments. If a work of art is powerful enough to positively change perceptions of marginalized persons, its use for that purpose is warranted.

The ethical authentication processes of dialogue and justification are vital to the development of consensus in the discipline, the development of mutual understanding of the adequacy of the knowledge on which nursing is based, and understanding which knowledge expressions have development priority. Nurses who come together to discuss the ethical merits of nonethical forms of knowledge expression, such as empiric evidence related to fatigue associated with cancer chemotherapy, bring about awareness of different perspectives of what is right, wrong, and responsible as together they pursue a more responsible basis on which to recommend chemotherapy.

Communal dialogue from the perspective of ethical knowing contributes to personal knowing because it is through dialogue with others that your own personal knowing can be reflected and responded to. In this way you begin to understand where your personal strengths lie as well as how your Self has come to contribute to empowerment of others and social justice promotion. Dialogue and justification is also implied. Works of art, such as a sculpture or a play performance, are examined in relation to whether they have potential to inspire a deeper understanding of experiences that nurses manage in the course of client care.

The authentication ideals of appreciation and inspiration brought to bear on all forms of knowledge expression lead to a deeper level of understanding. Knowledge expressions, regardless of the pattern they are associated with, will have more or less potential to inspire the user. A well-constructed theory or ethical argument may be seen to be aesthetically inspiring when compared to one that is poorly constructed. Emancipatory action plans and visions for the future, as well as personal stories, can be examined by asking if they do inspire, and can be appreciated for what they represent. In this way formal expressions within the emancipatory and personal pattern can be made more adequate to guide nursing actions.

The empiric approaches of confirmation and validation cannot be used directly to authenticate emancipatory, ethical, personal, or aesthetic knowledge expressions. However, empirical evidence, confirmation, and validation-like processes do inform and shape knowledge that arises from all of the other patterns of knowing. For example, empirical evidence is often essential in determining if a particular social program is indeed effective in overcoming injustice. Sound empirical evidence is helpful in facing one's own personal attitudes. When a person harbors beliefs that are patently false by empirical evidence, it suggests that it is incumbent on the person to face the evidence and find ways to overcome false beliefs. Empiric evidence that is integral to confirmation and validation within empirics is important, for example, to understand the measurable features of care that is just and ethical and which needs to be commended. The degree to which critics who examine works of art for inspirational qualities agree is also a form of empiric knowledge.

In summary, while we have developed authentication processes for each pattern of knowing, it is not only possible, but helpful, to ask if authentication processes associated with other patterns might be useful to examine and improve formal expressions of knowledge.

CONCLUSION

In this chapter we have detailed authentication processes that are associated with each pattern of knowing. Additionally, we have shown how authentication processes within any pattern may be useful for authentication of knowledge in any other pattern. Numerous examples and case studies have been used to clarify the meaning of authentication processes.

References

Btoush, R., & Campbell, J. C. (2009). Ethical conduct in intimate partner violence research: challenges and strategies. *Nursing Outlook, 57*, 210–216. http://search.ebscohost.com/login.aspx?direct=true&db=rzh&AN=2010365552&site=ehost-live. Publisher URL www.cinahl.com/cgi-bin/refsvc?jid=272&accno=2010365552.

Creswell, J. W. (2013). *Qualitative inquiry and research design: choosing among five approaches* (3rd ed.). Thousand Oaks, CA: Sage. https://market.android.com/details?id=book-Ykruxor10cYC.

Denzin, N. K., & Lincoln, Y. S. (2012). *Collecting and interpreting qualitative materials* (4th ed.). Thousand Oaks, CA: Sage.

Drew, N. (1997). Expanding self-awareness through exploration of meaningful experience. *Journal of Holistic Nursing: Official Journal of the American Holistic Nurses' Association, 15*, 406–424.

Dubin, R. (1978). *Theory building* (rev. ed.). New York, NY: The Free Press.

Freire, P. (1970). *Pedagogy of the oppressed.* New York, NY: Seabury Press.

Freysteinson, W. (2009). The twins: a case study in ethical deliberation. *Nursing Ethics, 16*, 127–130. http://search.ebscohost.com/login.aspx?direct=true&db=rzh&AN=2010170653&site=ehost-live. Publisher URL www.cinahl.com/cgi-bin/refsvc?jid=863&accno=2010170653.

Frost, R. (n.d.). *Nothing gold can stay.* https://www.poets.org/poetsorg/poem/nothing-gold-can-stay.

Glaser, B., & Strauss, A. (1967). *The discovery of grounded theory.* Chicago, IL: Aldine Publishing Co.

Lincoln, Y. S., & Guba, E. G. (1985). *Naturalistic inquiry.* Newbury Park, CA: Sage Publications.

Newman, M. A. (1979). *Theory development in nursing.* Philadelphia, PA: F.A. Davis Co.

Polit, D., & Beck, C. T. (2016). *Nursing research: generating and assessing evidence for nursing practice* (10th ed.). Philadelphia, PA: Lippincott, Williams and Wilkins.

Quaghebeur, T., & Gastmans, C. (2009). Nursing and euthanasia: a review of argument-based ethics literature. *Nursing Ethics, 16*, 466–486. http://search.ebscohost.com/login.aspx?direct=true&db=rzh&AN=2010337352&site=ehost-live. Publisher URL www.cinahl.com/cgi-bin/refsvc?jid=863&accno=2010337352.

Reynolds, P. D. (2007). *A primer in theory construction.* Needham, MA: Allyn & Bacon.

Sitzman, K., & Watson, J. (2013). *Caring science, mindful practice: Implementing Watson's human caring theory.* New York, NY: Springer Publishing Company. https://market.android.com/details?id=book-2QM4AAAAQBAJ.

Swanson, K. M. (1990). Providing care in the NICU: sometimes an act of love. *ANS. Advances in Nursing Science, 13*(1), 60–73. https://www.ncbi.nlm.nih.gov/pubmed/2122802.

Wright, M. R. (1966). Research and research. *Nursing Research, 15*, 244.

Integrated Expression of Knowledge in Practice

The product of nursing is patient care; it is a process, not a physical thing and, not an outcome measurable except as a process. That product is no less beautiful, nor less finely tuned than a Steinway piano – just harder to get one's hands on.

Donna Diers (2004, p. 189; paraphrased)

*Nursing is not just an art, it has a **heart;** nursing is not just a science, it has a **conscience**.*

Anonymous

In this chapter we consider the integration of formal expressions of knowledge within the context of providing nursing care. Indeed, the whole reason for focusing on the patterns of knowing and their formal knowledge expressions is to improve patient and client care and create conditions where best care can be consistently provided. We believe that mindfully integrating knowledge in the context of care will benefit care in dramatic and beneficial ways. We say mindfully because whether or not nurses realize it, as they provide care, they are integrating multiple knowledge expressions that shape and create their approach to care. The integration of knowledge within the care context is necessary for the realization of the goals that support the best care practices.

A focus on mindfully integrating knowledge associated with all patterns of knowing in nursing practice also serves to make the patterns visible. It would be the unusual practitioner who would not recognize that integrating personal, ethical, aesthetic, emancipatory, and empiric knowledge does occur in the immediate context of care. Recognition is one thing, but deliberately focusing on the knowing patterns in the context of care and understanding how they operate to create care is another. As care is rendered, in retrospect, each pattern can be discerned, but the ongoing expression of knowledge in practice is an integrated whole—we call this the whole of knowing.

This chapter focuses on the whole of knowing that occurs when knowledge integration in practice occurs. Knowing emerges in the moment of care when the critical questions are "asked and answered," perhaps just below the surface of awareness. It is the "answers" to these questions that direct the ongoing knowing that forms and guides care. Knowing in the context of care is an ongoing process. What nurses know in the context of care depends on the totality of knowledge they have acquired through education and experience. The better the quality and the more complete knowledge in the discipline is, the more likely it will guide the nurse to appropriate actions in the moment of care.

In Chapter 9, we emphasized the importance of ensuring the formal expressions of knowledge are as authentic as possible in representing what they are intended to represent. This chapter proceeds from the premise that the ultimate means of authenticating nursing knowledge lies in the outcomes that are expressed in practice.

> ### ❗ Why Is This Important?
>
> It is important to remember that we have defined *knowledge* as the formal expressions within each of the patterns, expressions that differ within each pattern that can be tangibly represented and examined. *Knowing*, on the other hand, is in-the-moment understanding, interpretation, and internally "addressing" or "getting" the nature of the experience one is in. Knowing is complex and, in clinical contexts, depends on the ongoing, all at once, integration of knowledge within all-knowing patterns. Knowing is fluid and changing, and emerges as one moves through the care encounter. It is intangible, yet we believe the most productive or "best" knowing is grounded in quality formal expressions of knowledge within each of the patterns.

As this chapter addresses knowledge integration in practice keep in mind that as you work in a nursing context you are returning again to elements of the model we have proposed. You are asking, not aloud or deliberately, but subconsciously and intuitively all at once: "What is this? What does it mean? Do I know what I do and do I do what I know? Is this right? Who benefits here?" That is, you are asking those same critical questions that provide direction for knowledge development. You are setting the stage for revisiting those knowledge expressions and strengthening them depending on the outcomes of knowledge integration—for example, care outcomes. The animation of the knowing patterns in action that can be accessed by scanning the QR code on the inside front cover or by visiting http://booksite.elsevier.com/9780323530613 which is extremely useful in illustrating what we mean by pattern integration.

Table 10.1 shows an overview of the knowledge development processes that we have addressed in previous chapters, with an emphasis, on the integrated forms of expression for each pattern of knowing. Fig. 10.1 is a pictorial representation of the integration processes. Overlap among and between the patterns' integrated expressions in practice (along the figure top) underscores that best care practices reflect these qualities and intentions in nurses.

The overlapping cloudlike spheres (along the figure bottom) represent the knowledge authentication processes within each pattern. This emphasizes that the ongoing authentication of knowledge both flows from and creates best nursing practice.

PATTERNS GONE WILD

In order to more fully appreciate the importance of integration of knowledge and knowing, we have found it helpful to consider examples of each pattern "gone wild." When knowledge within any one pattern is not integrated into the whole of knowing, distortion—rather than understanding—is produced. Knowledge that is developed in isolation without the consideration of all patterns of knowing leads to uncritical

TABLE 10.1 Dimensions Associated With Each of the Patterns of Knowing With Emphasis on Integrated Expressions in Practice

Dimension	Emancipatory	Ethics	Personal	Aesthetics	Empirics
Critical questions	Who benefits? What is wrong with this picture? What are the barriers to freedom? What changes are needed?	Is this right? Is this responsible?	Do I know what I do? Do I do what I know?	What does this mean? How is this significant?	What is this? How does it work?
Creative processes	Critiquing Imagining	Clarifying Exploring	Opening Centering	Envisioning Rehearsing	Conceptualizing Structuring
Formal expressions	Action plans Manifestoes Critical analyses Visions for the future	Principles and codes	Personal stories Genuine Self	Aesthetic criticism Works of art	Facts Models Formal descriptions Theories Thematic descriptions
Authentication processes	Social equity Sustainability Empowerment Demystification	Dialogue Justification	Response Reflection	Appreciation Inspiration	Confirmation Validation
Integrated expression in practice	Praxis	Moral and ethical comportment	Therapeutic use of self	Transformative art/acts	Scientific competence

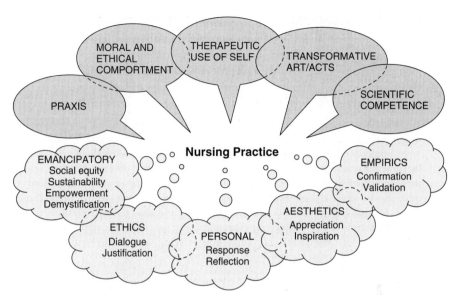

FIG. 10.1 Integrated Expressions in Practice and Underlying Nursing Knowledge.

acceptance, narrow interpretation, and partial use of knowledge. We call this situation "patterns gone wild." When this occurs, the whole of knowing disintegrates and the patterns are used in relative isolation from one another, and the potential for the synthesis of the whole is lost.

>> *Consider This...*

To illustrate the patterns gone wild in practice, imagine Ruth, an elderly woman who is living in an extended care facility. Ruth's life has been rich in experience and activities, and she verbally explores her past to make sense of what it means and how it relates to her present life. She has always been physically active, and she takes a nightly stroll before going to bed. She walks the halls, unsteady but determined, smiling and peering into other rooms. When she hears other residents talking or moaning, she sometimes goes into their rooms and tells them stories or talks with them to ease their troubled nights. She does not willingly retire to her own room, and her nightly excursions often disturb others who are trying to sleep or who want to be left alone.

Consider what might happen if any one of the patterns of knowing were isolated from the context of the whole of knowing. Emancipatory knowing alone might lead you to defend Ruth's individual right to do as she wishes, regardless of how this affects others, on the basis of a liberal political philosophy of the primary rights of the individual. Ethics taken alone might impose your view of what is good for Ruth, which may lead to a prescription in her care plan that would confine her to bed after the lights are out, thus creating a rigid, rule-oriented atmosphere that is insensitive to what others see as right or good for Ruth or that Ruth sees as being beneficial for herself. Personal knowing in isolation could impose your bias that Ruth is a nuisance who is interfering with the time needed to complete the charting for the night. Aesthetics alone would impose your own tastes, preferences, and meanings on the situation. You might attempt to confine Ruth to her room and play your favorite new age music without considering whether Ruth can hear the music or whether she finds the music soothing or appealing. Empirics isolated from the other patterns of knowing might require giving Ruth a sleep-inducing drug, thereby controlling the situation and manipulating Ruth into compliance, regardless of other concerns.

When you, being the best nurse you can be, act so that emancipatory knowing, ethics, aesthetics, personal knowing, and empirics come together as a whole, your purposes for developing knowledge and your actions based on that knowledge become more responsible and humane and create liberating choices. A whole understanding of Ruth and the meaning of her life means that you have taken into account the social and political prescriptions for long-term care, Ruth's safety, the needs of other residents, Ruth's personal life history and what gives her pleasure, the ethical dimensions of moral development and caring for others, the aesthetic meanings of Ruth's actions in the cultural context of aging, and the personal perspectives of the nurses who care for Ruth. Many choices remain open when addressing Ruth's situation, but all these considerations together would lead you to nursing approaches that would differ from any of the approaches taken from one knowing perspective alone.

As Ruth's story illustrates, emancipatory knowing removed from the context of the whole of knowing produces an extreme political standpoint that is unjustly imposed on others. Even when a particular political system has the potential to benefit people and to create a more equitable social order, if it is imposed on others in the extreme, it has the potential to create another form of oppression and injustice. Freire referred to this phenomenon as becoming sectarian, meaning a person becomes fanatically aligned with one point of view. Failure to question and subsequently imposing your own political standpoint is counter to emancipatory knowing and may lead to this pattern of knowing going wild. Instead, remaining critically reflective and open to empiric, ethical, personal, and aesthetic insights is central to emancipatory knowing.

Empirics removed from the context of the whole of knowing can lead to control and manipulation. Ironically, these have been the explicit traditional goals of the empiric sciences. When the validity of empiric knowledge is not questioned, one danger is its potential use in contexts where it does not question "What is this?" and "How does it work?" but rather assumes the answer is known. When you recognize how all the patterns contribute to empiric knowing, you begin to see the fallacy of valuing empiric knowledge over all others, resulting in control and manipulation—a distortion or misuse of empiric knowledge.

Ethics removed from the context of the whole of knowing can result in the imposition of rigid doctrine and insensitivity to the rights of others. This happens when you simply set forth or hold to your personal ideas about what is right or good and advocate a position on the basis of reasoning derived from your own perspective alone. You may present a justification for a perspective to others but not take seriously the processes of dialogue that the justification invites. In the absence of this integrating process, an individual's position remains isolated and unknown, with little or no opportunity for empiric, personal, or aesthetic insights to give meaning and social relevance to the ideas.

Personal knowing removed from the context of the whole of knowing produces self-distortion. When this happens, the individual self remains isolated and truncated, and knowledge of the Self comes only from what is known internally. Self-distortions can take a wide range of forms, from aggrandizement and the overestimation of the self to destruction and the underestimation of the self.

Aesthetics removed from the context of the whole of knowing produces a lack of appreciation for the fullness of meaning in context. Without aesthetic knowing, actions emerge from and are represented by the meanings and desires of the individual alone, without taking into account the cultural meanings that are inherent in an authentic art/act. Your attempts to enact art/acts are not artful but rather grow out of a failure to comprehend the deeper cultural, historical, and political significance of the art/act itself. Inauthentic meanings are assigned to another's experience, or a self-serving posture is assumed with respect to another person.

Let us emphasize that we do not presume that nursing care takes place in a context where the knowing patterns are totally absent. Rather we do believe that without some attention to knowledge within all-knowing patterns, the potential for some of the patterns to "go wild" is more likely. In other words, being aware of what the patterns imply and what integration means improves the likelihood of best practices in nursing. In the example of Ruth, when the nurse relies almost entirely on one pattern of knowing, the whole of knowing is unbalanced. In fact, each of these "gone wild" scenarios is plausible, demonstrating how easily nursing practice can be compromised when one pattern prevails.

Much of what informs the integration of knowledge into a whole of knowing remains in the background of awareness. What remains in the background usually can be brought to awareness when attention turns to the reasoning process itself. In other words, when engaged in care situations, the seasoned nurse is not deliberatively thinking about the knowledge that justifies what is done in the moment. The nurse likely could, in retrospect, provide information about knowledge within each of the patterns that informs what is done as the patterns are integrated.

Think About It...

Bring to mind a significant encounter that you experienced in your practice—one that remains vivid in your memory. Identify the knowledge that informed you as you moved through the situation.

- Did you consider all patterns of knowing? How were they important?
- Did you "stop and think" deliberatively about what you were doing?
- Was there some pattern that was neglected that should have been more prominent? If so, what part of your nursing care would have changed?
- Are there any aspects of the situation where you feel that the existing knowledge associated with any pattern is not adequate to inform your actions—that is, areas of knowledge that need further development?
- Can you describe everything you "knew" as you experienced the encounter?

In summary, we claim there is a need for mindful integration of formal expressions of knowledge within each pattern to form a whole of knowing that aims to accomplish quality care. This assumes a certain quality of integration as well as quality of knowledge upon which knowing is based. Remember that knowing is fluid and ongoing, instantaneous and in the moment—much of which is intangible. In the background of this knowing, however, should be a strong basis of knowledge within each of the patterns of knowing. The following sections consider the integrated expressions in practice for each of the knowing patterns.

INTEGRATION OF KNOWLEDGE WITH A FOCUS ON EMANCIPATORY KNOWING: PRAXIS

Specifically, there is a need to further explore the political, economic, and social forces in communities around the country that influenced the growth of both nursing and medicine during this century. The rigidities and inflexibilities of mythical conceptions about the roles of men and women in health care and the resulting responses of community members need examination also.

J. Ashley (1976, p. X)

All the processes within the dimension of emancipatory knowing—critical questions, creative processes of imagining and critiquing, and formal expressions of emancipatory knowing—contribute to the creation of a new lens with which to view the world. This lens reveals something that is not perceived because it may seem natural, or because it is difficult to see beyond those things that are assumed to be true. When what has not been perceived before is seen, it then seems to become perfectly obvious. Ways to effectively change the situation begin to make sense, and action occurs. As each action is taken, other insights and understandings begin to come to awareness, and new actions are taken. This circular emerging process of acting, gaining new insights, and acting again is *praxis*. The process of praxis is ongoing and begins as soon as critical questions are asked; it gains momentum as creative process and formal expressions are critically reflected and acted upon and more critical questions are generated. The lines between the processes of emancipatory knowing are blurred and blend together in experience, but we identify and name them here as a way to explain the nature of praxis. Praxis, as an integrated expression of emancipatory knowing, depends on credible knowledge expressions within each of the patterns of knowing.

Emancipatory knowing tends to focus heavily on the global context of care. Recall from Fig. 1.1, our model representing the whole of knowing depicts emancipatory knowing as surrounding and encompassing all other patterns. The integrated expression of emancipatory knowing as praxis encompasses and addresses such things as accessibility to care and insurance availability. It also is concerned with eliminating racial and gender bias that affect the quality of care individuals receive within clinics and other care facilities. The practitioner who notices bias and hatred toward a certain group or individuals can and should return again to the global context of care and ask: "What is wrong with this picture?" As this emancipatory process becomes integrated within nursing care, a nursing praxis emerges that moves nursing toward overcoming injustices.

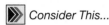 *Consider This...*

> The life and work of Karen Silkwood (portrayed by Meryl Streep in the 1983 film *Silkwood*) reflect emancipatory knowing processes, including praxis. Silkwood was employed at a facility that manufactured radioactive materials for nuclear power plants. She became a union representative and was requested to investigate (ask critical questions) regarding health and safety at the plant. As a result of this "critical questioning," poor respiratory equipment, improper storage facilities, and violations of health rules were uncovered (were imagined and critiqued, and requestioned) that should have protected workers from radioactive contamination. Silkwood testified (a form of action plan) along with other union members to the U.S. Atomic Energy Commission (AEC). Ultimately, in an effort to publicize the radioactive contamination of herself and other workers, she compiled a document (manifesto, action plan, critical analysis) that detailed violations at the plant. Driving to meet with a newspaper reporter, she was killed in an automobile crash of questionable origin, and the documents she planned to share were not found. After her death, the plant was federally investigated, and Silkwood's allegations were found to be true. Subsequently, the facility was closed (Legacy.com staff, 2010).
>
> In this example, all knowing patterns would be integrated as praxis occurred. A few examples of how the patterns might operate follow: **Empirics** would be called upon to verify the facts about the extent to which regulations were violated, as well as for understanding the pathophysiological basis by which the violations and subsequent radiation exposure would affect worker's health. **Ethics** would be implicated as Silkwood knew what was happening was unfair and unjust. How to react to that unfairness would be framed around whether to "obey company rules" and just let the situation persist, or to work toward the "greater good for the workers." Ethics would also be implicated in relation to how data was obtained to justify actions—whether worker confidentiality would be respected and how. **Aesthetics** would be required to know how to best gather information so as not to be "found out" and how to question both workers and authorities who might be suspicious of Silkwood's motives, or in the case of workers, who might fear losing their jobs. Certainly **personal knowing** would be integrated as Silkwood did what she knew—and knew what she did—and in the end it allegedly cost Silkwood her life.
>
> What other aspects of all knowing patterns, from a nursing perspective, would be integrated as Silkwood worked toward her goal?

Although Karen Silkwood was not a nurse, her activism illustrates the process of praxis that can inspire nursing action. It is important to note that praxis was occurring throughout the example. Her story illustrates the integrated expression of knowledge with a focus on emancipatory knowing in practice. Empiric knowledge of details of exposure such as numbers of violations and morbidity due to exposure to radiation was important for change. Silkwood also used ethical knowledge to justify and determine what her position about the exposure would be. Undoubtedly she had a strong sense of personal self that energized her actions and she certainly integrated aesthetic knowledge related to the art/act of transforming this politically charged unsafe situation into one where workers were safe. In this example Silkwood began to recognize, understand, analyze, solve, and publicly act to expose and mitigate the radioactive contamination, an unjust practice that exploited plant workers. Although the closing of the facility might be considered the final event, the process embedded in this example continues in relation to similar unjust and unfair circumstances.

A contemporary example of praxis as the integrated expression of emancipatory knowing is the formation of the Rebellious Nursing group. Having recognized and critically questioned unjust practices in their experiences as nurses and in health care, the nurses involved came together as a group to interact and plan (imagine, critique, formulate action plans and visions for the future) for changes that could eliminate those injustices. In 2012, the group convened in Philadelphia outside their ongoing practice environment to contemplate barriers, changes, and problems in health care and who benefits, undoubtedly returning to the context of care, raising more critical questions, and making changes in the work environment. The group continues to network across the United States, with groups meeting locally to focus on local actions. The group in the San Francisco Bay area, for example, participated in a 2016 community-wide demonstration to stop the threat of coal being transported by rail into Oakland for export overseas—a project that would involve the construction of a massive coal terminal in Oakland that would threaten the health of the Oakland community ("Our Campaign," 2016).

The following statement describing the purpose of the Rebellious Nursing group illustrates the emancipatory intent of their work:

We believe that Nursing is an inherently political profession and that all nurses are rebellious.

We seek to create a world where all people receive and have a say in competent, compassionate, and respectful care in their communities. As opposed to a world where nurses are divided by education and training, as well as structural forms of oppression that pervade society, such as racism and sexism, we seek to include all nurses in our organizing on equal footing, by confronting what divides us. As opposed to a world where a wall is placed between healthcare providers and patients and their friends and families, we envision a world where caregiving is a communal activity. As opposed to a world where access to care and education is determined by money, we seek a future where we all contribute according to our abilities, and everyone receives care according to their needs.

We seek to create networks of nurses committed to addressing these issues and nurturing these projects. If you're interested in working with us, we'd LOVE your input and ideas! ("Rebellious Nursing: About Us," 2012)

 Discuss This...

Read a personal report of the Philadelphia 2012 Rebellious Nursing conference on Peggy Chinn's blog (https://peggychinn.com/2013/10/07/report-on-the-rebel-nursing-conference/; or download the conference program by clicking on the program image). Then with a group of your peers, discuss your responses to this report. Focus on ways in which each of the patterns of knowing and knowledge have or can inform and shape the activism of nurses who seek to create the changes envisioned by the Rebellious Nursing group.

In summary, the integrated expression of emancipatory knowing is praxis. Praxis is ongoing reflection and action; it is both an individual process and an interactive process. As nurses practice, they notice (critically question) situations that are not just or fair (reflection) and then begin to take whatever steps needed and possible to eliminate those injustices (action). When this begins to happen, other nurses, health care providers, and persons in the situation are called on to participate. Nurses can initiate change in groups by coming together to share and explore the nature of an unjust situation (reflection) and begin to initiate changes (action). Fundamental changes in social structures cannot occur without collective participation. No matter how the process begins, it sets into motion an ongoing cycle of reflection and action, which is the hallmark of integrated expression in practice. Social change requires that, as each step toward change is taken, reflection on what is happening leads to the next stage of action.

INTEGRATION OF KNOWLEDGE WITH A FOCUS ON ETHICS: MORAL/ETHICAL COMPORTMENT

> *We do not act morally unless we act from a sense of conviction and reason, guided by our own conscience.*
>
> **Isabel Stewart (1921, pp. 906, 909)**

The integrated expression of ethics in practice is moral/ethical comportment. The term *comportment* basically refers to how people behave and, in this case, how they behave in relation to what they do morally and what they know ethically. Moral/ethical comportment requires the consideration of all other knowing patterns in the moment of practice. The moral/ethical challenges that nurses encounter typically involve the relationship that nurses have with other people as individuals, families, and groups—situations in which it is not easy to determine the right, morally just, or ethically sound action. In order to comport one's self with moral integrity, knowledge within all patterns must be brought to bear on a situation. Emancipatory knowing provides insight into the social and political context in which the situation resides. Personal knowing provides the foundation for a nurse's capacity for therapeutic use of Self. Aesthetic knowing guides bringing all elements into a cohesive whole that shapes a desired future. Empiric knowing provides facts and probabilities that inform difficult choices.

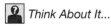 *Think About It...*

In thinking about ethics in the context of the knowing patterns it is useful to consider everyday situations versus the more weighty life and death situations that often frame discussions about ethics. For example, suppose you are a nursing student who is caring for Sam, who is in critical but stable condition following a ruptured aneurysm. Sam is not expected to live and Justine, his daughter, is visiting. In the course of care for Sam, Justine asks you if her dad is going to survive because she needs to take care of some financial and legal matters if he is not. You have noticed that Justine is extremely anxious and you have been told by your instructor it is important not to upset her. While you busy yourself adjusting Sam's IV settings, Justine asks again. In making a decision about how and if to answer you are integrating all patterns of knowing around whether or not this is information about which you should share your opinion and whether Justine has a right to that information. **Empirics** arises in relation to the knowledge that indeed, Sam will likely die but the course his death will take is unclear. **Aesthetics** enters the mix as you realize you cannot fully discern the meaning of the situation before you—you have never been in this situation before and you are not sure the best way to handle it, especially because your instructor has told you not to upset Justine. **Personal** knowing comes into play because even though you have been told to be cautious and not upset Justine by your instructor, you do feel that her interest is not nefarious and she should know the best truth available despite your lack of confidence in your ability to impart that information well. **Emancipatory** knowing is also implicated as you believe Sam probably has not received the health care that might have prevented this situation, given that he did not have the help he needed to choose appropriate insurance coverage and his family faces serious financial hardship. Access to a health care advocate might have prevented this situation in the first place.

How would you handle this situation? What other expressions of knowledge within the knowing patterns would be integrated as you decide how to answer Justine?

Integration of ethical knowing in practice requires, and is based on, the formal expressions of ethical codes that emerge from professional processes of dialogue and justification. Many agencies have an active ethics committee or board that engages in these processes for cases that defy resolution at the point of care. But even in the absence of such a review committee, nurses who are faced with a difficult situation in the moment need to act based on their best understanding of the situation and what they know to be sound ethical knowledge. However, after the situation passes, it is important to reflect on it, to refine your own ethical knowing and contribute to the development of nursing knowledge.

 Consider This...

"Mike's Story" as told by Parker (1990) illustrates the contribution to ethical knowledge that can arise from deliberative reflection on practice experiences that challenge ethical knowing. In this story, Parker describes the difficult choices she faced when caring for Mike, who was not able to communicate with words and was experiencing life-threatening, painful complications after a long struggle with severe diabetes, emphysema, and stroke. Parker integrates the art of storytelling, the context of biomedical ethics, empirical facts about Mike's condition and his treatment, and her own inner reflections that informed her choices of moral action.

- Consider this story and reflect on ways in which your own ethical challenges are informed by all patterns of knowing.

INTEGRATION OF KNOWLEDGE WITH A FOCUS ON PERSONAL KNOWING: THERAPEUTIC USE OF SELF

Trust yourself. Create the kind of self that you will be happy to live with all your life. Make the most of yourself by fanning the tiny, inner sparks of possibility into flames of achievement.
Golda Meir (Read more at: http://www.brainyquote.com/ quotes/keywords/self.html)

The genuine Self is conveyed most explicitly in nursing practice when the nurse engages in the therapeutic use of the Self. The therapeutic use of the Self is the integrated expression in practice that is at the heart of nursing's healing art. Although it is a somewhat elusive concept, the therapeutic use of the Self suggests the ability to engage authentically with the Self and the other to facilitate health and healing. At the heart of the therapeutic use of the Self is the assumption that it is critical to know the nature of the Self, to acknowledge the Self, and to put aside or change biases and attitudes that interfere with understanding and caring for others. As you come to understand yourSelf more fully, the therapeutic use of the Self in the context of nursing care is more fully actualized. Empiric knowledge about the characteristics of Self as revealed in a self-assessment tool might provide information that affects integration as the Self examines what it knows and does. Ethical knowledge related to a Self's moral and ethical foundation will be part of knowledge integration that affects the transformative art/acts of aesthetics. Emancipatory knowledge about one's relative situation of privilege, or lack thereof, will also enter into knowledge integration and create a need to understand Self and its ability to be therapeutic in the context of care.

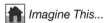 *Imagine This...*

Consider Edson who has been a paraplegic for most of his adult life. Edson is quite obese and basically keeps himself homebound. Edson spends most of his day watching television from his bed, although he does verbalize that he knows he should be out and about more. Edson is in dire need of a ramp into his residence which would allow him easier access to the outdoors but he cannot afford to have one built. Ruth Ann, his neighbor, is a nurse who has maintained a long-term personal interest in Edson. Ruth Ann has helped him and his family navigate the health care system and provided information and advice from time to time. Over the years Ruth Ann has watched Edson become more and more reclusive and she knows that he needs the ramp. Ruth Ann's cousin is a builder and would build a ramp for Edson at reduced cost, and Ruth Ann has the means and could pay for it if Edson did not have the funds. She does not have a good sense, however, if the ramp would lead to more socialization for Edson or not.

All knowing patterns integrate around personal knowing as she makes her decision about whether to pay for Edson's ramp. While she knows Edson would benefit from a ramp she recognizes that **personally** she is a bit angry at him for not being more aggressive about his well-being. He seems willing to spend money on things she feels are unnecessary like alcoholic beverages and lottery tickets. Over the years, she reasons, Edson could have saved enough money to pay for a ramp. Moreover, Edson has a son who is capable of building the ramp but can't seem to get himself together to do it. Ruth Ann realizes her priorities are not those of Edson or his son who seems to not understand the importance of the ramp. She also wonders if she might be like Edson if she were in his situation. As Ruth Ann considers what to do, **empirically**, she knows that easier access to the outdoors could be beneficial for Edson both physically and emotionally. **Ethically** she questions her duty to care, knowing she has the means to help Edson but spending money this way would limit her charitable giving to other causes she supports. **Aesthetically**, should she offer to build Edson's ramp she faces a delicate situation in approaching the landlord to make a case for the ramp as adding to the property's value. Her previous dealings with the landlord have not been positive and the landlord has seemed unwilling to authorize any improvements or changes. **Emancipatory** knowing comes into play when Ruth Ann considers what to do about the enforcement of laws that keep homebound persons in a rental where there is no easy egress available.

Imagine what you would do in this situation if you were Ruth Ann. What other aspects of all knowing patterns would be integrated as you decide what to do about Edson and his ramp?

Intentionality, from the perspective of holistic nursing theories, is an important perspective that can contribute to integrating the therapeutic use of Self with all knowing patterns. Intentionality includes the conscious choice that persons make in terms of how they want to "be" in the world, and in any particular situation. Your choice, your intention, is conveyed to others in subtle ways that can dramatically influence the nature of your interaction. In the context of what is known as "holistic healing modalities," even the intention to seek the very best for those in your care will place you in an energetic mode to support whatever is best in each situation you encounter. Intentions can expand your heart and your awareness, bringing about a dimension to the whole of nursing practice that is open, receptive, and ready to respond to whatever comes from the people with whom you interact. Without this type of intention, your concerns, worries, and focus tend to narrow down to mere tasks and the burdens of a situation, instead of seeing and attending to what is possible. You become ready and open to offer the therapeutic potential that resides within your Self.

 Think About It...

The idea of "therapeutic use of Self" is the least understood, yet perhaps the most important dimension of nursing in any context. Spend a few minutes thinking about what this means to you. Consider situations in which you believe you made a real difference for others because of who you are—that is, what you brought to the situation as a person. Consider if you set an intention to use your Self therapeutically in the situation. The situation could be a one-to-one interaction with a patient or a colleague, or a group situation in which your presence made a difference. Consider all aspects of the situation and ways in which your presence—your intentions, actions, words, ways of being—reflected the integration of all patterns of knowing.

INTEGRATION OF KNOWLEDGE WITH A FOCUS ON AESTHETICS: TRANSFORMATIVE ART/ACTS

Nurses create a transformative future by being with others in life-giving ways...
Paula Kagan (2009, p. 19)

Transformative art/acts are in-the-moment expressions of the art of nursing. Transformative art/acts require a certain quality of being and doing that is grounded in an intention to create a possibility for the future—a possibility of health and well-being. The words and actions of the nurse reflect a deep comprehension of what is happening, and responds to the moment in ways that bring about what is not yet real, but possible. What the nurse says and does may not seem dramatic or particularly notable, but it is transformative art/acts, emerging from the situation to move it toward an ongoing future that would not otherwise be possible. Art/acts guide the experience of those involved from one moment to the next and help them to envision and create possibilities for the future. During the transformative art/act, everything about the situation comes together in synchrony, like a dance that works for everyone in the situation. The art/act has an element of mystery; it is perceived in the moment but not consciously or analytically understood. It creates a possibility that can never be deliberately planned or anticipated but that is sensed as being right for the moment.

Integration of formal knowledge expressions with aesthetics considers empirics, for example, the pathophysiology of a condition or illness; ethics in relation to whether a treatment approach is likely to produce valued (for the person or society) results and whether full information is disclosed; personal knowing in relation to an understanding of the level of comfort you feel and why as you approach care; and emancipatory knowing in relation to whether or not the condition presented is due to social conditions that might be particular to a marginalized group.

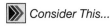 *Consider This...*

Jake is a PNP who works in a pediatric practice. Callie brings her 5-year-old twins in for their yearly checkup and immunizations. As Jake moves through the routine of the visit he notices that Emily, unlike her twin Ellie, is quite difficult to understand when she speaks. At their 4-year-old visit, Jake had documented his recommendation to Callie that she explore programs available through the public school system that would begin speech therapy. Callie became quite incensed and vocal that a nurse would be capable even of making such an assessment and declared: "She is just fine!" Given the hostile response, Jake contacted the speech therapy department of the public school system and asked that they contact the Montessori school that Ellie and Emily attend and work with the faculty there to get Emily the therapy needed. Considering **empirics**, Jake knew that the longer the speech difficulty persisted the more time and effort it would take to correct. In relation to **emancipatory** knowing he also knew resources for such services are limited as a function of the limited value placed on social programs for children. Thus, he understood that probably the call never happened because he was not able to continue making the contact. **Ethically** he felt that he needed to do something to try and get the child into treatment so the condition would not worsen and require even more time and resources to correct. **Personal** knowing came into play with the knowledge that his original advice to Callie may not have been taken seriously because of his dark skin and long hair, and the fact that he is a nurse and perceived as not having authority. Thus, all knowing patterns come into play as Jake considers the **aesthetics** of if, when, or how, to again suggest to Callie that Emily's speech should be of concern to her.

What other aspects of all knowing patterns would be integrated as Jake considered how to get help for Emily?

Transformative art/acts in practice often arise from the nurse's knowledge of what is possible in a situation—a possibility that is not immediately apparent to those who are experiencing the challenges of a health crisis. Knowledge of what is possible comes from what the nurse has learned in educational programs, and through experience with others in a similar situation. What is possible is envisioned but is certainly far from guaranteed. The nurse's experience in similar situations reinforces that the envisioned possibility could occur, and actions that support moving toward it are created.

Consider the challenge of helping someone regain motor skills they have lost as a result of a stroke. You know, as a nurse, that there is a strong possibility of moving beyond the debilitating loss experienced just after the stroke, so you can engage in interactions that support this movement. By integrating your intentional therapeutic use of Self, your empiric knowledge of the situation, a clear ethical commitment to do the right thing, your understanding of the social context that shapes what is possible, and your vision of what might be possible, you are able to provide the best quality of nursing care possible.

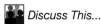 *Discuss This...*

Visit "The Art of Nursing" website (https://artofnursing.squarespace.com/#overview) with a group of your colleagues. As you browse through several of the pages on the site, discuss ways in which all patterns of knowing in nursing are reflected, either implicitly or explicitly. Discuss in particular the use of the phrase, "the art of nursing," as the central theme for this organization.

INTEGRATION OF KNOWLEDGE WITH A FOCUS ON EMPIRICS: SCIENTIFIC COMPETENCE

Practice is goal directed. Clinical testing of theory is therefore essential. Choose your theory—it does not hold in all circumstances. The professional must not be just a simple user of theory, but a developer, a tester and expander of theory. Not for the purpose of scholarship, but for intelligent practice.

Rosemary Ellis (1969, p. 1435)

Empiric knowing is expressed in practice within the whole of knowing as scientific competence by means of action grounded in empiric knowledge, including theory. Scientific competence involves conscious problem solving and logical reasoning, as the questions "What is this?" and "How does it function?" are continuously asked and answered. As with the other patterns, the knowledge informing these questions and their answers remains in the background as they are integrated into a knowing whole. Empiric knowing draws upon ethics to know which actions are justified; upon aesthetic knowing as the nurse makes care adjustments based on physical characteristics of the person; on personal knowing as one's own biases are understood in relation to the ethnicity of the person; and on emancipatory knowing as the client's marginalized status might mean they expect some degree of misjudgment or mistreatment.

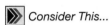 *Consider This...*

Sally is a nurse on an orthopedic unit where Jill is hospitalized. Jill has had extensive surgery to repair broken bones following a bicycle accident. Coming home from her university classes she was struck by a distracted driver who was texting. Jill has begged Sally to let her roommate Betsy bring in her new puppy for a visit. Sally questions if this is a good idea or not as animals have not been permitted on the unit and the puppy is a large and very energetic golden Labrador. Yet, Sally thinks it might be possible to do. **Empirically**, Sally needs to consider such things as risk of infection given Sally's recent surgeries; the possibility of a puppy's exuberance damaging equipment or injuring Jill, and evidence of the beneficial effect of pets. She also considers potential dander allergies in the person Jill is sharing the hospital room with. Her decision will also consider **ethically** whether to break or test rules in place, or consider care **ethics**; and whether the good to Jill from the visit will outweigh any potential harm to Jill's environment or operative sites. As for **aesthetics**, she envisions how she could create a healing encounter, integrating her own love of pets with nursing interactions to contribute to the emotional healing that Jill desperately needs. She also considers how she might present the research evidence supporting pet visitation to the supervisor, and soften the supervisor's concern about infection by laying out a plan to reduce the risk of any compromise on sanitary conditions on the unit. **Personal** knowing comes into play when she realizes that her love for dogs might affect the reasonableness of her actions, but her intention is to bring the best of herself to the situation so a pet can encourage Jill's healing of mind, body, and spirit without interference. She also cautions herself not to do anything stupid without going through proper channels. Finally, **emancipatory** knowing helps Sally realize that with better laws and law enforcement this accident, and the cost to Jill personally and to society in general, would not have happened. Sally vows to let her elected officials know that texting while driving needs to be a primary offense and that a public service campaign around bicycle safety is needed. Because Jill is in this position through no fault of her own, Sally is more inclined to work toward facilitating a visit with the new puppy as part of her nursing care plan.

Empiric knowledge is essential to the provision of excellent nursing care. However, as illustrated in the story of Sally caring for Jill, empiric knowledge alone is not adequate to guide practice decisions, in part because empiric evidence often yields conflicting ideas about the best course of action, or is not yet clearly conclusive. Evidence related to the benefit of pets, theoretically, dates back to Nightingale's "Notes on Nursing," in which she notes the beneficial effects of pets for the sick (1860/1969). For decades, the benefits of animals to assist those who are sick or disabled has been well documented. This evidence gives an opening to move in that direction, but other empiric factors also need to be taken into account such as risks of infection, contamination, or injury. In order to make a decision and create a plan for visitation, all patterns of knowing need to enter into consideration.

 Think About It...

> Bring to mind a nursing situation that you have encountered, for which the empiric evidence that you have on hand was not sufficient to guide your practice, or one in which the empiric evidence was contradictory. Make a list of the nursing actions that the empiric evidence does suggest, and a note of what evidence could be helpful. Now consider how the patterns of personal, aesthetic, ethical, and emancipatory knowing might provide insight as to how to respond to such a situation, given the limitations of the empiric evidence.

CONCLUSION

In this chapter we illustrated how the integration of knowledge expressions within all patterns occurs in nursing practice. Our view is based on the premise that practice is the ultimate basis on which both knowing and knowledge are shaped, revised, and refined. As knowledge across all patterns integrates, the whole of knowing continuously emerges. During the whole of knowing processes, the critical questions are asked, not openly or deliberately, but intuitively and subconsciously in order to form, create, and move through the care encounter. The critical questions of care encounters are useful to point to where knowledge expressions need strengthening. As nursing moves toward a more deliberate consideration of knowledge development across all patterns the profession is strengthened and the goals and intentions of nursing are better achieved. In the next chapter, we expand discussion of integrated expressions of knowledge in practice by considering a variety of nursing roles and the professional environments in which nursing is taught and practiced.

References

Aghebati, N., Mohammadi, E., Ahmadi, F., & Noaparast, K. B. (2015). Principle-based concept analysis: Intentionality in holistic nursing theories. *Journal of Holistic Nursing: Official Journal of the American Holistic Nurses' Association, 33*(1), 68–83. https://doi.org/10.1177/0898010114537402.

Ashley, J. (1976). *Hospitals, paternalism, and the role of the nurse.* New York, NY: Teachers College Press.

Benner, P. A., & Wrubel, J. (1989). *The primacy of caring: stress and coping in health and illness.* Menlo Park, CA: Addison Wesley.

Diers, D. (2004). *Speaking of nursing: Narratives of practice, research, policy, and the profession.* Sudbury, MA: Jones and Bartlett.

Ellis, R. (1969). The practitioner as theorist. *The American Journal of Nursing, 69*, 1434.

Kagan, P. N. (2009). Historical voices of resistance: crossing boundaries to praxis through documentary film-making for the public. *ANS. Advances in Nursing Science, 32,* 19–32.

Legacy.com staff. (2010). *The mysterious death of Karen Silkwood.* http://www.legacy.com/news/celebrity-deaths/article/the-mysterious-death-of-karen-silkwood.

Nightingale, F. (1860/1969). *Notes on nursing: what it is and what it is not.* New York, NY: Dover Publications, Inc.

O'Conner-Von, S. (2013). Animal-assisted therapy. In R. Ruth Lindquist, M. Snyder, & M. F. Tracy (Eds.), *Complementary & alternative therapies in nursing* (7th ed.) (pp. 229–253). New York, NY: Springer Publishing Company.

Our Campaign. (2016). http://nocoalinoakland.info/our-campaign/.

Parker, R. S. (1990). Nurses' stories: the search for a relational ethic of care. *ANS. Advances in Nursing Science, 13,* 31–40.

Rebellious Nursing: About Us. (2012). http://www.rebelnursing.org/about-us/.

Stewart, I. M. (1921). Some fundamental principles in the teaching of ethics. *The American Journal of Nursing, 21,* 906–913.

Webster, A. (2016, January 3). *How intention works.* http://reikirays.com/29013/how-intention-works/.

Integrated Expressions in Practice: Strengthening the Discipline

Finally, it is worth reiterating the point that compared with atheoretical actions, those that are conceptually grounded have a higher probability of achieving their intended consequences. Not just because they are contemplated more intentionally but because the vast majority of population-focused theories/frameworks pay heed to the important messiness of context and the use of power.

Patricia Butterfield (2017, p. 9)

In this chapter we extend the discussion of practice as the ultimate basis on which and for which knowing and knowledge are developed. Importantly, we continue to emphasize as we have throughout this text the importance of paying attention to the deliberative thought that undergirds what we do. The opening quote by Butterfield expresses our concern well—conceptual, theoretical thought is basic to truly understanding the nature of the practice, political, and educational world that nursing inhabits.

In this, the final chapter, we consider the effect of various nursing roles and the professional environments in which nursing is taught and managed. We describe how evidence that informs practice contributes to pattern integration and the whole of knowing. We also consider how the professional focus on the Professional Nursing Doctorate has potential to contribute to evidence-informed nursing. Finally, we suggest how the contexts in which nursing care, leadership, policymaking, scholarship, and education is provided affects pattern integration and the whole of knowing. Many things can both interfere with and benefit from thought and action that serve to strengthen the profession and, thus, improve health care. In this chapter we examine ways to strengthen the profession and to strengthen knowledge integration in practice.

CONCEPTUALIZING FEATURES OF YOUR PRACTICE IN RELATION TO DISCIPLINARY KNOWLEDGE

We begin with you, as an individual practitioner. A look at how you and your colleagues integrate knowledge in practice and the ease and/or difficulty with which it is done can provide clues about how knowledge needs to change or be strengthened. Following are key questions you can pose to examine the relationship between the disciplinary knowledge you integrate as you practice. Your answers form a basis for improving integration of knowledge in practice, as well as improving the knowledge expressions being created within the discipline.

Goal Congruence: Are Your Practice Goals and the Goals Embedded in Nursing's Formal Expressions of Knowledge Congruent?

Since practice goals are often quite explicit and relatively easy to identify, start by identifying goals you are likely to have for individual clients or patients in your practice. Then think about the empiric, emancipatory, ethical, personal, and aesthetic forms of knowledge that are relevant to your practice goals and challenge the extent to which the formal expressions reflect, implicitly or explicitly, outcomes that are congruent with your practice. Consider if the goals implied in the expressions of knowledge can be implemented and might improve existing standards of practice. Consider how your practice experience could shed light on ways to improve the expressions of nursing knowledge. How might you communicate your thoughts to those in a position to improve the knowledge expression? How can you improve the knowledge expression directly?

One often cited nursing goal is self-care. Self-care is a concept of central importance in a number of nursing conceptual frameworks or models. Although this goal might be appropriate for some situations, it is probably not the best goal for a situation in which a person is not capable of independent, rational self-care due to physical or mental limitations or conditions. Another example is the goal of "compliance," which in many practice situations has been demonstrated to be unrealistic. Some practitioners prefer to work toward a mutually determined approach that involves patients and families in determining realistic individualized goals rather than compliance with directives issued by health care providers. You also might find that some of the conceptualizations of adaptation are unrealistic in a health care setting where your goal is to help people leave abusive or unhealthy situations, not adapt to them. In examining directives for outcomes found in current nursing literature, you may find that some are appropriate for your situation, whereas others might potentially be appropriate if changes in the work environment were made.

Context: Are the Contexts Embodied in Nursing Knowledge Congruent With Your Practice Situation?

This question addresses how well the context wherein knowledge was developed is suitable for your practice situation. As an example, nursing knowledge that focuses on pain alleviation in the context of adulthood may not adequately address caring for children. You might explore how well the ideas expressed in theories, stories, works of art, and codes of ethics might transfer to your own situation and also explore what implications your context offers for further knowledge development. If context seems to be inappropriate for your situation, then integration of knowledge to form a whole of knowing can be improved by further development of the knowledge expressions that address pain management.

Suppose you find a research article that suggests pre-surgery patients have better outcomes if they are familiarized with aspects of the post-op experience. The research reports that patients who were familiarized with the operative suite and recovery room area by visiting it, and were shown the devices they might be attached to, were less fearful and experienced less pain. You believe the young children you work with might benefit from such an approach but recognize the context of normal adults having surgery is much different than children awaiting surgery. You decide to modify the approach the research used and change the context to be appropriate for young children. This might include using dolls or stuffed animals and simulating some of the equipment and experiences used in the research but in relation to doll or animal play. In this way, the goal of alleviating fear and pain is appropriate for young children but the context within which the research was completed needs to be modified (and potentially subjected to research) before use in a pediatric population.

Concepts and Assumptions: Is There or Might There be Similarity Between the Concepts and Assumptions as Expressed in Nursing Knowledge, and What You Experience in Practice? This question compares the ideas structured within knowledge expressions as concepts, with what you encounter in your practice situation. What you experience in practice provides insights to refine the meanings of the concepts that are used in formal expressions of knowledge and helps to differentiate between ideas that are similar. Your experiences in practice, and your reflection on your experience, can lead to language that expresses experiences you know to be real. When what you experience has not yet been adequately conceptualized in formal knowledge expressions, your ability to integrate that knowledge in practice is limited.

For example, an empiric theory about learning that potentially might guide patient teaching may not explicitly provide a definition for the learner, but you notice it has conceptualized the learner as a healthy individual. If in your practice you know the people you teach are under considerable stress, perhaps having just been given a diagnosis of type 1 diabetes, you know they are not at that moment "healthy" in the way that is assumed in the theory. Because they are not stress free, and are living with untreated diabetes, you know that a theory that has a basic assumption of health in the learner may not be as useful as it could be. This affects your ability to integrate the theory in your practice. If you know the unique approaches that you have developed in teaching moments often result in real changes for the people with whom you work, but in all of the nursing knowledge you examine, you find nothing that reflects your experience, you have a basis for contributing to the development of new knowledge that more adequately expresses your experience. This, in turn, ultimately serves to strengthen disciplinary knowledge, and the profession as a whole.

An ethical theory that conceptualizes disclosure as the "open and honest communication about the risks and benefits" of, for instance, a procedure, a medication, or genetic testing may be inappropriate for persons with mild dementia. While it may be tempting to "follow the rules of disclosure" and proceed, it would be important to recognize that disclosure is not conceptualized appropriately for this population.

The importance of conceptual meaning and assumptions within research reports as well as other formal expressions cannot be overemphasized. It is tempting to jump to conclusions or directives offered that may seem useful without looking at whether or not the way concepts are defined and the assumptions made are operating in your situation.

Sufficiency: Are Formal Expressions Sufficient as a Basis for Nursing Action?
Responses to this question require expert judgment about the particular nursing actions that are implied within formal knowledge expressions, whether anything of importance has been omitted, or if any distortions or inaccuracies are perpetrated. Is the knowledge form complete in relation to the context for which it was developed? As an expert nurse, you may find it difficult to describe the basis on which you would judge knowledge to be sufficient or not sufficient, perhaps because the context of care is fluid. If, however, factors you deal with on a day-to-day basis are not addressed by the knowledge expression, you might judge the knowledge form to be insufficient for your purposes. In these instances, you might examine in what ways a formal expression seems to cover what is important in light of your practice. You may feel tentative about your conclusions, but if you determine that additional factors need to be considered in order for the formal expression to be maximally useful, then providing your thoughts for others to consider can serve to improve knowledge expressions and thus improve care.

Let's say, for example, that a theory of uncertainty which you might find useful enumerated a list of factors or variables that are associated with the experience of uncertainty in adults undergoing chemotherapy for cancer. The presence of these factors, and the degree to which they are scored as important, is linked to the degree of expressed uncertainty of outcomes of chemotherapy. In reviewing the research report and the schematic of the theory you notice that certain social stability factors have not been accounted for. You are working with a population of unemployed individuals and the population on which the theory was developed were not unemployed. The omission of information about how job status, and perhaps factors associated with unemployment affect uncertainty, may make the theory insufficient for your use.

You will notice that many of the above-mentioned factors to be examined in knowledge expressions do overlap. If context differs from yours, this may make a theory or formal expression insufficient; if concepts are defined inappropriately for your situation, that also affects sufficiency. If a formal expression is not inclusive enough, it may be related to assumptions basic to the research process, and so forth. When a knowledge expression is deemed not useful for your practice, it does not mean the knowledge is faulty or bad, it just means it doesn't work for you. Thus, you are left with revising or adapting the formal expression to meet your needs, or perhaps creating a new one that does fit your situation. What is important here is to examine the conceptual basis and understand how and why any formal expression of knowledge does or does not work in a clinical context. The goal is to avoid unintended consequences of using formal knowledge without examining it carefully in relation to your practice situation.

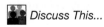 *Discuss This...*

> Consider a theory of parent–child interaction, which has undergone extensive development and refinement through the work of Dr. Kathryn Barnard (Barnard, 1981, 1996; Barnard, Eyres, Lobo, & Snyder, 1983). The Barnard theory has been refined through a program of theory development and research that has spanned several years and that still is active.

In the Barnard model, the following three-way conceptual relationship is central to the theory of how (1) the child, (2) the caregiver or parent, and (3) specific environmental factors interact. The interaction of these three elements determines how a parent or caregiver and a child will relate interpersonally. For example, features of the child (fussy? docile?), features of the caregiver or parent (oversolicitous? nonattentive?), and features of the environment (child care classes available? other individuals available for care relief?) create interpersonal interaction patterns. The practice value of Barnard's model comes from research describing which factors and combinations of factors interfere with normal infant development.

Because normal infant development is a goal in which nurses have much interest, the theoretic relationships justify the importance of assessing caregiver/parent–child interactions and providing early intervention when interactions are problematic. Checklist scales have been developed that a nurse can use to observe and assess parent–child interaction during activities of feeding or when caregivers or parents teach the child a developmentally appropriate skill. There are accompanying assessment tools that have been used extensively to benefit families and children. This empirical theory can be used widely because research was employed to identify, confirm, and validate the factors that were significant in creating problematic parent/caregiver–child interactions. Furthermore, factors of significance were represented in a way that could be easily assessed in clinical practice. Research evidence that is generated with an insensitivity to whether variables and assessments are practical for nurses to use runs the risk of creating theories and models that require further development before they can be used in practice.

With a group of your colleagues, examine, in relation to a real or imagined situation of pediatric nursing, whether Barnard's theory (or a theory or research of choice) adequately meets the following conditions in a way that would make it useful for nurses practicing in the situation.
- Goal congruency
- Context and assumption congruency
- Concept adequacy
- Sufficiency

How would the theory or research need to be changed in order for a nurse to integrate it into practice?

INTEGRATION OF KNOWLEDGE AND EVIDENCE INFORMED PRACTICE

Clearly, when we talk about integrating knowledge characterized as "evidence" the nature of that evidence will affect how well it can be integrated into practice. In the previous section the focus was on the individual practitioner and how formal knowledge expressions, including forms of evidence, might be evaluated for conceptual adequacy in relation to particular situations. In this section we consider how evidence as focused on by the profession can be integrated into practice.

By practice, we mean the experiences a nurse encounters during the process of caring for people, interacting with families and groups, enacting leadership roles in health care, and advocating for justice, equity, and protection of health in public policy. Experiences can be those of the client, the community, the nurse(s), or others such as families and friends. Some experiences are more interactive than others, and some focus more on the immediate and broader environment. Practice experiences occur in many settings, but when they occur in the context of providing nursing care, or in contexts that affect nursing care, they are considered part of nursing practice.

The current professional trend to embrace evidence-based practice as a standard for professional nursing has potential to significantly influence how knowledge is and can be developed and, therefore, integrated in practice. A view of "evidence" that is narrowly defined as research evidence alone leaves a substantial gap in the foundation that is needed for nursing (Porter, 2010; Thorne & Sawatzky, 2014). As Betts (2009) claims, many concerns must be addressed for the best nursing care, including philosophic and theoretic perspectives along with the evidence provided by empirical research. We would add that best nursing care requires a practical perspective that considers the broad context within which evidence is used. In other words, evidence that can be integrated in practice should be created in consideration of all patterns of knowing.

The emergence of proposals for developing practice-based evidence (rather than evidence-based practice) highlights the need to take a view of evidence that considers the context and goals of practice. Thinking about practice-based evidence underscores the importance of all knowing patterns more clearly than a focus on more narrow views of evidence-based practice. Practice-based evidence is an approach that acknowledges the significance of the environment of practice in determining practice recommendations. Practice-based evidence values knowledge that generates from practice, versus knowledge that conforms to hierarchies of evidence and is created apart from the context of practice. Practice-based evidence is not decontextualized, universal knowledge—rather, it is quite the opposite (Fox, 2003; Horn & Gassaway, 2007; Porter, 2010; Simons, Kushner, Jones, & James, 2003). This is not to say that practice-based evidence is a panacea, or that it might, in fact, perpetuate problematic situations. Rather, it is to say that a view toward practice-based evidence might have potential to shed light on why some evidence is better integrated in some practice situations and not in others.

▷▷ *Consider This...*

Although some evidence-based recommendations are reasonable, some may not be practical or useful. For example, evidence may support providing multiple individualized sessions to teach families how to best communicate with a family member who has had a stroke. The need to consider what contributed to the stroke as a result of access to health care (emancipatory); how many resources to bring to bear on rehabilitation (ethical); which approaches might work better with the person and how those approaches should be tailored (aesthetic); and the nurses' feelings about self-responsibility for health (personal) are operating. Without thinking about such factors (and there are many more) evidence-based recommendations may make sense on the surface, but may not be practical for a specific situation in the standard health care setting.

DiCenso, Guyatt, and Ciliska (2005) proposed a definition of evidence-based practice that we favor because it requires meaningful connections between empiric knowledge including theory, research, and practice. Furthermore, it acknowledges that a comprehensive range of situational factors that address the knowing patterns other than empirics need to be taken into consideration for evidence-based practice to be accomplished. For these authors, evidence-based practice integrates best research evidence, health care resources, patient preferences and actions, clinical setting and circumstances, and the clinician's judgment in clinical decision making (pp. 4–5). Thus, evidence-based practice is not simply the utilization of research in practice as it is sometimes characterized. Evidence-based practice requires considering of an array of circumstances, including concerns not only arising from empirics but from aesthetic, personal, ethical, and emancipatory knowing. DiCenso and colleagues focus on evidence-based practice and the use of research evidence in nursing in consideration of a broad array of other factors affecting practice integration. They promote a focus on knowledge expressions within all patterns of knowing when developing and utilizing research evidence. They acknowledge that research and inquiry particular to all knowing patterns will affect clinical nursing care. If evidence-based practice as described by DiCenso and colleagues is taken seriously, evidence that is increasingly suitable for integration in practice will emerge.

For empirical researchers a significant challenge related to evidence-based practice is to develop knowledge around questions that are clinically important and to complete research in ways that generate evidence that can be integrated in practice. This requires communication between researchers and clinicians. Clinicians have knowledge of situational factors that require attending to if evidence is going to be useful in clinical care. Meaningful communication that acknowledges all-knowing patterns are important has potential to more fully enmesh the roles of nurse researcher and nurse clinician and subsequently result in the creation and use of knowledge that can, and will, be integrated into practice and strengthen the profession.

As clinicians strive to locate best research evidence appropriate to managing care and attempt to use that knowledge within their practice environment, the extent to which that evidence is available and usable will become more obvious. The difficulties and benefits of various methodological approaches to generating empiric research evidence will be made more visible. When clinicians discover well-conceived and well-carried-out research evidence that requires, for example, use of assessment tools that are impractical clinically, researchers will begin to understand the importance of considering how research is conducted in order for it to be well integrated into practice. Structuring clinically important concepts into meaningful theoretical relationships and representing those relationships in ways that allow clinicians to make use of findings in practice will become clearer.

Because we believe research evidence needs to be developed in consideration of all knowing patterns, we use the term "evidence-informed practice." This terminology puts emphasis on the important role research evidence has in care provision while counteracting the idea that practice is best directed by evidence as portrayed by evidence hierarchies. Thinking of evidence as informing practice has potential to illuminate areas where even well-conceived and well-developed empirical evidence cannot be integrated into practice because of lack of resources, patient or client considerations, and other contextual factors. Research evidence may be appropriate for practice, and concepts in relationship may have been studied in a way that makes them well suited for use in practice. However, features of context such as nurse–patient ratios, insurance reimbursement patterns, or institutional policies around security, if not considered, may make it difficult to use that evidence in practice. These situations bring to light the need to integrate emancipatory, personal, ethical, and aesthetic knowledge to create a care context that will allow and encourage the use of best evidence.

The emergence of the Doctorate of Nursing Practice (DNP) as the basic educational credential for advanced nursing practice is well underway. This trend has significant potential to strengthen integration of all knowledge forms in practice, in a way that supports evidence- informed practice. The DNP was conceptualized as a path to prepare nurses to contribute to the development of nursing knowledge by integrating knowledge developed by nurse researchers, into the clinical setting ("The Essentials of Doctoral Education for Advanced Nursing Practice," 2006). When these practitioners facilitate the integration (or themselves integrate) research findings and formal knowledge expressions in practice in the face of expectations for evidence-informed practice—the nature of evidence needed and subsequent implications for inquiry, including research and knowledge development should become increasingly evident. While the ongoing benefit of the DNP on nursing practice remains to be seen, these practitioners have potential to evaluate how easily empiric evidence can be integrated in practice. When integration is difficult, then a focus on improving empiric evidence by further development that considers all-knowing patterns may be needed. When factors addressed by other patterns are considered the possibility of research evidence actually informing practice is strengthened. It follows that knowledge integration is strengthened and professional goals are better attained.

In summary, evidence-informed practice requires much more than simply the "application" of research in practice. Embracing a view of empiric knowledge expressions that truly inform and improve practice will, of necessity, strengthen the linkages between empiric knowledge and all patterns of knowing. Evidence that informs practice requires communication among nurses in a variety of roles. More specifically evidence-informed practice does the following:

- Strengthens the practitioner's and researcher's ability to collaborate in framing important practice issues and the clinical questions that need to be addressed (Chesla, 2008)
- Improves the skills of practitioners in determining the quality and limitations of research evidence and in synthesizing research (Copnell, 2008; Fawcett & Garity, 2008)
- Supports a decision-making infrastructure and database development that is appropriate for the context of nursing practice (Burkhart & Androwich, 2009; Porter, 2010)
- Makes visible the challenges inherent in utilizing knowledge developed outside the realm of practice (Canam, 2008), especially knowledge that does not consider all knowing patterns

- Provides researchers with information about the types of knowledge structures that are required to meet health care goals (Doane & Varcoe, 2008; Fawcett, Watson, Neuman, Walker, & Fitzpatrick, 2001; Porter, 2010)
- Creates approaches to developing theory that are relevant in practice (Doane, Browne, Reimer, MacLeod, & McLellan, 2009)
- Brings to light contextual factors related to resources and setting that affect evidence-based practice (Chesla, 2008)
- Energizes theory and research practices that are intended to address social issues such as health care disparities and cultural diversity (Betts, 2009; Chesla, 2008; Chung, Cimprich, Janz, & Mills-Wisneski, 2009)
- Enhances the potential for academic researchers and clinicians in all disciplines to work together and share roles—in fact, dissolving distinctions among research, practice, and theory (Lenz, 2007; Ryan, 2009)

When evidence is developed using research processes that are sensitive to the context and goals of practice, and that deliberately consider inquiry in relation to all patterns of knowing, transformation of practice is possible.

QUALITY CARE AND KNOWLEDGE INTEGRATION

The context of modern nursing emphasizes empirical evidence when evaluating care quality, and the methods of empirics are important in achieving quality in health care. In the following sections, we discuss empiric approaches to evaluating quality care outcomes, and consider how accounting for all patterns of knowing when assessing care quality can contribute to knowledge integration and, thus, achieving desired outcomes and effectiveness of care. This is not to claim that knowledge within all patterns will directly affect outcomes, but only that it is wise to at least consider how all knowing patterns might affect the design and implementation of quality care research and outcomes and how best outcomes might improve knowledge integration

Quality assurance research draws on traditional evaluation research methods (Posavac, 2010; Schroeder & Maibusch, 1984; Smeltzer, Hinshaw, & Feltman, 1987). In evaluation research, the method is designed to provide evidence about the overall well-being of people who receive care, the scientific competence of those who practice nursing, and the practice setting itself. Usually, this type of investigation involves assessing quality outcomes when a different approach to care is implemented in an effort to demonstrate what changes from previous care approaches have been attained.

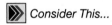 *Consider This...*

If you believe implementing a theory of pain alleviation would improve quality care outcomes, you might design a study that would first estimate the quality of nursing care and patients' experiences of pain before the theory is used in practice. Your assessment could include the perspectives of nurses, people receiving nursing care, and others involved in caring for people who experience pain. After you have this information, you would begin to use the theory in practice and over time continue to observe the same outcome indicators of quality of care. On the basis of your findings, you could make recommendations for practice and for revisions in the theory. If you designed your research without considering how important the time and effort needed for already overburdened nurses to implement the theory (emancipatory knowledge), your quality outcomes are less likely to be achieved.

If it is not possible to obtain data directly from your population before changing a care approach that is designed to improve quality outcomes, alternative approaches may be used. These include obtaining population or epidemiologic data from a comparable population or group of people. In this instance you would compare quality outcomes to quality outcomes derived from population statistics of a comparable group.

This approach is useful in many types of situations. One such circumstance is nursing care that is directed toward the prevention of negative outcomes, such as child abuse. If you intend to implement an approach that will decrease the incidence of child abuse by mothers, you are unlikely to obtain reliable preimplementation data for the outcomes you are seeking to achieve. The mothers that you are working with may not be willing to divulge information about the part they have played in child abuse for a number of legal and socially stigmatized reasons. Moreover, they may not want to divulge information about factors in their lives that predispose them to abusing their child. In this case factors within the emancipatory knowing pattern (job discrimination related to their ethnicity) or empirics (mental/emotional condition) might be important to recognize in designing methods for obtaining data as well as outcomes you want to achieve.

Again, when you are unable to get data needed to assess outcomes within your population, you would obtain population statistics regarding the incidence of child abuse. You might monitor the incidence of abusive behaviors among the parents for whom you are providing care, and compare your outcomes with the population statistics. You might change your set of desired outcomes altogether. When it is not possible to assess extent of child abuse directly, you might look at assessing outcomes that contribute to child abuse by mothers, rather than incidence of abuse itself. In this instance you might gather information about the income level or the family job status of mothers, religious affiliations, available support systems, recreational or prescription drug use, or other factors known to contribute to potential child abuse. You would assess these factors prior to implementing an educational program designed to familiarize mothers with support services available to them as well as general education about the factors that promote child abuse. You would then assess these same factors after the program as a way to indirectly assess the incidence of child abuse. In this instance you would want to think about the importance of ethical and aesthetic knowing (how to get reliable data about a forbidden activity—abusing a child), personal knowing (Do the mothers know that they should not abuse?), and emancipatory knowing (Does anger felt from pressure to conform to societal ideals fuel anger directed at their child?).

These are just a few examples of how a nod to all knowing patterns might operate to strengthen evaluation research. If outcomes that are not seen practical or possible when all knowing patterns are considered, then data resulting from quality outcome evaluation research is not going to reflect what is really operating. It follows that care changes made on the basis of quality outcomes that are not carefully conceived, are not going to improve care and professional practice.

In general, evaluation research to improve quality care depends on knowing what outcomes you want to achieve and on having a well-planned approach for achieving your goal. It requires assessing by some means those pertinent goals or outcomes before implementation of evaluation research, and then reassessing those same goals or outcomes for changes.

The following sections describe quality-related outcomes you might consider when examining quality of care. These outcomes, when assessed, and when deficiencies are addressed, have potential to further improve quality care outcomes.

Scientific Competence of Nurses

Although the primary aim when considering quality care assurance is improving the outcomes of those who receive care by assessing accepted practice standards, it is also important to assess the scientific competence of nurses. When scientific competence is evaluated and subsequently improved this will ultimately improve knowledge integration and care quality. Standards of nursing practice accepted by your nursing practice unit often form the basis for much quality care assessment research. These may be limited and not demand a high degree of scientific competence of nurses because standards of care generally reflect only minimum acceptable practice. As you plan for evaluating care standards, you may need to consider what extensions of the standards reflect scientific competence.

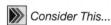 Consider This...

> If, in your unit, certain caring behaviors are to be implemented, your standards of care should reflect or require these caring behaviors as part of scientific competence for nurses. Examining scientific competence in relation to these outcomes might suggest a need to strengthen caring behavior of nurses as a way to improve their scientific competence.
>
> In this example, improving the scientific competence of nurses requires assessing more than minimal care standards that are basic to patient safety. Rather it suggests evaluating features of the nurses' scientific competence basic to care excellence. Once evaluated, areas that need strengthening can be addressed. As scientific competence is improved, nurses are likely to more easily notice how, for example, features of Self and environment affect care.

Functional Outcomes

Quality care outcomes are also affected by how efficiently the work of nursing is done, how cost effective it is, or how smoothly the work of each individual coordinates with others' work. If environmental factors that impede quality outcomes have been identified as needing improvement for a particular unit, the changes suggested and the factors indexing improvement need to be specified, assessed, and subsequently changed. Once baseline data assessing environmental factors have been obtained, measures of functional effectiveness can be obtained and compared. If a unit is not functioning effectively, and factors related to effectiveness are not assessed, the results of quality outcome research will not be as useful as it might be. When functional outcomes are not assessed, the smooth functioning of the unit cannot be known or improved upon if that is needed. In many ways, functional outcomes reflect the aesthetic quality of the unit—and when a unit is inefficient in its functioning less effective knowledge integration follows.

Nurse Satisfaction

Satisfaction with respect to job responsibilities in nursing can be clearly linked to improved knowledge integration. The job satisfaction of nurses can be assessed by factors such as working conditions, relationships with colleagues, personal fulfillment, various types of perceived benefits, and perceived dissatisfactions. Thus, a premise that underlies the inclusion of this outcome in evaluation research is that, if nurses are more satisfied with their work situations, integrated expression of knowledge in practice is more likely to occur, and quality of care provided will improve.

Quality of Care Perceived by Those Who Receive Care

People who receive care can be interviewed or surveyed to ascertain their perceptions of the quality of their care before, during, and after quality assurance research processes. Aspects of perceived quality of care that can be assessed include satisfaction with specific dimensions of care, perceived benefits obtained from the care, and perceived dissatisfactions. Responses that recur significantly generally indicate strengths or areas needing attention.

How those we serve perceive our care can point to multiple areas for improvement of knowledge expressions that are integrated as care is provided. Genuine selves that need to be commended and maintained may be revealed or deficiencies in aesthetics as nurses approach care might be noted. The care system may be difficult to navigate or many instances of appropriate treatment may be revealed.

> **!** *Why Is This Important?*
>
> Many factors at a variety of levels influence the extent to which integration of knowledge across all patterns can occur in practice settings. We believe that the best quality of nursing practice in any setting depends on the integration of all patterns of knowing—empirical, emancipatory, ethical, aesthetic, and personal.
>
> Nursing has a strong base in honoring knowledge as important for quality care, and current trends in practice and education continue to not only significantly strengthen empirical knowledge for practice, but also bring into focus the need to strengthen knowledge expressions across all knowing patterns. These trends include the focus on evidence-informed practice (also termed evidence-based practice), the DNP, the call for translational research, and growing emphasis on additional measures of quality assurance that strengthen the profession in ways that promote best practices.

It also merits mention that it is not just practitioners and developers of disciplinary knowledge that have a significant role in health care provision. Those who support nursing scholarship, education, and practice are important in helping ensure professional goals can be met and our nursing practice promotes health for those we serve.

IT TAKES A VILLAGE

The contexts within which nursing operates—the environments that support and affect direct care—have a significant influence on the quality of knowledge that, in practice, integrates to form the whole of knowing (Galuska, 2012). Context can provide the conditions that energize, guide, and provide support for knowledge development within all patterns of knowing. Contexts can also create and support disvalue for knowledge and knowledge development across the patterns of knowing. If nursing is to productively contribute to achieving optimal health care we believe that every nurse in an active nursing role needs to conceptually understand and integrate the knowing patterns in their various practices. In some ways a focus on the whole of knowing places a focus on nursing's roots prior to its turn toward the dominance of science and traditional research approaches that came about in the 1950s. There is evidence that a focus on the whole of knowing is taking hold more strongly in nursing (Jacobs, 2013; Kagan, Smith, & Chinn, 2014; Thorne & Sawatzky, 2014). In this section we consider the broader context that supports care and consider how educators, administrators, researchers, and policymakers can, and must, address all knowing patterns.

Educators and Educational Considerations

Educational considerations include formal curricular considerations as well as day-to-day interactions with students in the clinical and classroom environments. We propose that all participants in a teaching/learning situation can claim ownership of the need to address the whole of knowing. Nursing education programs perpetuate the emphasis on empirics, and often sustain a medical perspective that neglects due consideration of multiple ways of knowing. Students and teachers alike can call forth approaches that integrate learning experiences related to ethical, aesthetic, personal, and emancipatory knowing.

Nursing care plans can include assessments related to each of the patterns. In reflecting on clinical learning experiences, students and teachers can identify how knowledge derived from each of the patterns of knowing can contribute to improving nursing care. If there is a template for nursing care plans, assess the extent to which the template accommodates each knowing pattern.

It is important to examine the statements of philosophy, purpose, and formal objectives in your education program, and consider the extent to which these statements promote the inclusion of all knowing patterns. Teaching and learning approaches that develop and impart knowledge within all-knowing patterns lead to a more comprehensive form of nursing care based on the whole of knowing. Because human health experiences by definition are "whole" experiences that encompass more than simply a diagnosis or empirical "presenting complaint," each learning experience provides an opportunity for faculty and students alike to call forth all-knowing patterns, increasing their skills and abilities in knowledge integration.

Faculty who publish and otherwise share information around the implementation of the patterns of knowing in the classroom and clinical environments have potential to significantly improve a focus on all knowing patterns in the discipline of nursing. In addition to broadly sharing information around their experience of teaching across all patterns, faculty should avail themselves of information already in the literature about the importance of all patterns in relation to health and illness care as a way to improve their teaching approach.

When addressing the basis for making decisions in nursing, learners and faculty can assess the value of empiric evidence, and the extent to which that evidence is applicable in a particular situation. Broadening the focus, using the language of evidence-informed practice, and drawing on personal, aesthetic, ethical, and emancipatory knowledge to determine the best approach to care in a particular situation points both learners and faculty to decisions that encompass the whole of the situation (Thorne & Sawatzky, 2014) . A focus on evidence-informed practice promotes understanding of all factors within all of the knowing patterns that will affect not only how knowledge is generated, but how it is used.

Finally, it is important to encourage and support learners and faculty who have an interest in alternative or nontraditional research. Giving permission to faculty and learners to explore knowledge that falls outside the realm of traditional or even nontraditional empirics can be seen as promoting knowledge within nonempiric knowing patterns. This, in turn, strengthens the breadth of knowledge available for practice integration. It also is important for faculty with an interest in alternative knowledge development to educate higher level administrators about the nature of nursing practice, and the importance of a broad inquiry focus. Often nonnurses who control the nature of nursing education devalue such inquiry and have a stereotypical understanding of what nurses do and the basis on which our practice is founded.

Administration and Administrative Considerations

Administrative considerations are directed toward nurses and nursing allies who support and maintain the environment within which nurses and nursing students function. Our recommendations for strengthening focus on all knowing patterns for managers, administrators, and those who assume leadership roles in health care.

Whenever possible, administrators within nursing should advocate for the importance of all knowing patterns. This is shown through support for research and inquiry that generates, evaluates, or otherwise considers all patterns of knowing. Advocacy would include budgeting for the support of nontraditional research and ongoing programs that address all-knowing patterns, and formally assessing features of care that reflect the breadth of knowing both in relation to quality assurance and during routine personnel reviews.

Ongoing efforts to support and encourage all patterns of knowing are vital for the best quality of care within an institution. Ethics committees, composed of representatives from all groups employed in an institution as well as individuals with expertise in ethics, can have a major influence on and support ethical comportment. Because the work of nursing is emotionally demanding, drawing on nurses' personal, aesthetic, emancipatory, and ethical sensibilities, nurses can benefit immensely by having time dedicated to debriefing, to reflect and share their experiences in order to deepen their capacity to care. Administrative support is critical for nurses to be at the table for all discussions and decisions that affect their ability to provide care based on the whole of nursing

Nurses who approach research, administrative, and educational responsibilities with the lens of a broad view of nursing that includes knowledge within all patterns should be supported and encouraged. An open discussion of the importance of seeing professional responsibilities with a lens that includes all patterns of knowing is also important for creating both sharing and understanding (Galuska, 2012).

Administrators who maintain a working relationship with educational institutions help create shared pathways that support integration of all patterns within clinical environments. Shared seminars and continuing education opportunities that consider the ways of knowing need to be nourished. Finally, it is important for administrators of nursing to familiarize themselves with the literature around the knowing patterns as a way to understand their significance and strengthen their commitment to their practice significance for quality outcomes.

Policymaking and Community Organizing

Policy considerations include factors to be addressed within organizations and institutions that provide direction for nursing curricula, research, and practice. Nurses in all roles, as well as nursing students, can promote grassroots organizing that assist and support people in communities who are working on projects and taking political action directed at supporting fair and just public health policies. As awareness of health policies that promote health for all people and eliminate injustices for marginalized groups is shared, the importance of all patterns is promoted, but importantly the significance of emancipatory knowing emerges.

Policymakers within professional organizations such as the American Association of Colleges of Nursing, American Nurses Association, and the National League of Nursing need the support of all nurses to strengthen their voices and use their authority to actively resist policies and decisions that blunt quality care and professional goals. By becoming involved in any of the many professional organizations, nurses and students can participate in efforts to form and strengthen policy statements and recommendations for curricula and practice that promote the visibility and significance of all ways of knowing.

Nurses in positions of influence within National Institutes of Health and National Institute of Nursing Research working to increase funding for nontraditional forms of inquiry have potential to increase the availability of funding for inquiry related to all knowing patterns. Education of elected officials as well as for board members of private foundations that support research can also be a means of promoting alternative inquiry methods that support knowledge related to the patterns of knowing. As a nurse—whether a student, practitioner, educator, researcher, administrator, or other professional role—you can become involved in organizations, serve on boards, run for public office, or lend your voice in support of the development of the whole of nursing knowledge in varied ways (Ellenbecker & Edward, n.d.).

CONCLUSION

In this chapter our major focus was the importance of supporting the context within which direct nursing care exists in ways that support a focus on all knowing patterns. We discussed how, as a nurse, considering what you do in relation to disciplinary knowledge is important. Such things as reviewing knowledge for appropriateness of goals, context, concepts, assumptions, and sufficiency help ensure knowledge is not inappropriately integrated. We have discussed the nature of evidence-informed practice, and how advanced practitioners can support the generation of clinically appropriate knowledge that supports pattern integration. How quality care research can be modified to include indicators supporting pattern integration was also addressed. Finally, the idea that features of context that surround direct clinical care have a role in ultimately promoting the integration of knowledge across all patterns as health care is provided by nurses.

References

Barnard, K. E. (1981). An ecological approach to parent-child relations. In C. C. Brown (Ed.), *Infants at Risk: Assessments and interventions.* Madison, CT: Johnson & Johnson Pediatric Round Table.

Barnard, K. E. (1996). Influencing parent-child interactions for children at risk. In M. J. Guralnick (Ed.), *The effectiveness of early intervention* (pp. 249–265). New York, NY: Brookes.

Barnard, K. E., Eyres, S., Lobo, M., & Snyder, C. (1983). An ecological paradigm for assessment and intervention. In T. B. Brazelton, & B. M. Lester (Eds.), *New approaches to developmental screening of infants* (pp. 199–218). New York, NY: Elsevier.

Betts, C. E. (2009). Nursing and the reality of politics. *Nursing Inquiry, 16*, 261–272.

Burkhart, L., & Androwich, I. (2009). Measuring spiritual care with informatics. *ANS. Advances in Nursing Science, 32*, 200–210.

Butterfield, P. G. (2017). Thinking upstream: a 25-year retrospective and conceptual model aimed at reducing health inequities. *ANS. Advances in Nursing Science, 40*(1), 2–11. https://doi.org/10.1097/ANS.0000000 000000161.

Canam, C. J. (2008). The link between nursing discourses and nurses' silence: implication for a knowledge-based discourse for nursing practice. *ANS. Advances in Nursing Science, 31*, 296–307.

Chesla, C. A. (2008). Translational research: essential contributions from interpretive nursing science. *Research in Nursing & Health, 31*, 381–390.

Chung, L. K., Cimprich, B., Janz, N. K., & Mills-Wisneski, S. M. (2009). Breast cancer survivorship program: testing for cross-cultural relevance. *Cancer Nursing, 32*, 236–245.

Copnell, B. (2008). The knowledgeable practice of critical care nurses: a poststructural inquiry. *International Journal of Nursing Studies, 45*, 588–598.

DiCenso, A., Guyatt, G., & Ciliska, D. (2005). *Evidence based nursing: a guide to clinical practice.* St Louis, MO: Mosby.

Doane, G. H., & Varcoe, C. (2008). Knowledge translation in everyday nursing: from evidence-based to inquiry-based practice. *ANS. Advances in Nursing Science, 31*, 283–295.

Doane, G. H., Browne, A. J., Reimer, J., MacLeod, M., & McLellan, E. (2009). Enacting nursing obligations: public health nurses' theorizing in practice. *Research and Theory for Nursing Practice, 23*, 88–106.

Ellenbecker, C. H., & Edward, J. (n.d.). Conducting nursing research to advance and inform health policy. *Policy, Politics & Nursing Practice, 0*(0). https://doi.org/10.1177/1527154417700634.

Fawcett, J., & Garity, J. (2008). *Evaluating research for evidence-based nursing practice.* Philadelphia, PA: F.A. Davis.

Fawcett, J., Watson, J., Neuman, B., Walker, P. H., & Fitzpatrick, J. J. (2001). On nursing theories and evidence. *Journal of Nursing Scholarship: An Official Publication of Sigma Theta Tau International Honor Society of Nursing/Sigma Theta Tau, 33*, 115–119.

Fox, N. J. (2003). Practice-based evidence: toward collaborative and transgressive research. *Sociology, 37*, 81–102.

Galuska, L. A. (2012). Cultivating nursing leadership for our envisioned future. *ANS. Advances in Nursing Science, 35*(4), 333–345. https://doi.org/10.1097/ANS.0b013e318271d2cd.

Horn, S. D., & Gassaway, J. (2007). Practice-base evidence study design for comparative effectiveness research. *Medical Care, 45*, S50–S57.

Jacobs, B. B. (2013). An innovative professional practice model: adaptation of Carper's patterns of knowing, patterns of research, and Aristotle's intellectual virtues. *ANS. Advances in Nursing Science, 36*(4), 271–288. https://doi.org/10.1097/ANS.0000000000000002.

Kagan, P. N., Smith, M. C., & Chinn, P. L. (2014). Introduction. In P. N. Kagan, M. C. Smith, & P. L. Chinn (Eds.), *Philosophies and practices of emancipatory nursing: social justice as praxis* (pp. 1–20). New York, NY: Routledge Taylor & Francis Group.

Lenz, E. R. (2007). Impact on knowledge development and use in practice. In C. Roy, & D. A. Jones (Eds.), *Nursing knowledge development and clinical practice* (pp. 61–77). New York, NY: Springer Publishing.

Porter, S. (2010). Fundamental patterns of knowing in nursing: the challenge of evidence-based practice. *ANS. Advances in Nursing Science, 33*, 1–12.

Posavac, E. J. (2010). *Program evaluation: methods and case studies* (8th ed.). Englewood Cliffs, NJ: Prentice Hall.

Ryan, P. (2009). Integrated theory of health behavior change: background and intervention development. *Clinical Nurse Specialist: The Journal for Advanced Nursing Practice, 23*, 161–172.

Schroeder, P. C., & Maibusch, R. M. (1984). *Nursing quality assurance.* Rockville, MD: Aspen.

Simons, H., Kushner, S., Jones, K. D., & James, D. (2003). From evidence-based practice to practice-based evidence: the idea of situated generalization. *Research Papers in Education, 18*, 347–364.

Smeltzer, C., Hinshaw, A., & Feltman, B. (1987). The benefits of staff nurse involvement in monitoring the quality of patient care. *Journal of Nursing Quality Assurance, 1*, 1–7.

The Essentials of Doctoral Education for Advanced Nursing Practice. (2006). http://www.aacn.nche.edu/DNP/pdf/Essentials.pdf.

Thorne, S., & Sawatzky, R. (2014). Particularizing the general: sustaining theoretical integrity in the context of an evidence-based practice agenda. *ANS. Advances in Nursing Science, 37*, 1–10.

Interpretive Summary: Examples of Broad Theoretic Frameworks Defining the Scope, Philosophy, and General Characteristics of Nursing

The summaries provided here include writings published before 1989. The summaries are not complete descriptions or critical reflections of the theorists' works. Rather they are interpretive descriptions of key features of the frameworks. A notation of the theoretic writing that we used in preparing the summary precedes the summary. The original terminology of the theorists has been retained. Users are cautioned that some of the theorists summarized here have continued to evolve their ideas and certain elements within the theories have changed. For the most part, however, the essential nature of their work has not altered significantly. These summaries are included as a way to keep intact the major theoretic ideas that form nursing's historical theoretic core. Additional work of contemporary theorists who are still actively developing their work as well as the original writing of any theorist of interest should be accessed, described, and critically reflected in order to attain a more complete understanding.

H. E. PEPLAU
Interpersonal Relations in Nursing, 1952
The Art and Science of Nursing, 1988
The patient is an individual with a felt need, and nursing is a process that is both interpersonal and therapeutic. Nursing is the simultaneous application of art and science. The overall goal or purpose of nursing is to educate and be a maturing force so that personality development (a new view of self) occurs. This purpose is achieved when the nurse, as a medium for change, enters into a personal relationship with an individual, the patient, when a felt need presents itself. The personal relationship in nursing provides for meeting the individual patient's needs and assists the two persons (nurse and patient) with different goals to develop or assume congruent goals. The nurse–patient relationship occurs in phases, during which the nurse functions as a resource person, a counselor, and a surrogate. The following four phases take place: orientation, identification, exploitation, and resolution. When a person with a need seeks help, the nurse assists in orientation to the problem. During phase 1 the illness event is integrated. The person learns the facets of the difficulty and the extent of the need for help. Orientating to use of services, productively exploiting anxiety and tension, and learning the limits of necessary space and freedom also occur. This helps to ensure that the illness event is not repressed. When orientation is completed to a given degree, the phase of identification begins. In phase 2 the patient assumes a posture of interdependence, dependence, or independence in relation to the

nurse. The nurse assists the patient during this phase by taking into consideration the services needed and the patient's history. Identification helps assure the patient that the nurse can understand the interpersonal meaning of the patient's situation. When identification is accomplished, phase 3, exploitation, begins. In this phase, the patient derives full value from the relationship by using the services available on the basis of self-interest and needs. Resolution, the final phase, occurs as old needs are met. With resolution of older needs, newer and more mature needs emerge. When needs are resolved, the person is freed from dependence on others. The maturing force of nursing is realized as the personality develops through the educational, therapeutic, and interpersonal process of nursing. The phases of the relationship are serial, and the patient assumes an active role.

During the dyadic nurse–patient relationship and the more extensive nursing relationships with communities, nurses assume many roles, including stranger, teacher, resource person, surrogate, leader, and counselor. Multiple roles occur as a result of multiple problems and needs in individual interpersonal relationships, team functions, and varying social and professional expectations. The overall goal for professional nursing is the same as for the nurse–patient dyads—to implement a process that facilitates personality development by helping people use forces and experiences to ensure maximum productivity.

F. G. ABDELLAH, I. L. BELAND, A. MARTIN, AND R. V. MATHENEY
Patient-Centered Approaches to Nursing, 1960

The patient or family presents with nursing problems that the nurse helps them address through the professional function. The nurse addresses the following 21 problem categories: (1) hygiene and physical comfort, (2) activity and rest, (3) safety, (4) body mechanics, (5) oxygenation, (6) nutrition, (7) elimination, (8) fluid and electrolytes, (9) responses to disease, (10) regulatory mechanisms, (11) sensory function, (12) feelings and reactions, (13) emotions and illness interrelationships, (14) communication, (15) interpersonal relationships, (16) spirituality, (17) therapeutic environment, (18) awareness of self, (19) limitation acceptance, (20) resources to resolve problems, and (21) role of social problems in illness.

Nursing problems are both overt or obvious and covert. Nurses must be aware of covert problems to meet care requirements. Overt and covert problems must be identified to make a nursing diagnosis. Identification of problems precedes solution. The nursing process is the method nurses use to establish and focus on a nursing diagnosis. The overall goal is a patient's fullest possible functioning.

Individualized patient care is important for nursing. Both patients and nurses should be aware of the wholeness of each person and the need for continuity of care from before hospitalization to afterward. Individualized care will require changes in the organization and administration of nursing services and education.

I. J. ORLANDO
The Dynamic Nurse-Patient Relationship: Function, Process, and Principles, 1961
The Discipline and Teaching of Nursing Process: An Evaluation Study, 1972

The patient is an individual with a need that, if supplied, diminishes distress, increases adequacy, or enhances well-being. Needs include requirements for implementing physicians' plans or other innate requirements. The nurse acts to meet needs and thus alleviates distress.

Patients with needs behave verbally and nonverbally in a given manner. The nurse reacts to patient behavior by ascertaining both the meaning of the distress and what would alleviate the distress. Finally the nurse acts to alleviate the distress. Distress can be a result of the following: (1) physical limitations, either temporary or permanent; (2) adverse reactions to the setting, such as being misinterpreted or misinterpreting; and (3) inability to communicate.

Three elements—patient behavior, nurse reactions, and nurse actions—comprise a nursing situation. Patient behavior and nurse reactions relate to the assessment phase of the nursing process and involve ongoing interaction with the nurse. Having clearly ascertained the need through assessment, the nurse acts automatically or deliberatively. Automatic actions are those carried out for reasons other than resolving an immediate need, whereas deliberative actions seek to meet assessed needs. Automatic actions make problems by creating situational conflict that is evidenced through lack of resolution of needs and cooperation (i.e., distress is not alleviated).

Deliberative action yields solutions to problems and also prevents problems. Once the nursing action occurs, the nurse evaluates patient behavior to determine whether the need has been met and the resultant distress has been alleviated. The overall goal is to meet needs and, in that way, to alleviate distress.

E. WIEDENBACH

Clinical Nursing: A Helping Art, 1964

The patient is an individual under treatment or care who experiences needs. Needs are requirements for maintenance or stability in a situation that may be perceived by the individual as a requirement for help and may be met by the person or others. Also, people may have needs and not seek help or may help themselves without recognizing a need. Needs for help are defined as "measures or actions required and desired, which potentially restore or extend ability to cope with situational demands" (p. 6). Nursing is concerned with patients' needs for help. What nurses do and how they do it make up clinical nursing. Clinical nursing has the following four components: (1) philosophy, (2) purpose, (3) practice, and (4) art.

Philosophy is a personal stance of the nurse that embodies attitudes toward reality, and purpose is the overall goal. The purpose of clinical nursing is "to facilitate efforts of individuals to overcome obstacles which interfere with abilities to respond capably to demands made by the condition, environment, situation or time" (p. 15). This purpose is the embodiment of meeting needs for help, which implies goal-directed, deliberate, patient-centered practice actions that require the following: (1) knowledge (factual, speculative, and practical), (2) judgment, and (3) skills (procedural and communication). Practice includes the following four components: (1) identification of the perceived need for help, (2) ministration of help needed, (3) validation that help given was the help needed, and (4) coordination of help and resources for help (i.e., reporting, consulting, and conferring). The art of clinical nursing requires individualized interpretations of behavior in meeting needs for help.

The helping process is triggered by patient behavior that the nurse perceives and interprets. In interpreting behavior the nurse compares the perception to an expectation or hope. Nursing actions may be rational, reactionary, and deliberative. A rational response by the nurse is based on the immediate perception without going beyond to explore hidden meaning. A reactionary response is taken in reaction to strong feelings. Deliberative actions—the desirable mode—intelligibly fulfill nursing's purpose. Identification of needs for help involves the following: (1) observing inconsistencies, acquiring information about how patients mean the cue given, or determining the basis for an observed inconsistency; (2) determining the cause of the discomfort or need for help; and (3) determining whether the need for help can be met by the patient or whether assistance is required. Once needs for help are identified, ministration and validation that help was given follow.

The practice of clinical nursing is bounded by professional, local, legal, and personal constraints. Clinical nursing practice is supported by nursing administration, nursing education, nursing organizations, and nursing research. The clinical goal is to meet needs for help, integrating the practice and process of nursing. Greater professional goals include conservation of life and promotion of health.

L. E. HALL
Another View of Nursing Care and Quality, 1966

The patient is a unity composed of the following three overlapping parts: (1) a person (the core aspect), (2) a pathologic condition and treatment (the cure aspect), (3) and a body (the care aspect). The nurse is a bodily caregiver. Provision of bodily care allows the nurse to comfort and learn the patient's pathologic condition, treatment aspect, and person. Understanding, resulting from the integration of all three areas, allows the nurse to be an effective teacher and nurturer. The patient learns and is nurtured in the person (i.e., in the core aspect). Nurturance leads to effective rehabilitation, greater levels of self-actualization, and self-love.

Nursing occurs during one of two phases of medical care. Phase 1 medical care is the diagnostic and treatment phase; phase 2 is the evaluative, follow-up phase. The professional nurse's role is in phase 2, and professional nursing practice requires a setting in which patients are free to learn. In phase 2 the nurse's goal is to help the patient learn. Motivation to learn is ensured by advocating the patient's learning goals and not the doctor's curative goals. Once patient learning goals are co-determined with the nurse and motivation is therefore ensured, the patient will learn, and nurturance, rehabilitation, and self-love will follow. The overall goal for the patient is rehabilitation, which inspires a greater measure of self-actualization and self-love.

V. HENDERSON
The Nature of Nursing, 1966

The patient is an individual who requires help toward independence. The nurse assists the individual, whether ill or not, to perform activities that will contribute to health, recovery, or peaceful death—activities that the individual who had necessary strength, will, or knowledge would perform unaided. The process of nursing strives to do this as rapidly as possible, and the goal is independence. The nurse manages this process independently of physicians. Help toward independence is given autonomously by the nurse in relation to the following: (1) breathing, (2) eating and drinking, (3) elimination, (4) movement and posture, (5) sleep and rest, (6) clothing, (7) maintenance of body temperature, (8) cleaning and grooming of the body and integument protection,

(9) avoidance of environmental dangers and injury of others, (10) communication, (11) worship, (12) work, (13) play and participation in recreation, and (14) learning and discovery. Nursing can be evaluated as a profession on the basis of the extent to which it enables the individual to achieve each of these functions autonomously.

The role and functions of professional nursing vary with the situation. If the total health care team could be seen as a pie graph in health care situations, in some situations no role exists for certain health care workers. Although there is always a role for family and patients, the pie wedges for team members would vary in size according to the following: (1) the problem of the patient, (2) the patient's self-help ability, and (3) the help resources. Central to nursing's goal to help patients toward independence are empathetic understanding and unlimited knowledge. Empathetic understanding grounded in genuine interest will lead to helping the family understand what a patient needs. The ultimate goal for the nurse is to practice autonomously in helping patients who lack knowledge, physical strength, or strength of will in growth toward independence. Because of this function, nurses seek and promote research, education, and work settings that facilitate this goal.

J. TRAVELBEE
Interpersonal Aspects of Nursing, 1966, 1971
Nursing is an interpersonal process aimed at assisting individuals, families, or communities to prevent or cope with the processes of illness and suffering and, if necessary, to find meaning in the experiences. Nursing's purpose is achieved through human-to-human relationships, which are established by a disciplined intellectual approach to problems, combined with therapeutic use of self. Human-to-human relationships require transcending roles of nurse and patient to establish relatedness and rapport and respond to the humanness of others. Nursing activities are a means to establishing relatedness and rapport and achieving nursing's purpose. Nurses' values and beliefs determine the quality of nursing care provided and thus the extent to which nurses are able to help the ill find meaning in their situation.

Illness and suffering are spiritual, emotional, and physical experiences. The nurse assists the ill patient to experience hope as a means of coping with illness and suffering. Communication, a central concept for Travelbee, implies guiding, planning, and purposely directing interaction to fulfill nursing's purpose. Communication is instrumental in establishing relatedness and rapport (knowing persons), ascertaining and meeting nursing needs, and fulfilling nursing's purpose. Communication also implies that exchanged messages are understood. Communication techniques should enable the nurse to explore and understand the meaning of the person's communication. Establishment of the human-to-human relationship is phasic. The phases are (1) the original encounter, (2) emerging identities, (3) empathy, and (4) sympathy (1971). In such a relationship the needs of the person are met. Achievement of a human-to-human relationship requires openness to experiences and freedom to use personal and experiential background to appreciate and understand the experiences of others.

Health and illness may be defined subjectively and objectively. Objective criteria depend on cultural and societal norms, whereas subjective criteria are peculiar to the human being. The meaning of the symptoms of illness (or criteria for health) for the person is more significant than affixing a label of health or illness to its results.

M. E. LEVINE

The Four Conservation Principles of Nursing, 1967
Introduction to Clinical Nursing, 1973
The Conservation Principles: Twenty Years Later, 1989

A person is a holistic being whose open and fluid boundaries coexist with the environment, which may be perceptual, operational, and conceptual, and is a unity who is to remain conserved and integral. Patients send messages that reflect their current adaptive state. Adaptation is a method of change, and change is life process. When adaptation fails, conservation is threatened, and adaptation needs occur. Adaptive needs are reflected in sent messages.

Nursing occurs at the interface between the open and fluid boundaries of whole persons and environments. The nurse receives and interprets messages and intervenes supportively or therapeutically. Intervention is guided by the following four principles of conservation: conservation of energy, structural integrity, personal integrity, and social integrity. Conservation, based on an assessment of a person's adaptive needs, aids adaptation. When a patient's energy and structural, personal, and social integrity are conserved—that is, when the nurse acts therapeutically—adaptation can better occur, and the person achieves a state of unity and integrity. When conservation cannot be effected in the face of overwhelming adaptation needs, death ensues. Supportive interventions, such as assisting a patient toward peaceful death, are appropriate when adaptation is failing without hope of reversal. The goal for nursing is the wholeness of the patient, brought about by conservation in the four areas when adaptive needs are manifested.

M. E. ROGERS

An Introduction to the Theoretical Basis of Nursing, 1970
Nursing: A Science of Unitary Man, 1980
Science of Unitary Human Beings: A Paradigm for Nursing, 1983
Nursing: A Science of Unitary Human Beings, 1989

A unitary human being is an energy field co-extensive with the universe. Human–environment boundaries are only conceptually imposed and are arbitrary. The unity of human beings and environment is plausible, considering the sameness of matter and energy. Humans are more than and different from the sum of their parts, and generalities about the whole cannot be made from a study of the parts. The energy composing unitary human beings and the environmental field is characterized by four dimensions, in which a given point in time is not tenable. The four concepts—energy fields, openness, pattern and organization, and four-dimensionality—are used to derive principles that postulate how human beings develop. These principles are (1) integrality (formerly complementarity), (2) resonancy, and (3) helicy. According to the principle of integrality, the human and environmental fields interact mutually and simultaneously. Resonancy postulates the nature of wave pattern changes as continuous from lower-frequency to higher-frequency patterns. Helicy asserts that field changes are innovative, probabilistic, and characterized by increasing diversity of field patterns.

Nursing seeks to care for unitary human beings in accordance with its science and art. Science is emergent and based on research and logical analysis of the principles of homeodynamics. Nursing science seeks to describe, explain, and predict. Art is the imaginative and creative use of knowledge and science. Nursing's goal is maximization of health potentials of individuals, family, and groups consistent with health's ever-changing nature. It is achieved by artfully applying emerging science, based on the principles of homeodynamics.

D. E. OREM

Nursing: Concepts of Practice, 1971, 1980, 1985

Orem's self-care deficit theory of nursing includes theories of (1) self-care deficit, (2) self-care, and (3) nursing system. Self-care deficit theory postulates that people benefit from nursing in that they have health-related limitations in providing self-care. Self-care theory postulates that self-care and care of dependents are learned behaviors that purposely regulate human structural integrity, functioning, and development. Nursing systems theory postulates that nursing systems form when nurses prescribe, design, and provide nursing that regulates the individual's self-care capabilities and meets therapeutic self-care requirements.

Assumptions basic to the general theory are as follows:

- Humans require deliberate input to self and environment to be alive and to function.
- The power to act deliberately is exercised in caring for self and others.
- Mature humans sometimes experience limitations in their ability to care for self and others.
- Humans discover, develop, and transmit ways to care for self and others.
- Humans structure relationships and tasks to provide self-care.

Humans need continuous self-care maintenance and regulation and provide this by caring for self, which enables purposeful action. Self-care activities maintain life, health, and well-being. Health refers to the state of a person, which is characterized by soundness or wholeness of developed human structures and bodily and mental functioning. Well-being refers to a person's perceived condition of existence, which is characterized by experiences of contentment, pleasure, happiness, movement toward self-ideals, and continuing personalization.

There are three types of self-care requisites—universal, developmental, and health deviation. Universal requirements relate to meeting common human needs. Developmental self-care requisites relate to conditions that promote developmental processes throughout the life cycle. Health deviation self-care requisites relate to self-care that prevents defects and deviations from normal structure and integrity and those that control the extension and effects of such defects.

Adults care for themselves, whereas infants, the aged, the ill, and the disabled require assistance with self-care activities. When self-care action is limited because of the health state or needs of the care recipient, nursing responds and provides a legitimate service. Thus patients are people with health-related self-care deficits. The following two variables affect these deficits: self-care agency (ability) and self-care demands.

Self-care agency is a learned ability and is deliberate action. Given their focus on care of patients with health-related limitations in self-care abilities, nurses must accurately diagnose self-care agency. Thus they must have information about deficits and their reasons for existing. Such information is basic to selecting helping methods.

Nursing agency regulates or develops patients' self-care agency and ability to meet therapeutic self-care demand. Nursing is a helping service that involves acting or doing for another, guiding and supporting another, providing a developmental environment, and teaching another. Nursing agency varies with educational preparation; orientation to practice situations; mastery of technologies of practice; and ability to accept, work with, and care for others.

Nursing systems may be wholly compensatory, partially compensatory, or supportive-educative. Wholly compensatory systems are required for patients unable to monitor their environment and process information. Such patients are unable to control their movement and position and are unresponsive to stimuli. Partially compensatory systems are designed for patients with limitations in movement as a result of their pathologic condition or injury or who are under medical orders to restrict their movements. Supportive-educative systems are designed for patients who need to learn to perform self-care measures and need assistance to do so. Nursing systems are formed to regulate self-care capabilities and meet therapeutic self-care requirements.

I. M. KING
Toward a Theory for Nursing: General Concepts of Human Behavior, 1971
A Theory for Nursing: Systems, Concepts, Process, 1981
King's General Systems Framework and Theory, 1989
The patient is a personal system within the environment who coexists with other personal systems. Individuals form groups that comprise interpersonal systems, and interpersonal systems contribute to social systems. Thus patient and nurse are composed of personal systems as subsystems within interpersonal and social systems. The nurse must understand given aspects of all three systems. Concepts identified for each system affect total system function. There are three comprehensive concepts: (1) perception for the personal system, (2) organization for the social system, and (3) interaction for the interpersonal system. Personal system concepts related to perception include self, body image, growth and development, time, space, and learning. The nurse also must have knowledge of role, communication, transaction, and stress to understand interactions central to interpersonal system function. Because interaction occurs within social systems—including family, belief, educational, and work systems—nurses require knowledge or organizational concepts of power, authority, control, status, and decision making to function adequately.

The focus for nursing is the human being in the system context. The goal is health. Health implies helping people in groups attain, maintain, and restore health; live with chronic illness or disability; or die with dignity. Interactions of the individual with the environment are significant in influencing life and health. Nurse and patient meet in a health care organization—a patient who needs help and a nurse who offers help. Nurse and patient perceive one another, then act and react, interact, and transact. In this process, presenting conditions are recognized, goal-related decisions are made, and motivation to exert control over events to achieve goals occurs. Transactions are basic to goal attainment and include social exchange, bargaining and negotiating, and sharing a frame of reference toward mutual goal setting. Transactions require perceptual accuracy in nurse–patient interactions and congruence between role performance and role expectation for nurse and patient. Transactions lead to goal attainment, satisfaction, effective care, and enhanced growth and development. The goal of nursing process interaction is transaction, which leads to attainment of goals set in relation to health promotion, maintenance, and recovery from illness.

C. ROY
Introduction to Nursing: An Adaptation Model, 1976, 1984
The Roy Adaptation Model, 1980, 1989
Theory Construction in Nursing: An Adaptation Model, 1981 (with S. Roberts)
The person is an adaptive system. System inputs include the following: (1) three classes of stimuli (focal, contextual, residual) that arise from within the person and the external environment and (2) the adaptation level. The adaptation level is fluid, is composed of all three classes of stimuli, and represents the person's standard or range of stimuli in which responses will be adaptive.

Inputs are mediated by the control process subsystems of cognate and regulator coping mechanisms. The regulator mechanism is an automatic neuroendocrine response, whereas the cognator subsystems represent perception, information processing, and judgments influenced by learning and emotions. Coping activity may or may not be adequate to maintain integrity. A system difficulty is present when coping activity is inadequate as a result of need excesses or deficits.

The system effectors are the adaptive modes. These modes (physiologic, self-concept, role function, and interdependence) are the form in which regulator and cognator subsystems manifest their activity. The adaptive system (person's) output is a response that may be adaptive or ineffective. Adaptive responses are those that contribute to adaptation goals (i.e., responses that promote growth, survival, reproduction, and self-mastery). Adaptation is an ongoing purposive response. Adaptive responses contribute to health and the process of being and becoming integrated; ineffective responses do not.

Using nursing process, the nurse promotes adaptive responses in the adaptive modes during health and illness; thus energy is freed from inadequate coping to promote health and wellness. System responses in each mode are assessed (i.e., described according to objective and subjective data; first-level assessment). Behaviors can be assessed by observation, measurement, and interviews. A tentative judgment about whether the behavior is adaptive or ineffective is then made, and stimuli influencing the adaptive system are then identified (second-level assessment). A nursing diagnosis follows, goals are set, and interventions are selected. Goals are mutually agreed on, and a goal-setting hierarchy is proposed. Survival is a priority goal, followed by goals that promote growth, ensure continuation of the species or society, and promote attainment of full potential. Factors precipitating ineffective behavior are changed, and coping behavior (i.e., adaptation level) is broadened. The person's level of coping is revised continuously. Evaluation of interventions requires returning to the first steps in the nursing process (i.e., noting behaviors manifested by the adaptive system or person).

J. G. PATERSON AND L. T. ZDERAD
Humanistic Nursing, 1976
The person is a unique being, extant in all nursing situations, who innately struggles—to know. Humanistic nursing is an existential experience of being and doing so that

nurturance with another occurs. Fundamentally, nursing is a response to human need that can be described to build a humanistic nursing science.

Humanistic nursing requires that the participants be aware of their uniqueness, as well as their commonality with others. Authenticity is required—an in-touchness with self that comes in part with experiencing. Humanistic nursing also presupposes responsible choices. The ability of an individual to make choices based on authentic awareness and knowledge of such choices is a concern of humanistic nursing and cultivates moreness. Also, a commitment to the value of humanistic nursing must be present.

A nurse with the foregoing attitudes and qualities can offer genuine presence to another. Humanistic nursing concerns the basic nursing act: the response of one human in need to another. At this level, nursing is related to the health-illness quality of the human condition: nurturance toward more being.

M. M. LEININGER

Transcultural Nursing: Concepts, Theories, and Practices, 1978
Caring: A Central Focus of Nursing and Health Care Services, 1980
The Phenomenon of Caring: Importance, Research Questions and Theoretical Considerations, 1981
Leininger's Theory of Nursing: Cultural Care Diversity and Universality, 1988

Caring is postulated as the central and unifying domain for nursing knowledge and practices. Diverse factors influence patterns of care and health or well-being in different cultures. Caring includes assistive, supportive, and facilitative acts for another individual or a group with evident or anticipated needs. Caring serves to ameliorate or improve human conditions through behaviors, techniques, processes, and patterns. Professional nursing care embodies scientific and humanistic modes of helping or enabling receipt of personalized service to maintain a healthy condition for life or death.

Caring emphasizes healthful, enabling activities of individuals and groups that are based on culturally defined ascribed or sanctioned helping modes. Caring behaviors include comfort, compassion, concern, coping behavior, empathy, enabling, facilitating, interest, involvement, health-consultative acts, health-instruction acts, health-maintenance acts, helping behaviors, love, nurturance, presence, protective behaviors, restorative behaviors, sharing, stimulating behaviors, stress alleviation, succorance, support, surveillance, tenderness, touching, and trust (1981). Culture determines personal life or world views that are mediated through language. Contextual factors such as technology, religion, philosophic beliefs, social and kinship lines and patterns, values and life ways, political and legal factors, economic factors, and educational factors all influence care patterns. Likewise, these factors affect care patterns and the health of individuals and families, as well as groups. Diverse health systems mediate the expression of health. Nursing is one health system that overlaps with folk systems and professional health care systems.

Human caring is a universal phenomenon, and every nursing situation has transcultural nursing care elements. Caring is essential to human development, growth, and survival, and caring behaviors vary transculturally in priorities, expression, and needs satisfaction. Caring plays a more important role in recovery than in cure but receives less reward. If effective, caring reflects professional concern, compassion, stress alleviation, nurturance, comfort, and protection. Nursing should provide care consistent with its emergent science and knowledge, with caring as a central focus. Caring and culture are inextricably linked, and nursing care should be culturally congruent and aimed at preserving, maintaining, accommodating, negotiating, repatterning, and restructuring care patterns.

J. WATSON

Nursing: The Philosophy and Science of Caring, 1979
Nursing: Human Science and Human Care, 1985
New Dimensions of Human Caring Theory, 1988
Watson's Philosophy and Theory of Human Caring in Nursing, 1989
The following are assumptions underlying human care values in nursing: (1) care and love comprise the primal and universal psychic energy and (2) care and love are requisite for our survival and the nourishment of humanity. Caring for and loving self is a requisite to caring for others. Curing is not the end to be sought but is a means to care. Nursing's ability to sustain its caring ideology and translate it into practice will determine its contribution to society. Nursing traditionally has held a caring stance in relation to patients with health and illness concerns, and caring is the unifying focus for practice in nursing. Caring has received little emphasis in the health care system, and the caring values of nursing are critical to sustaining care ideals in practice. Preservation of human care is a significant issue; human care can be practiced only interpersonally; and nursing's social, moral, and scientific contributions lie in its commitment to human care ideals. The foregoing assumptions provide a rationale for developing nursing as a human science.

Humans are capable of transcending time and space, and each possesses a spirit, soul, or essence that enables self-awareness, higher degrees of consciousness, and a power to transcend the usual self. Human life is a continuous (with time and space) being in the world. Caring, an intersubjective human process, is the moral ideal of nursing. Human care processes have an energy field and involve engagement of mind-body-soul with another in a lived moment. Illness, not necessarily disease, is a state of subjective turmoil in which the self as "I" is separated from the self as "me." Conversely, health is a harmony within mind-body-soul in which the "I" and "me" are aligned. A healthy person is open to increased diversity. The goal of nursing is to help people increase harmony within mind-body-soul, which leads to self-knowledge, self-reverence, self-healing, and self-care.

Theoretic premises identified include the following: at nursing's highest level, the nurse makes contact with the person's emotional and subjective world as the route to inner self; mind and soul are not confined in time and space and to the physical universe; and a nurse can access inner self through the mind-body-soul, provided the physical body is not perceived separate from the higher sense of self. The geist (spirit or inner self) exists in and for itself and relates to the human ability to be free; love and caring are universal givens; and illness may be hidden from the "eyes" and requires finding meaning in inner experiences. Finally, the totality of experiences at the moment constitutes a phenomenal field or the individual's frame of reference.

Humans strive to satisfy needs experienced in the perceived phenomenal field, including being cared for, loved, and valued and experiencing positive regard, acceptance, and understanding. People also strive to achieve union, transcend individual life, and find harmony with life. All needs are subservient to a basic striving toward actualizing spiritual self and establishing harmony within mind-body-soul. Harmony is consistent with a sense of congruence between "I" and "me," between self as perceived and self as experienced, and between subjective reality (phenomenal field) and external reality (world as is).

Caring occasions involve action and choice by the nurse and individual. If the caring occasion is transpersonal, the limits of openness and human capacities are expanded. Transpersonal caring relationships depend on the following: (1) moral commitments to enhance human dignity to allow people to determine their own meaning, (2) the nurse's affirmation of the subjective significance of the person, (3) the nurse's ability to detect feelings of another's inner condition and feel a union with another, and (4) the nurse's history of living and experiencing feelings and human conditions and imagining others' feelings (i.e., personal growth, maturation, and development of the nurse's self).

Nursing interventions related to human care are referred to as carative factors and include nurturing, forming, cultivating, and using the following: (1) a humanistic-altruistic system of values; (2) faith–hope; (3) sensitivity to self and others; (4) helping-trusting human care relationships; (5) expressed positive and negative feelings; (6) a creative problem-solving caring process; (7) transpersonal teaching–learning; (8) support-ive, protective, and/or corrective mental, physical, societal, and spiritual environments; (9) human needs assistance; and (10) existential-phenomenologic spiritual forces. Carative factors are actualized in the human care process.

M. A. NEWMAN

Theory Development in Nursing, 1979
Newman's Health Theory, 1983
Health as Expanding Consciousness, 1986
Individuals are subsumed by a greater whole and are part of multiple system levels in space. Explicit assumptions are made in relation to health, pathologic conditions, and patterns. Health can encompass pathology and disease; therefore, disease and health are not continuous variables or opposites. Pathology is manifested according to a preexisting unitary pattern; thus disease gives clues to the pattern of a person's life, and pattern is reflected in energy exchange within humans and between humans and the environment. Personal patterns manifesting as disease are part of larger patterns, which are not altered when the disease is eliminated. Disease as a pattern manifestation may be considered health. The existence of disease may evoke ten-sion, an important evolutionary ingredient. Disease is not advocated as a desirable state, but the significance of attending to the meaning of the disease is highlighted. Health is an expansion of consciousness, and pattern-manifesting disease expands consciousness.

Consciousness, the informational capacity of the system, is reflected in both the qual-ity and quantity of responses to stimuli. Health involves developing awareness of self and environment, coupled with increased ability to perceive and respond to alternatives.

Movement is a central concept, a property of life. The concepts of consciousness, time, movement, and space are interrelated in that movement reflects consciousness and is an identifiable and specific individual characteristic. Time is an index of consciousness and a function of movement. Movement is the means by which time and space become reality, and space and time have a complementary relationship. Without movement, time and space are not real, and there is no change at any system level. Movement reflects the organization of consciousness and therefore reflects health. The implied goal is consciousness expansion and therefore health and life. Health is not a state but an experienced process.

D. E. JOHNSON
The Behavioral System Model for Nursing, 1980
The individual patient is a behavioral system composed of subsystems. As a behavioral system, the patient's subsystems strive to maintain balance by making adjustments to factors impinging on them. Humans seek experiences that may disturb balance and require behavior modifications to reestablish balance. Behavioral systems are essential and reflect adaptations that are successful. The behavioral system is composed of behaviors that form an integrated unit. Behavioral systems maintain their own integrity, link individuals with environment, and are self-perpetuating if environmental conditions remain orderly and predictable. The multiple tasks of behavioral systems require continual system changes, including subsystem evolution. Subsystems also must be protected, nurtured, and stimulated.

Behavioral system subsystems are formed from responses or response tendencies that share a common goal and are modified by maturation and experience. Each subsystem of the overall behavioral system has a specialized task or function that can be described on the basis of that structure and function. The following are the four structural elements in each subsystem: (1) drive stimulated or goal sought; (2) set or predisposition to act in a given way; (3) choices, or scope of action alternatives; and (4) behavior. Only the last structural element is observable. The following seven subsystems are identified: (1) attachment or affiliative, (2) dependency, (3) ingestive, (4) eliminative, (5) sexual, (6) aggressive, and (7) achievement. The attachment subsystem responses provide security, and dependency provides for nurturance responses. The ingestive and eliminative subsystems relate to eating and excretion of waste. The sexual subsystem relates to the dual responses of procreation and sexual fulfillment. The aggressive subsystem functions to preserve the person, and the achievement system functions so that mastery of self and the environment is fostered.

Nursing problems are manifested when subsystems cannot maintain a dynamic stability or when the subsystem has not achieved an optimum level of function. Anticipated problems in subsystems can be prevented, and manifested problems can be solved. The nurse acts to impose a regulatory mechanism, change structural units, and fulfill functional requirements of subsystems. The nursing act seeks to "preserve the organization and integration of the patient's behavior at an optimal level under those conditions in which the behavior constitutes a threat to physical or social health, or in which illness is found" (p. 214).

B. NEUMAN
The Betty Neuman Health Care Systems Model: A Total Person Approach to Patient Problems, 1980
The Neuman Systems Model, 1982, 1989
The person is a unique, holistic system yet possesses a common range of normal characteristics and responses. Persons are a dynamic composite of physiologic, psychologic, sociocultural, developmental, and spiritual variables. These variables interact with internal and external environmental stressors. The holistic system of the person is open. As an open system it interacts with, adjusts to, and is adjusted by the environment. The external environment is defined as all that interfaces with the person's system. The internal and external environments are a source of stressors that have different potentials to disturb the normal line of defense and disrupt the system. The normal line of defense essentially is the usual steady state of the individual and is composed of the normal range of responses to stressors within people that evolve over time. The flexible line of defense cushions and protects individuals from stressors. Lines of resistance are conceptualized as internal factors that help people defend against stressors, and they protect the core structure and stabilize and return individuals to a normal line of defense when stressors break through.

The system's model is based on an individual's relationship to stress, reaction to it, and reconstitution factors that are dynamic in nature. The nurse assesses, manages, and evaluates patient systems. Nursing's focus is the variables that affect a person's response to stressors. Assessment of individuals considers knowledge of factors influencing a patient's perceptual field, the meaning stressors have to a patient as validated by patient and caregiver, and factors the caregiver believes influence the patient situation. Basically, nursing focuses on the occurrence of stressors, the organism's response to them, and the state of the organism. Primary prevention identifies and allays risk factors associated with stressors; it focuses on protecting the normal line of defense and strengthening the flexible line of defense. Secondary prevention is related to symptomatology, intervention priorities, and treatment; it helps to strengthen internal lines of defense. Death occurs if the basic core structure of the system fails to support the intervention. Tertiary prevention protects reconstitution or return to wellness after treatment.

Nursing acts to impede or arrest an entropic state or a state of disorder and disorganization. Health is a state of movement toward negentropy or evolution; it is a state of inertness free from disrupting needs. Health implies a homeostatic balance. This balance depends on free energy flow between the organism and the environment. In health the system's normal line of defense is maintained, and the lines of resistance are intact; the basic structural elements of the system are preserved.

R. R. PARSE
Man-Living-Health: A Theory of Nursing, 1981, 1989
Nursing Science: Major Paradigms, Theories, and Critiques, 1987
The person is unitary—that is, an indivisible being who interrelates with the environment while co-creating health. Theoretic assumptions synthesize the concepts of energy field, openness, pattern and organization, four-dimensionality, helicy, integrality, co-constitution, coexistence, and situated freedom with tenets of human subjectivity and intentionality. Assumptions (nine in the 1981 book were reduced to three in the 1987

chapter) state that man is a recognizable pattern who evolves simultaneously with environment. Man–environment relationships are such that a continuity of what was and what will be unfolds in the now. Man chooses the meaning given to co-created situations and is responsible for choices made. Unitary man is recognized by individual patterns of relating, which are co-created in man–environment interchange. There is mutual man–environment interrelatedness as man chooses to move toward irreversible possibilities. Man experiences in multiple dimensions simultaneously and relatively. The negentropic interchange of man–environment both enables and limits becoming.

Health is an open process of becoming, an incarnation of man's choosing. As man and environment connect and separate, health is co-created. Thus health is a synthesis of values co-created in open interchange with environment. Health is a continuous process of transcending with the possibles—that is, reaching beyond the actual. Health is an emergent—a negentropic unfolding. The theory of man-living-health emerges from the stated assumptions, and the following three principles are notable: (1) structuring meaning multidimensionally is co-creating reality through the languaging of valuing and imaging, (2) co-creating rhythmic patterns of relating is living the paradoxical unity of revealing-concealing and enabling-limiting while connecting-separating, and (3) co-transcending with the possibles is powering unique ways or originating in the process of transforming (1987).

Principle 1 asserts that reality is continually co-created by assigning meaning to all-at-once experiences occurring multidimensionally. Imaging, valuing, and languaging serve to structure meaning multidimensionally. Principle 2 asserts that there is an unfolding cadence of co-constituting ways of being. Ways of being are recognized in the man–environment interchange and are lived rhythmically. Rhythms of revealing-concealing, enabling-limiting, and connecting-separating are integral in the principles. The final principle asserts that concepts of co-transcending with the possibles—powering, originating, and transforming—are man's ways of aspiring toward the "not-yet." The following three theoretic structures are posited: (1) powering is a way of revealing and concealing imaging, (2) originating is a manifestation of enabling and limiting valuing, and (3) transforming unfolds in the languaging of connecting and separating (1981).

NOLA J. PENDER
Health Promotion in Nursing Practice, 1982, 1987
The Health Promotion Model describes sets of variables that determine the likelihood that individuals will engage in health-promoting behavior. These include cognitive-perceptual factors, modifying factors, and cues to action. The model is linear in nature and identifies seven cognitive-perceptual factors and five modifying factors that determine an individual's likelihood of participation in health-promoting behavior. Cognitive-perceptual factors have a direct effect on the likelihood of engaging in health-promoting behaviors. Cognitive-perceptual factors include perceptions of the individual in relation to health status, importance of health, control over health, and meaning of health, along with perceived self-efficacy and benefits/barriers to health-promoting behavior. Situational, behavioral, interpersonal, biologic, and demographic factors indirectly affect engagement in health-promoting behaviors by modifying cognitive-perceptual factors. Cues to action also directly affect a person's likelihood of engaging in health-promoting behaviors. The model focuses on individual persons and assumes that individuals have

potential to exhibit behavior that promotes or deters health. The function of the nurse is inferred to be that of positively influencing health-promoting behavior. It is assumed that health-promoting behaviors are useful to promote health states. Thus the goal for the individual person is to exhibit behavior that promotes health.

P. BENNER AND J. WRUBEL
The Primacy of Caring, 1989

Caring is primary because it determines and constitutes what matters to people. Subsequently caring creates possibilities for coping, enables possibilities for connecting with, and concern for, others, and allows giving and receiving help. Caring determines what is stressful to people and how they will cope.

Drawing on Heideggerian phenomenology, Benner and Wrubel posit a phenomenologic view of the person central to this view of caring. The person is a self-interpreting being who is defined by the process of living and being in the world. Through the process of living, people come to possess a nonreflective view of the self and immediately can grasp the meaning of a situation; that is, people understand the meaning of a context without conscious, deliberative reflection. This immediate grasping of situational meaning—self-interpretation—is possible because of the following human characteristics: (1) embodied intelligence, (2) acquisition of background meaning, and (3) concern.

Embodied intelligence is the capacity of being in a situation in meaningful ways and effortlessly understanding it in relation to self. Background meanings are the cultural traditions "given" to a person from birth. These two features account for how people are in the world. Concern, the third characteristic of self-interpreting beings, accounts for why people are involved in the world in certain ways. These three characteristics are central to involvement with the world in ways that ensure people will grasp the meaning of situations in relation to the situation's meaning for them. Both nurse and patient are self-interpreting beings. This view of the person as self-interpreting is central to understanding how caring and concern in nursing relate to understanding and facilitating stress-coping situations in patients.

People have both freedoms and constraints that result from the assumption that people are self-interpreting (i.e., their being is contextual or situational, and they interpret contexts in relation to self). In this view, ordinary life experiences both create and determine stress and coping patterns of people. When illness and disease inevitably occur in the course of living, life contexts change and situational meanings alter. Old self understandings do not work, a qualitatively different form of stress occurs, and the need for new patterns of coping emerges. New coping possibilities do exist in current situations, but these are understood in the context of old habits, skills, practices, and expectations. These new possibilities and freedoms within the present contexts and situations (like the old possibilities and freedoms that no longer work) are not readily understood by the person.

Nursing is a process of helping people cope with the stress of illness, not by following sets of prescribed rules but by contextually dependent caring and concern. Understanding the illness experience of the patient is central to concern and caring. Illness is a central focus of nursing. Illness is not reducible to disease (cellular pathology), but it connotes human loss experiences and dysfunction precipitated by human loss. Because nursing concerns itself with the relationship between the disease process and the illness experience of self-interpreting beings, a concept of mind–body dualism is not possible.

Caring in the context of nursing depends on discerning problems; recognizing solutions; and helping patients implement, and live, a solution. Thus nursing is a moral act that goes beyond mere application of scientific knowledge. Understanding the illness experience of the person is central to helping an individual come to live meaningful coping processes and return to health. Being present for patients and using expert interpretive skills facilitate concern as a vehicle for caring. Caring concern is central to human (nurse and patient) understanding of the situation of illness. Concern allows both nurse and patient to be in touch with the patient's lived experience. Emotions are a particular focus for concern because they are essential to patient and nurse understanding of the context of the patient, they provide clues to what is important in the situation, and they are linked to past experiences that need to be focused on and reinterpreted in the context of the present. This reinterpretation of past experiences and of old patterns of coping with life's inevitable stresses creates new contexts, and the situated freedoms and possibilities inherent in the present are more fully illuminated. New coping options result.

Because human beings can inhabit a common world with common meanings, common stress and coping patterns will exist. Phenomenologically grounded scientific study of stress and coping would reveal those common themes, meanings, and personal concerns as a basis for understanding caring practices in nursing.

References

Abdellah, F. G., et al. (1960). *Patient-centered approaches to nursing.* New York, NY: Macmillan.

Benner, P., & Wrubel, J. (1989). *The primacy of caring.* Menlo Park, CA: Addison-Wesley.

Hall, L. E. (1966). Another view of nursing care and quality. In K. M. Straub, & K. S. Parker (Eds.), *Continuity in patient care: the role of nursing.* Washington, DC: Catholic University Press.

Henderson, V. (1966). *The nature of nursing.* New York, NY: Macmillan.

Johnson, D. E. (1980). The behavioral system model for nursing. In J. P. Riehl, & C. Roy (Eds.), *Conceptual models for nursing practice* (2nd ed.). New York, NY: Appleton-Century-Crofts.

King, I. M. (1971). *Toward a theory for nursing: general concepts of human behavior.* New York, NY: Wiley.

King, I. M. (1981). *A theory for nursing: systems, concepts, process.* New York, NY: Wiley.

King, I. M. (1989). King's general systems framework and theory. In J. Riehl-Sisca (Ed.), *Conceptual models for nursing practice* (3rd ed.). Norwalk, CT: Appleton & Lange.

Leininger, M. M. (1978). *Transcultural nursing: concepts, theories, and practices.* New York, NY: Wiley.

Leininger, M. M. (1980). Caring: a central focus of nursing and health care services. *Nursing Health Care, 1,* 135.

Leininger, M. M. (1981). The phenomenon of caring: importance, research questions and theoretical considerations. In *Caring: an essential human need (proceedings of the three national caring conferences).* Thorofare, NJ: Charles B. Slack.

Leininger, M. M. (1988). Leininger's theory of nursing: cultural care diversity and universality. *Nursing Science Quarterly, 1,* 152.

Levine, M. E. (1967). The four conservation principles of nursing. *Nursing Forum, 6,* 45.

Levine, M. E. (1973). *Introduction to clinical nursing* (2nd ed.). Philadelphia, PA: FA Davis.

Levine, M. E. (1989). The conservation principles: twenty years later. In J. Riehl-Sisca (Ed.), *Conceptual models for nursing practice* (3rd ed.). Norwalk, CT: Appleton & Lange.

Neuman, B. (1980). The Betty Neuman health care systems model: a total person approach to patient problems. In J. P. Riehl, & C. Roy (Eds.), *Conceptual models for nursing practice* (2nd ed.). New York, NY: Appleton-Century-Crofts.

Neuman, B. (1982). *The Neuman systems model*. Norwalk, CT: Appleton-Century-Crofts.

Neuman, B. (1989). *The Neuman systems model* (2nd ed.). Norwalk, CT: Appleton & Lange.

Newman, M. A. (1979). *Theory development in nursing*. Philadelphia, PA: FA Davis.

Newman, M. A. (1983). Newman's health theory. In I. W. Clements, & F. B. Roberts (Eds.), *Family health: a theoretical approach to nursing care*. New York, NY: Wiley.

Newman, M. A. (1986). *Health as expanding consciousness*. St. Louis, MO: Mosby.

Orem, D. E. (1971). *Nursing: concepts of practice*. New York, NY: McGraw-Hill.

Orem, D. E. (1980). *Nursing: concepts of practice* (2nd ed.). New York, NY: McGraw-Hill.

Orem, D. E. (1985). *Nursing: concepts of practice* (3rd ed.). New York, NY: McGraw-Hill.

Orlando, I. J. (1961). *The dynamic nurse–patient relationship: function, process, and principles*. New York, NY: G. P. Putman's Sons (republished in 1990 by the National League for Nursing).

Orlando, I. J. (1972). *The discipline and teaching of nursing process: an evaluation study*. New York, NY: G. P. Putnam's Sons.

Parse, R. R. (1981). *Man-living-health: a theory of nursing*. New York, NY: Wiley.

Parse, R. R. (1987). *Nursing science: major paradigms, theories, and critiques*. Philadelphia, PA: WB Saunders.

Parse, R. R. (1989). Man-living-health: a theory of nursing. In J. Riehl-Sisca (Ed.), *Conceptual models for nursing practice* (3rd ed.). Norwalk, CT: Appleton & Lange.

Paterson, J. G., & Zderad, L. T. (1976). *Humanistic nursing*. New York, NY: Wiley (republished in 1987 by the National League for Nursing).

Pender, N. J. (1982). *Health promotion in nursing practice*. New York, NY: Appleton-Century-Crofts.

Pender, N. J. (1987). *Health promotion in nursing practice* (2nd ed.). Norwalk, CT: Appleton-Lange.

Peplau, H. E. (1952). *Interpersonal relations in nursing*. New York, NY: G. P. Putnam's Sons.

Peplau, H. E. (1988). The art and science of nursing: similarities, differences, and relations. *Nursing Science Quarterly*, *9*, 8.

Rogers, M. E. (1970). *An introduction to the theoretical basis of nursing*. Philadelphia, PA: FA Davis.

Rogers, M. E. (1980). Nursing: a science of unitary man. In J. P. Riehl, & C. Roy (Eds.), *Conceptual models for nursing practice* (2nd ed.). New York, NY: Appleton-Century-Crofts.

Rogers, M. E. (1983). Science of unitary human beings: a paradigm for nursing. In I. W. Clements, & F. B. Roberts (Eds.), *Family health: a theoretical approach to nursing care*. New York, NY: Wiley.

Rogers, M. E. (1989). Nursing: a science of unitary human beings. In J. Riehl-Sisca (Ed.), *Conceptual models for nursing practice* (3rd ed.). Norwalk, CT: Appleton & Lange.

Roy, C. (1976). *Introduction to nursing: an adaptation model*. Englewood Cliffs, NJ: Prentice-Hall.

Roy, C. (1980). The Roy adaptation model. In J. P. Riehl, & C. Roy (Eds.), *Conceptual models for nursing practice* (2nd ed.). New York, NY: Appleton-Century-Crofts.

Roy, C. (1984). *Introduction to nursing: an adaptation model* (2nd ed.). Norwalk, CT: Appleton-Century-Crofts.

Roy, C. (1989). The Roy adaptation model. In J. Riehl-Sisca (Ed.), *Conceptual models for nursing practice* (3rd ed.). Norwalk, CT: Appleton & Lange.

Roy, C., & Roberts, S. (1981). *Theory construction in nursing: an adaptation model*. Englewood Cliffs, NJ: Prentice-Hall.

Travelbee, J. (1966). *Interpersonal aspects of nursing*. Philadelphia, PA: FA Davis.

Travelbee, J. (1971). *Interpersonal aspects of nursing* (2nd ed.). Philadelphia, PA: FA Davis.

Watson, J. (1979). *Nursing: the philosophy and science of caring*. Boston, MA: Little, Brown (republished in 1988 by the National League for Nursing).

Watson, J. (1985). *Nursing: human science and human care*. Norwalk, CT: Appleton-Century-Crofts.

Watson, J. (1988). New dimensions of human caring theory. *Nursing Science Quarterly*, *9*, 175.

Watson, J. (1989). Watson's philosophy and theory of human caring in nursing. In J. Riehl-Sisca (Ed.), *Conceptual models for nursing practice* (3rd ed.). Norwalk, CT: Appleton & Lange.

Wiedenbach, E. (1964). *Clinical nursing: a helping art*. New York, NY: Springer.

Glossary

This glossary contains definitions that we have created for the purposes of this book. Some are common definitions that are consistent with the meanings that are generally found in the nursing literature. Other definitions are consistent with generally accepted meanings but adapted—we think appropriately—to suit our purposes and perspectives. We ask you to use the glossary with the understanding that we are not the final authority with regard to meanings. Our definitions are reasonable and carefully formulated, but other nuances of meaning for many of these terms are possible.

abstract concept Mental image derived largely from indirect evidence that is not easily presented by a specific empiric indicator.

accessibility Trait of theory that is useful for questioning and clarifying the degree to which concepts have indicators in observable reality and, subsequently, how attainable are the outcomes, goals, and purposes of the theory.

aesthetic criticism Form of knowledge within the aesthetics pattern that is a discursive representation of meaning for expressions of aesthetic knowledge; criticism is formed from aesthetic methods that are designed to deepen shared meanings for aesthetic knowing.

aesthetics Fundamental pattern of knowing in nursing related to the perception of deep meanings that call forth inner creative resources to transform experience into what is not yet real but is possible; expressed as knowledge through works of art and criticism and integrated in practice as transformative art/acts.

allies Persons who are not directly affected by a particular disadvantage, injustice, or unfair practice but who join those who are affected; allies honor the perspectives of the disadvantaged while they assist with efforts to rectify injustices and create more equitable situations.

appreciation Process of focusing and reflecting on aesthetic knowledge as it is understood and valued by members of the discipline; interacts with the process of inspiration to challenge and authenticate aesthetic knowledge.

assumption Structural component of theory that is taken for granted or thought to be true without systematically generated empiric evidence; theoretic assumptions may be value statements or may have the potential for empiric testing, but are assumed to be true within the theory because the assumptions are reasonable.

atomistic theory Theory that deals with a narrow scope of phenomena; the term often implies an assumption that the whole may be understood from a study of the parts.

authentication Processes within each of the patterns of knowing for evaluating and assessing the soundness of knowledge that is formally expressed; each pattern requires specific approaches for authentication that reflect the pattern's form of expression and knowing.

axiom Type of premise used in deductive logic that is often not tentative but relatively firm; axioms as premises are used for deducing theorems, especially in mathematics.

centering Process that involves a deliberate focus on inner feelings, perceptions, and experiences and that involves contemplation and introspection to form deep inner personal meaning from life experiences; interacts with the process of opening to create personal knowledge.

clarifying [values] Process that involves a deliberate focus on understanding the values undergirding ethical decisions and dilemmas and on bringing to full understanding those actions that are right and good; interacts with the process of exploring [alternatives} to create ethical knowledge.

clarity Trait of theory that is useful for questioning and understanding the degree to which a theory is semantically and structurally lucid and consistent.

codes Form of knowledge expression within the ethics pattern; codes are shorthand expressions of prescribed professional behaviors that are generally accepted as right and good; codes primarily describe behaviors that represent the nurse's accountability as expressed in rights, duties, and obligations.

components of theory Features of theory that are useful for describing theory and that form a template for critically reflecting theory; components include purpose, concepts, definitions, relationships, structure, and assumptions.

concept Complex mental formulation of experience; concepts are a major component of theory and convey the abstract ideas within the theory.

conceptual framework Logical grouping of related concepts or theories that is usually created to draw together several different aspects that are relevant to a complex situation, such as a practice setting or an educational program; term used synonymously with *theoretic framework;* knowledge form within the empiric pattern.

conceptualizing General process within the empiric pattern that focuses on identifying, defining, and creating meaning for concepts within theory; conceptualizing includes but is not limited to the focused process of creating conceptual meaning.

conclusions Relationship statements that are derived from premises in a deductive logic system; conclusions are a type of proposition and may take the form of a theorem or hypothesis.

confirmation In qualitative research, the processes of establishing the validity of empiric theory and research; in some qualitative methods, confirmation may be assumed as a result of the methodology used; confirmation may also require the theory and research to be used in additional settings.

consistency Theory trait related to clarity; consistency may be semantic or structural and refers to the general agreement, harmony, and compatibility of components within the theory.

construct Type of highly abstract and complex concept; constructs are formed from multiple less abstract or more empiric concepts.

creating conceptual meaning Theory development process of identifying, examining, and clarifying the mental images that comprise the elements, variables, or concepts within a theory; process that conveys the thoughts, feelings, and ideas that reflect the human experience of the concept.

criteria for concepts Essential features of a concept formed by examining conceptual meaning; criteria are designed with reference to the purposes for which the concept is being used and should be useful to identify the concept and to differentiate it from other concepts.

criteria for nursing diagnoses Essential features for a specific diagnosis to be used in a given instance or situation encountered in nursing practice.

critical analysis Form of formal expression of emancipatory knowledge; critical analyses illuminate meanings that would otherwise remain hidden and that can be informed by multiple perspectives, including feminist, liberal, poststructural, and postcolonial.

critical multiplism Approach to inquiry that integrates multiple methodologic processes within the research inquiry process; sometimes refers to the combining of qualitative and quantitative approaches to data collection to reduce bias.

critical reflection Process that questions the function, purposes, and value of empiric knowledge structures, especially theory, as reflected in the clarity, generality, simplicity, accessibility, and importance of the structure; the questioning process does not imply an expected response; for example, inquiring about clarity does not imply that clarity is desirable.

critical theory Broad term used to describe both the process and the product of analyses that take a historically situated and sociopolitical perspective; critical theory seeks to undermine dominant power structures that create inequities and that maintain oppression and other forms of social injustice.

critical thinking Deliberate use of clear, concise, and thorough thought processes that consider diverse elements of a broad array of existing problems with the intent of solving the problem; emancipatory knowing builds on critical thinking but focuses on problems related to social and political inequities; unlike critical thinking, emancipatory knowing requires the examination and understanding of how sociopolitical networks sustain unfair institutionalized practices.

critiquing Creative inquiry process for emancipatory knowing that exposes the hidden dynamics and meanings that are structured and institutionalized by social, cultural, and political practices and ideologies.

deconstruction Process of uncovering hidden and oppressive assumptions, ideologies, and frames of reference within text; deconstruction makes visible features of text that cannot be justified as a basis for truth; its purpose is to uncover conventions of language and social practices that promote and sustain inequities and injustices.

deduction Form of reasoning that moves from the general to the specific; in deductive logic, two or more premises as relational statements are used to draw a conclusion; in deductive research processes, an abstract theoretic relationship is used to derive specific questions or hypotheses.

definition   Component of theory that indicates the empiric basis for a concept; definitions are statements of meaning that provide a link between theoretic abstractions and empiric indicators; may be relatively general or specific.

deliberative utilization and validation of theory   Theory development process that refines and develops empiric knowledge in relation to practice; involves processes that refine conceptual meaning and validate theoretic relationships and outcomes within practice contexts.

demystification   Process of making things visible, especially oppressive social practices; the open disclosure of that which was formerly hidden from understanding.

descriptive relationships   Statements that provide an account of what something is; descriptive relationships provide an image or impression of the nature or attributes of a phenomenon.

dialogue   Process of exchanging various points of view concerning what is right, good, or responsible; interacts with the process of justification to challenge and authenticate ethical knowledge.

discipline   Group of individuals engaged in developing knowledge; the structured knowledge within an area of concern or a domain of inquiry.

discourse   Interconnected systems or patterns of language, symbols, and human communications that create meanings and behavior.

discourse analysis   Inquiry approach that focuses on understanding patterns of language as well as other symbolic systems of communication (e.g., television, artwork, advertisements) as constitutive of meanings and behavior; in discourse analysis, interconnected symbolic systems (i.e., discourses) are assumed to create historically situated meanings and behavior; critical discourse analysis focuses on decentering dominant discourses that perpetuate power and justice inequities.

emancipatory knowing   Pattern of knowing that makes social and structural change possible; the ability to recognize barriers that create unfair and unjust social conditions and to analyze complex elements of the sociopolitical context to change a situation to one that improves people's lives; praxis, which is value-motivated and constant reflection and action to transform the world, is the fundamental process of emancipatory knowing.

empiric indicators   Sensory experience linked to a concept; more empirically grounded concepts have more direct empiric indicators; abstract concepts require the construction of indirect measures or tools that provide an approximate empiric measurement of some feature of the phenomenon.

empiric-abstract continuum   Means of visualizing or representing the extent to which concepts have a basis in empiric reality; empiric concepts have a direct reality basis and are more directly experienced, whereas abstract concepts have an indirect basis in empiric reality and are more mentally constructed.

empirics Fundamental pattern of knowing in nursing that is focused on the use of sensory experience for the creation of mediated knowledge expressions; expressed as knowledge with the use of theories and formal descriptions and integrated in practice as scientific competence.

empowerment Growing capacity of individuals and groups to exercise their will, to have their voices heard, and to claim their full human potential; addressing and changing conditions to remove barriers that thwart an individual's or a group's ability to claim his/her/its full potential.

envisioning Process of imagining forms, ways of being, actions, and outcomes into a possible future; interacts with the process of rehearsing to create aesthetic knowledge.

epistemology Pertaining to the "stem" or basis of knowledge; perspectives regarding how knowing becomes knowledge or how knowledge is created.

ethics Fundamental pattern of knowing in nursing that focuses on matters of moral and ethical significance; expressed as knowledge by principles and codes and integrated in practice as moral and ethical comportment.

evidence-informed nursing practice Nursing practice that integrates empiric evidence that is appropriate for a specific situation, but that is also guided by ethical, personal, aesthetic, and emancipatory knowing and is responsive to the unique, particular situation and the people involved; this conceptual definition regards all sources of knowing as equally important in shaping nursing practice and differs from the concept of evidence-based nursing practice, which places empiric knowledge at a higher value than other sources of knowing.

explaining Statements that provide an account of how something came to be; explanatory relationships provide an image or impression of how the nature or attributes of a phenomenon interrelate.

explanatory relationships Statements that provide ideas about how events happen and that indicate how related factors affect or result in certain phenomena.

exploring [alternatives] Approach to understanding and analyzing the values inherent in situation as well as the various actions that flow from those values; a process that cultivates awareness of alternatives to personal values and facilitates recognition of the merits and pitfalls of different approaches to moral and ethical decision making; exploring interacts with the process of clarifying to create ethical knowledge.

fact Objectively verifiable event, object, or property; a phenomenon that is experienced and named similarly by others in a similar context.

feminism Philosophic perspectives and methods that focus on the oppression of women as a class; a perspective that values women and women's experiences; actions of feminist scholars and activists who are committed to a variety of social and political changes that improve women's lives and in turn the lives of all people.

formal descriptions Expressions of knowledge within the empiric knowing pattern; a rigorous and confirmable accounting of perceptions, inferences, and understandings expressed in a variety of written formats; some formal descriptions may not be structured as theory, but may reflect the components of theory.

formal expressions of knowledge Written documents that convey in systematic ways what is known, and that have content that can be examined and authenticated; each pattern of knowing has specific forms of expression that are appropriately suited to that pattern.

general definition Statement of the meaning of a term or concept that sets forth characteristics of the phenomenon or indicates with what the phenomenon is associated; by contrast, a specific definition states particular characteristics or indicators that name what the phenomenon is.

generality Trait of theory that is useful for questioning, clarifying, and understanding the range of phenomena to which the theory applies; generality in combination with simplicity yields parsimony.

generalizability Extent to which research findings can be applied to or used as a basis for making decisions in like situations; generalizability is affected by the soundness of the conceptualization process, the research design, and the analysis of the data.

genuine self Form of nondiscursive knowledge expression within the personal knowing pattern; refers to the whole and entire self as understood by the self and others.

grand theory Theory that deals with broad goals and concepts that represent the total range of phenomena of concern within a discipline; this term may be used to imply macro theory and molar and wholistic theory.

grounded theory Theory that is generated from inductive research processes; the source of data is empiric evidence.

hegemony Interconnected network of dominant views, values, assumptions, ideologies, and patterns of thought that benefit privileged groups; hegemonic structures are taken to be "the way things are" without question while they unfairly separate and continue to disadvantage certain groups; hegemony is difficult to challenge because of its institutionalization in the social order.

hermeneutic inquiry Inquiry approach for interpreting text (language based) that considers the historical situation in which the text was produced; approaches to hermeneutic inquiry vary but in general require movement between text and the historical context for the researcher to understand embedded meanings.

holism See *wholism.*

holistic theory See *wholistic theory.*

hypothesis Tentative statement of relationship between two or more variables that can be empirically tested; the term *hypothesis* generally is used to refer to a relationship statement that is tested with the use of specific research methods.

ideology Ideals and values that dominate the discourses of a culture or society, that are often unfair and unjust, and that typically go unquestioned.

imagining Creative development process for emancipatory knowing; focuses on envisioning and communicating how social and political structures must change to remove conditions of injustice and inequity, thereby creating conditions that enable full human potential.

importance Trait of theory that is useful for questioning, clarifying, and understanding the extent to which a theory is clinically significant or has value for the profession.

induction Form of reasoning that moves from the specific to the general; in inductive logic, a series of particulars are combined into a larger whole or set of things; in inductive research, particular events are observed and analyzed as a basis for formulating general theoretic statements (often called *grounded theory*).

inspiration Process of responding to aesthetic knowledge to imagine new possibilities and directions; interacts with appreciation to challenge and authenticate aesthetic knowledge.

interpretive research General inquiry approach that assumes that "truth" is constructed from the frame of reference of the knower, including both the research participants and the researcher; interpretive research approaches can be contrasted with objectivist research approaches, which assume that there exists an independent reality with truth values that are independent of the knower.

intersectionality Perspective that recognizes multiple sources of oppression and disadvantage based on sociopolitical factors (e.g., race, religion, gender, sexual and gender identities, economic status) and views these as multiplicative, not additive, when more than one factor are involved in a situation.

isolated research Research that is completed without recognized reference or linkage to theory.

justification Process of developing explicit descriptions of the values on which an ethical ideal rests and the line of reasoning toward which an ethical conclusion flows; justification interacts with the process of dialogue to challenge and authenticate ethical knowledge.

knowing Individual human processes of perceiving and understanding the Self and the world in ways that can be brought to some level of conscious awareness; not all that is comprehended during the processes of knowing can be shared or communicated, but what is shared, communicated, and expressed in words or actions becomes the knowledge of a discipline.

knowledge Awareness or perception acquired through insight, learning, or investigation expressed in a form that can be shared; knowledge is a reasonably accurate accounting of the world as it is known and shared by members of a discipline; it is a representation of knowing collectively judged by shared standards and criteria.

law Relationship between variables that has been thoroughly tested and confirmed; laws are said to be highly generalizable and relatively certain.

logic System of reasoning that deals with the form of relationships among propositions without specific regard to their content.

macro theory Theory that deals with a broad scope of phenomena; this term may be used to imply grand, molar, or wholistic theory.

manifesto Type of formal expression of emancipatory knowledge; action-oriented and impassioned portrayals of that which is problematic, descriptions of the ideals envisioned, and actions required to effect change.

metalanguage In general, language that encompasses or transcends other language; in nursing, the broad concepts of nursing, person, society, environment, and health often referred to as *nursing's metaparadigm*.

metatheory Theory about the nature of theory and the processes for its development.

methodolotry Idolization or "worship" of methodology in research; the adherence to rules of method as being primary without regard to the value or utility of a methodology for answering questions of importance to a discipline; methodolotry stands in contrast to other techniques for blending methodologies in relation to research questions.

micro theory Theory that is relatively narrow in scope or that deals with a narrow range of phenomena; this term may be used to imply atomistic or molecular theory.

middle-range theory Relative classification for theory that embodies concepts, relationships, and purposes that reflect limited aspects of broad phenomena; concepts in middle-range theory can be more easily linked to perceptible events and situations.

model Symbolic representation of empiric experience in words, pictorial or graphic diagrams, mathematic notations, or physical material (e.g., a model airplane); when represented in written language, models are a form of knowledge within the empiric pattern.

modernism In knowledge development, the period that began during the early 1900s after the widespread abandonment of metaphysical and religious explanations of knowing; modernism is characterized by the rise of traditional science with a focus on objectivism and a reliance on reason for the creation of knowledge.

molecular theory Theory that is relatively narrow in scope or that deals with a narrow range of phenomena; this term may be used to imply micro theory or atomistic theory.

moral distress Distress that results when ethically significant moral behavior is blocked (e.g., by institutional or legal factors).

moral and ethical comportment Expression of ethical knowledge and knowing in nursing practice that is integrated with emancipatory, personal, aesthetic, and empiric knowledge and knowing.

morals, morality Expression of ethical precepts in behavior and actions; ontologic or behavioral expression of what is good and right.

multivocality Use of many "voices" for methods, data sources, and interpretations in research and knowledge development; the gleaning of different interpretations from the same data set to form multiple understandings rather than a single "correct" interpretation.

narrative analysis Research approach that typically makes use of a story that is told chronologically as data; narrative analysis focuses on the meanings of interrelationships among elements in the story.

nursing practice Experiences that a nurse encounters during the process of caring for people, including those of the person receiving care, the nurse, others in the environment, and their interactions.

objectivity, objectivism Assumption on which methods of science are based in which truth is thought to exist apart from or outside of the person who knows; based on a dualistic view of the rational mind that involves the existence of a reality that is separate from the person who knows.

ontology Pertaining to ways of being in the world; perspectives on the existence and experience of being.

opening Process that involves the taking in of experience fully and with conscious awareness; interacts with the process of centering to create personal knowledge.

operational definition Statement of meaning that indicates how a term or concept can be assessed empirically; operational definitions are inferred from theoretic definitions and specify as exactly as possible the empiric indicators used to observe, assess, or measure the concept empirically; the standards or criteria to be used when making observations.

paradigm Worldview or overarching frame of reference directing knowledge development; a paradigm implies standards or criteria for assigning value or worth to both the processes and the products of a discipline as well as the methods of knowledge development.

parsimony Trait of theory that incorporates degrees of both simplicity and generality; a highly parsimonious theory is one that has a broad range or generality and that is stated in very simple terms.

patterns gone wild Distortion of understanding that occurs when one pattern of knowing is not critically examined and integrated with the whole of knowing; overemphasis on one pattern without integration leads to uncritical acceptance, narrow interpretations, and partial use of knowledge.

personal knowing Fundamental pattern of knowing in nursing that is focused on the inner experience of becoming a whole, aware self; expressed as knowledge through autobiographic stories and the genuine self and integrated in practice with other patterns as the therapeutic use of the self.

personal stories Tangible expressions of personal knowledge that are discursive in form and that can be shared within the discipline.

philosophy Form of disciplined inquiry for the purpose of discerning general traits of reality and principles of value.

postcolonialism Approach to understanding the relationship between culture and imperialistic colonization (i.e., takeover and domination of the powerless by the powerful); generally, postcolonial thought is concerned with reversing the effects of political or ideologic colonization.

postmodernism Period after modernism in which confidence in the achievement of objective knowledge through reason was eroded; postmodernism generally rejects universal truths and the idea that truth is possible and instead embraces multiple approaches to knowledge generation.

poststructuralism In linguistics, the view that language is not reflective but rather constitutive of meaning; for poststructuralists, there is no reality or truth, and the humanist idea of an autonomous knower is rejected; to these thinkers, we do not have language but instead language "has us" in the sense that it constructs our experiences and understandings.

practice-based evidence Evidence that comes from the validation of clinically used approaches and techniques that are known to be effective for promoting health-related goals; emphasizes investigating and confirming what seems to be effective in practice as a way to generate research evidence.

praxis Expression of emancipatory knowing and knowledge in nursing practice; value-grounded, thoughtful reflection and action that occurs in synchrony and that integrates ontology and epistemology; a value-motivated process that changes nursing practice and the larger sociopolitical environment to end injustices and inequities; praxis creates conditions in which all people can reach maximum well-being and full potential, and is integrated with ethical, aesthetic, personal, and empiric knowledge and knowing in nursing practice.

predicting Process used for the creation of empiric knowledge; prediction involves a focus on interrelating concepts and variables to create an understanding of when and how phenomena and events will occur and recur; used in conjunction with explaining.

predictive relationships Set of statements that interrelates variables so that a specified outcome can be expected when the theory is used.

premises Relationship statements that are used in deductive logic as a basis for forming a conclusion; in logic, the form of the argument must be valid, regardless of how sound the premises are; examples of types of premises are hypotheses and axioms.

principles Forms of knowledge expression within the ethics pattern; principles are general statements that reflect general and fundamental precepts of value or truths that are adhered to when providing nursing care, such as "do no harm."

problem solving Process of identifying a discrete difficulty or dilemma and finding situation-specific corrections or solutions.

processes for theory development In a practice discipline, the processes for theory development include creating conceptual meaning, structuring and contextualizing theory, refining and validating concepts and theoretic relationships, and deliberatively using and validating theory.

profession Vocation that requires specialized knowledge, provides a role in society that is valued, and uses some means of internal regulation of its members.

proposition Statement of a relationship between two or more variables; the term *proposition* is a general category that includes postulates, premises, suppositions, axioms, conclusions, theorems, and hypotheses; when a distinction in meaning is made among these various terms, it reflects the form or purpose of logic used or the context in which the proposition occurs; for example, the term *hypothesis* is generally used in the context of a research study, whereas the terms *axiom* and *theorem* are used to refer to the relationship statements that are made as part of a particular type of deductive logic.

purpose Component of theory that establishes the reasons that underlie a theory's development; the outcome or outcomes expected to emerge if the relationships of the theory are valid; the purpose of the theory also suggests the range of situations in which the theory is expected to apply.

qualitative methods Methods of data collection and analysis that depend on talk, language expressions of talk, or observations expressed in language, with interpretations presented by nonnumeric (usually language) means.

quantitative methods Methods of data collection and analysis that depend on measurement and that are expressed in numeric terms.

reductionism Philosophic stance that the whole can be partitioned and understood through generalizations that are made from a study of the parts.

refining concepts and theoretic relationships Process for linking research and theory that focuses on the correspondence between the ideas of the theory and the accessible experience that involves both qualitative and quantitative approaches; includes validating empiric indicators for concepts, grounding emerging relationships empirically, and validating relationships with the use of empiric methods.

reflection Process that requires integrating a wide range of perceptions to realize what is known within the Self; interacts with the process of response to challenge and authenticate personal knowledge.

reflective practice Necessary component of best practices that requires practitioners to thoughtfully consider and adopt ways to improve practice over time; part of the process of praxis, but praxis requires bringing oppressive social and political practices to the center of concern when transforming practice to end injustices and inequities.

rehearsing Process of creating and re-creating narrative, body movements, gestures, and actions in relation to an anticipated situation; interacts with the process of envisioning to create aesthetic knowledge.

relationship statement Any statement that sets forth a connection or association between two or more phenomena; this general term is used to denote both tentative and confirmed types of statements, such as propositions, laws, axioms, and hypotheses; as a more general term, it does not imply a particular form of logic or a particular context in which the statement is used.

relationships Component of theory that refers to the interconnections among concepts.

replication Process that draws on methods of science to determine the extent to which an observation remains consistent from one situation or time to another; interacts with the processes of validation and confirmation to challenge and authenticate empiric knowledge.

research Application of formalized methods of obtaining confirmable and valid knowledge about empiric experience.

response Process of interacting with one's own self and others to provide insight regarding the meanings that are conveyed in experience; interacts with the process of reflection to challenge and authenticate personal knowledge.

science As a product, the knowledge forms generated by the use of rigorous and precise empirically based methods (e.g., facts, formal descriptions, models, theories); as a process, the use of empirically based methods to generate theories, models, and descriptions of reality.

scientific competence Expression of empiric knowledge and knowing in nursing practice that is integrated with emancipatory knowing and knowledge, ethics, aesthetics, and personal knowing and knowledge.

simplicity Trait of theory used in critical reflection for questioning, clarifying, and understanding the degree to which a theory reduces complexity by utilizing a minimum number of descriptive components, especially concepts, to accomplish its purpose; simplicity in combination with generality yields parsimony.

situation-specific theory Theory that is developed with the sensitive consideration of context; assumes that theory (even middle-range formulations) generally cannot be used without taking into account important differences across populations; draws attention to the variables that significantly affect the successful use of theory.

social equity Criterion for the authentication of emancipatory knowledge; the demonstrable elimination or reduction of conditions that create disadvantage for some and advantage for others.

specific definition Statement of the meaning of a term or concept that names the associated object, property, or event and assigns it particular characteristics, as opposed to saying what the concept is like or associated with in reality.

structuralism In linguistics, the view that the meanings of words and language are not universally understood but rather derived from the language structure within which the words are found; more broadly, language practices are structured by the context of use and reflect the broader social and political environments.

structure Component of theory that refers to the overall morphologic arrangement of specific elements, especially concepts, within the theory.

structuring Process that involves forming empiric concepts into formal expressions, such as theories, models, and frameworks; interacts with the process of explaining to create empiric knowledge.

structuring and contextualizing theory Theory development process of forming relationships between and among concepts in a unique, creative, rigorous, and systematic way that is consistent with the purposes of the theory; this process also includes identifying and defining the concepts, identifying assumptions, clarifying the context of the theory, and designing relationship statements.

substantive middle-range theory In nursing, theory that tends to cluster around a concept (usually clinical) that is of interest to nursing; theories of pain alleviation, fatigue, or uncertainty represent theory in the middle range.

sustainability Criterion for the authentication of emancipatory knowledge; establishes how well the envisioned and implemented social change survives and thrives.

theoretic definition Statement of meaning that conveys essential features of a concept in a manner that fits meaningfully within a theory; a theoretic definition specifies conceptual meaning and implies empiric indicators for concepts; this term may be used synonymously with *conceptual definition.*

theoretic framework Logical grouping of related concepts that is usually created to draw together several different aspects that are relevant to a complex situation, such as a practice setting or an educational program; this term is used synonymously with *conceptual framework;* a knowledge form within the empirics pattern.

theory Expression of knowledge within the empirics pattern; the creative and rigorous structuring of ideas that project a tentative, purposeful, and systematic view of phenomena.

theory-linked research Research that is designed with reference or linkage to a theory; theory-linked research may be theory testing or theory generating; theory-testing research ascertains how accurately existing theoretic relationships depict reality-based events, whereas theory-generating research is designed to discover and describe relationships by observing empiric reality and then constructing theory on the basis of the empiric data observed.

therapeutic use of self Expression of personal knowledge and knowing in nursing practice that is integrated with emancipatory, ethical, empiric, and aesthetic knowledge and knowing.

transformative art/act Expression of aesthetic knowledge and knowing in nursing practice that is integrated with emancipatory, empiric, aesthetic, and personal knowing and knowledge.

translational research Research designed to move evidence into the clinical arena by evaluating outcomes in the practice setting; research to connect basic discoveries with patient/client care.

validation Process that draws on the traditional methods of science to substantiate the accuracy of conceptual meanings in terms of empiric evidence; interacts with replication to challenge and authenticate empiric knowledge; may also refer to newer methods for establishing the credibility or truth value of knowledge structures within the empiric pattern.

wholism Perspective that is based on the assumption that a whole is emergent and cannot be reduced to discrete elements or be analyzed without consideration of the sum of its parts; may also refer to an emphasis on the value of the whole but with consideration for discrete parts that are interrelated.

wholistic theory Theory that deals with a broad scope of phenomena; often implies an assumption that the whole is greater than the sum of its parts; this term may be used to imply macro or grand theory.

work of art Tangible expression of knowledge within the aesthetic patterns that is not discursive in form and that can be communicated and shared within the discipline; includes aesthetic expressions such as poetry, drawings, music, dance, and other forms that are generally understood to be art.

Index

Page numbers followed by *b, t,* and *f* indicate boxes, tables, and figures, respectively.